To
ELIZABETH
BEST WISHES
DANIEL MAN M.D

THE ART OF MAN

FACES OF PLASTIC SURGERY

BY DANIEL MAN, M.D. AND L.C. FAYE

SECOND EDITION

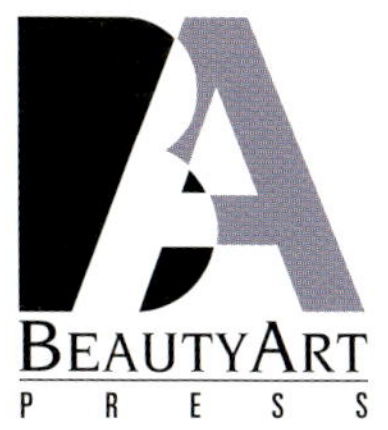

Printed in the United States of America

IMPORTANT READER INFORMATION:

The patients who are depicted here have kindly consented to have their photos used and to be interviewed for this book. The patients represented are actual patients treated by Dr. Man. Photos depict the patients before and after their surgery which was performed by Dr. Man. It should be noted that many patients may have more than one procedure performed by Dr. Man, and that some patients may have had procedures by other physicians prior to being treated by Dr. Man. Please note that the patient photos are not a guarantee as to individual results, as each patient is different and unique, and results may vary. Readers are strongly urged to consult with their physician and a board-certified plastic surgeon. The authors and the publisher do not intend this book as the primary source of information on plastic surgery, nor to dispense medical advice or prescribe the use of any technique or treatment, whether directly or indirectly, nor to diagnose or convey medical information which should be conveyed by a board certified plastic surgeon. Despite the best efforts of the authors, this book may contain mistakes and the reader should use the book only as general information and not as the ultimate source. The reader is encouraged to consult with a board certified plastic surgeon. In the event the reader uses any information in this book, the authors and publisher accept no responsibility.

Printing, graphics and typography: Gulfshore Communications, Inc., Naples, Florida
Second printing: R.R. Donnelley & Sons Company
Design concept: Benzi Rotman, Dagesh International
Cover Photography: Crazy Moon Photography, Boca Raton, Florida
Dr. Man and Patient Photography: Peter Lorber, Custom Photo Lab, Boca Raton, Florida
Max Kaufmann, The Photography Studio, West Palm Beach, Florida
Cover Makeup: Thomas Joseph, Boca Raton, Florida
Patient Hair Stylist: Marilyn Carlson, Boca Raton, Florida
Paintings and Sculptures: Daniel Man, M.D.
BSE Graphic Design, West Palm Beach, Florida

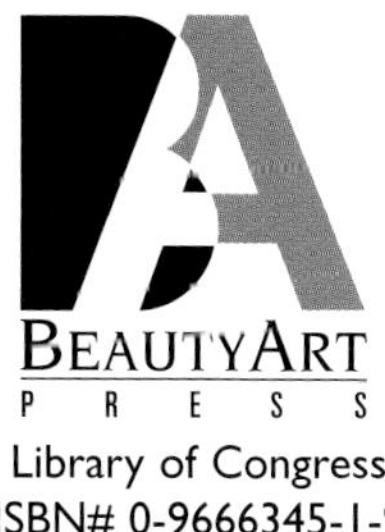

Library of Congress
ISBN# 0-9666345-1-9
Printed in the United States of America

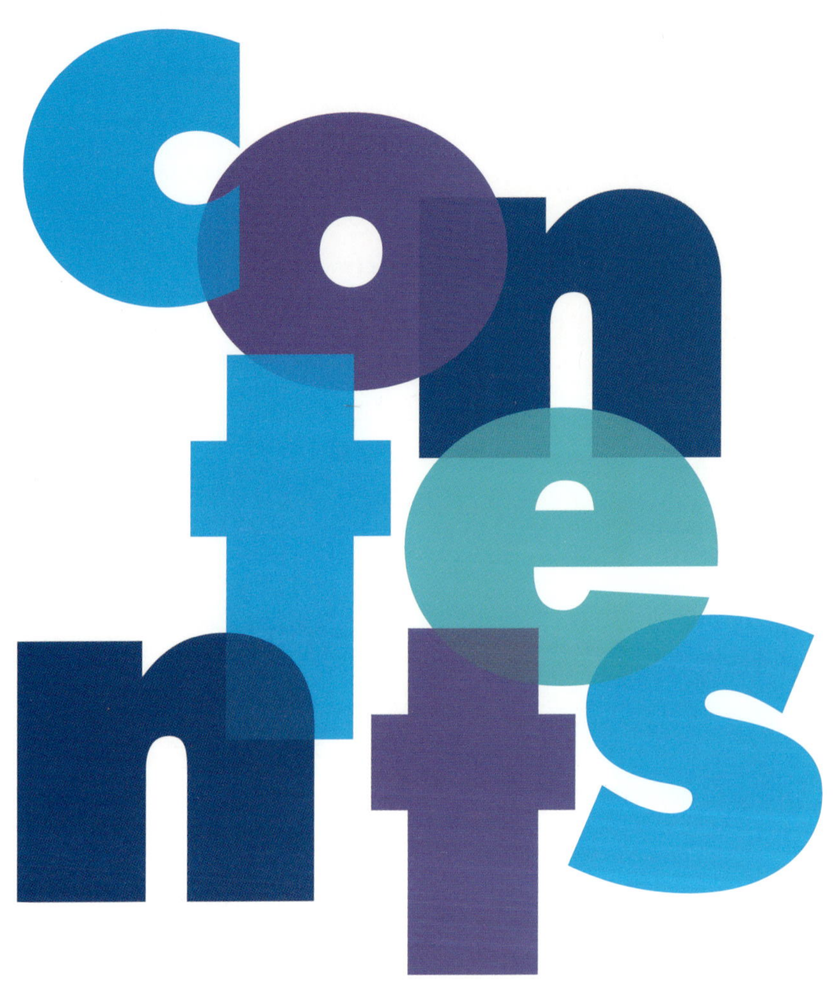
contents

PART 1

PART 2

PART 3

PART 4

acknowledgements

Every accomplishment no matter the size is usually attained through the efforts of many. This book is no exception, as it brings to life my work, my art and the people who share in it; my patients, my colleagues and my friends. I am grateful to you all. I give special thanks to the many patients who contributed to this work by sharing their wonderful stories. Without them, this book would not have been possible. To my staff and colleagues around the world, I give my appreciation for their encouragement . . . To my wife Dena, our parents and our sons, I offer my love and gratitude . . . To Peter Lorber and Courtenay Gilbert whose photographs captured the beauty of the many patients who shared their stories . . . To Sarah Weatherford, our staff esthetician, who worked with our many patients and contributed her valuable knowledge on skin care and makeup and . . . to "L.C." Faye whose writing helped bring these stories to life. I give my thanks and appreciation for your contributions and hard work. I also wish to acknowledge the American Society of Plastic & Reconstructive Surgeons for its support and dedication to the advancement and excellence of plastic surgery.

This book is dedicated to Dr. Leonard Weiner, professor of plastic surgery at the University of Louisville, who has always been there for me, giving me his friendship and his guidance.

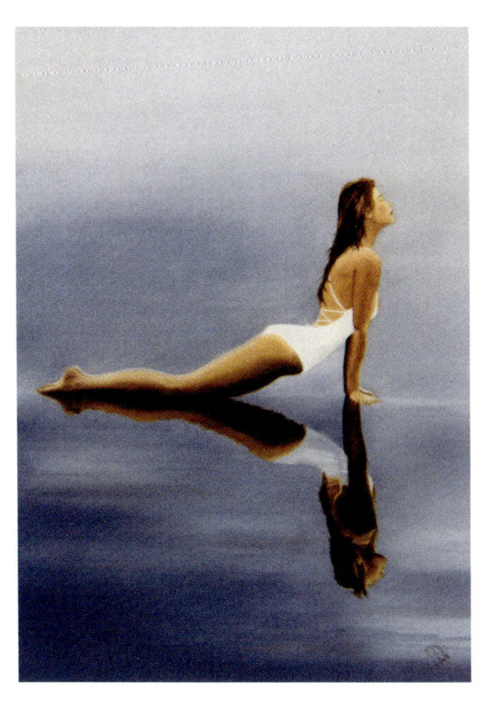

dedication

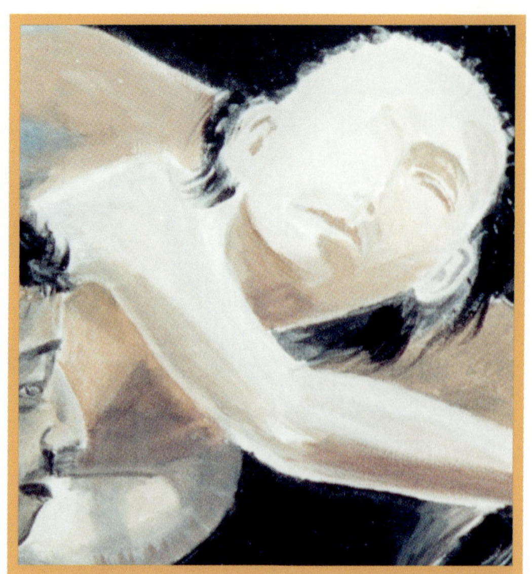

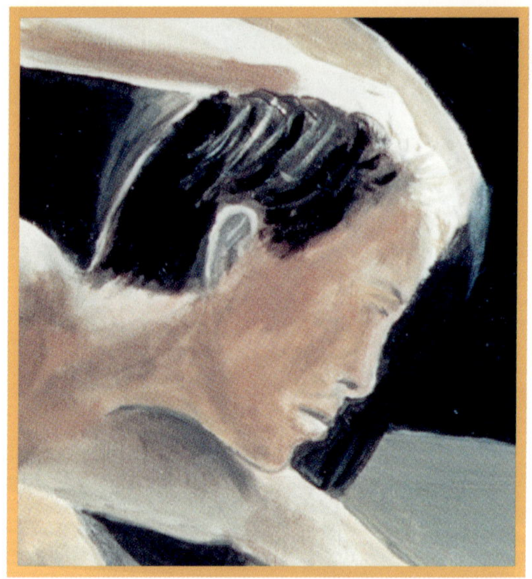

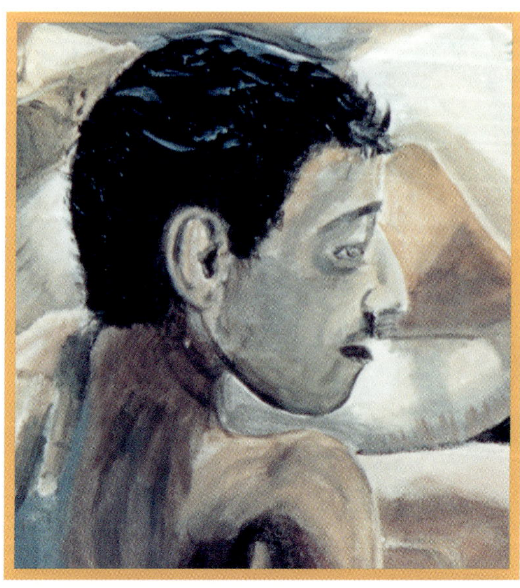

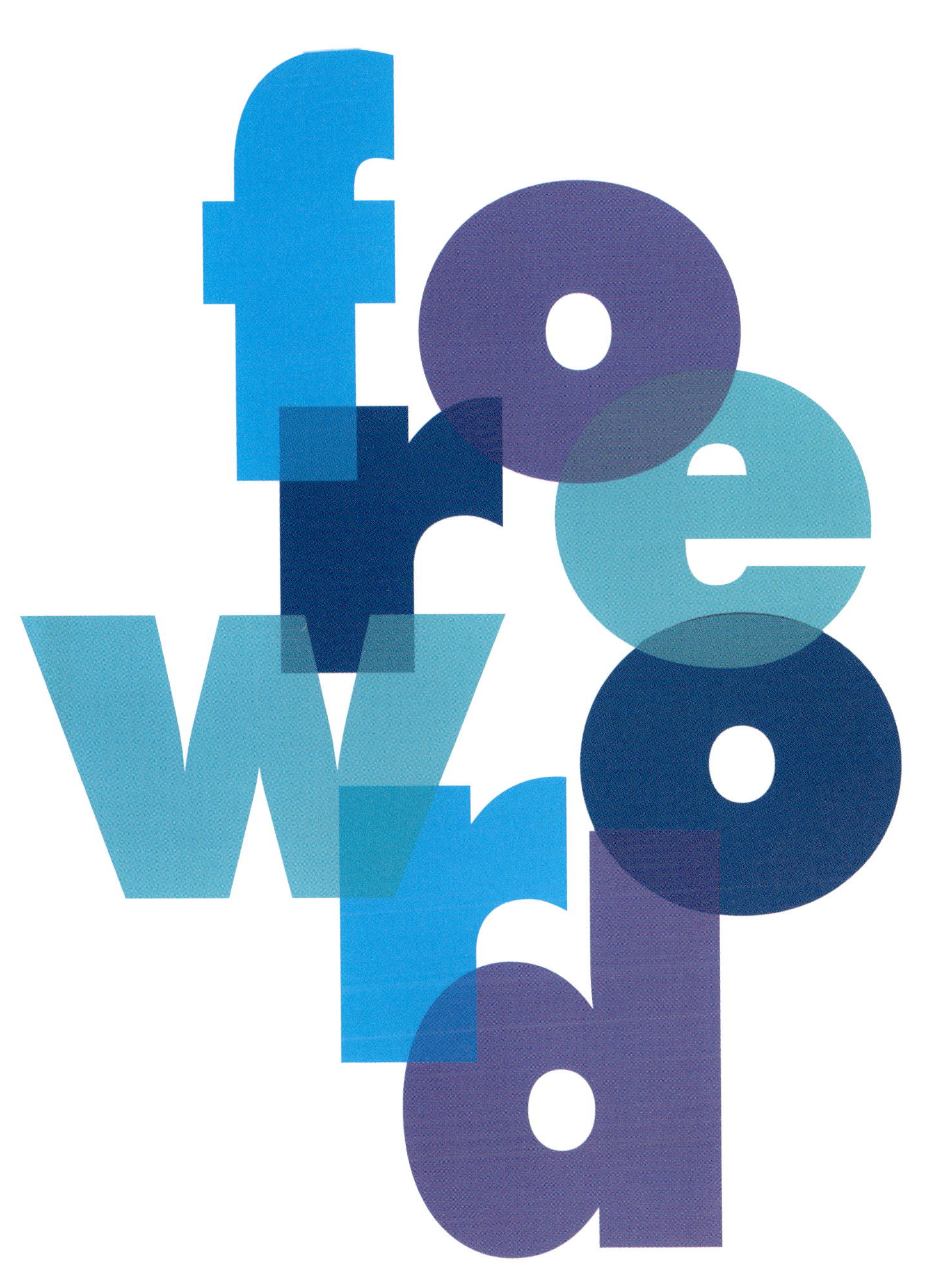
foreword

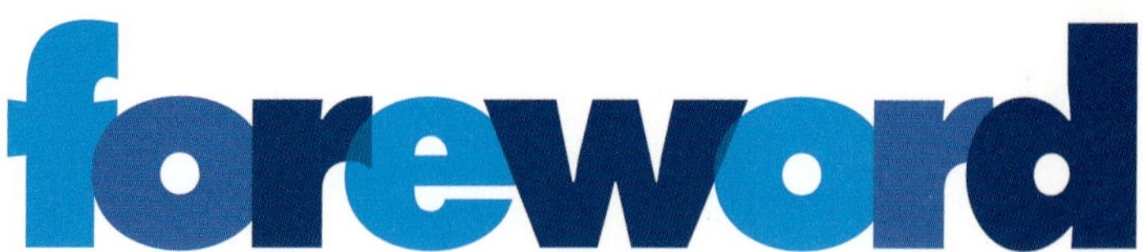

foreword

There are many books published on plastic surgery. One such book is the *American Society of Plastic and Reconstructive Surgeons' Guide To Cosmetic Surgery.* Books like this contain important information on electing a surgeon, evaluating options, the consultation, and getting ready for surgery.

The Art of Man: Faces of Plastic Surgery is very different. It is about choices and the people who make them. It does not attempt to represent the full spectrum of plastic surgery, dispense medical advice, or try to include all procedures. While it does describe the most popular procedures and advances, it is not a technical or "how to" book, nor does it endeavor to describe every detail of the procedures, treatments and risks. This is a book about my work as a plastic surgeon and as an artist, and the people who made the decision to change their lives through plastic surgery.

Hopefully, this book will answer many of the questions you have about cosmetic surgery — helping to serve as a resource and general guide book for those people who are considering plastic surgery. It will suggest important questions to ask your surgeon before you decide to have plastic surgery and will introduce you to many of the new and most popular procedures today. And, it will offer you an opportunity to meet patients who have undergone many of the procedures you may now be considering, so that you can hear their stories firsthand and judge for yourself.

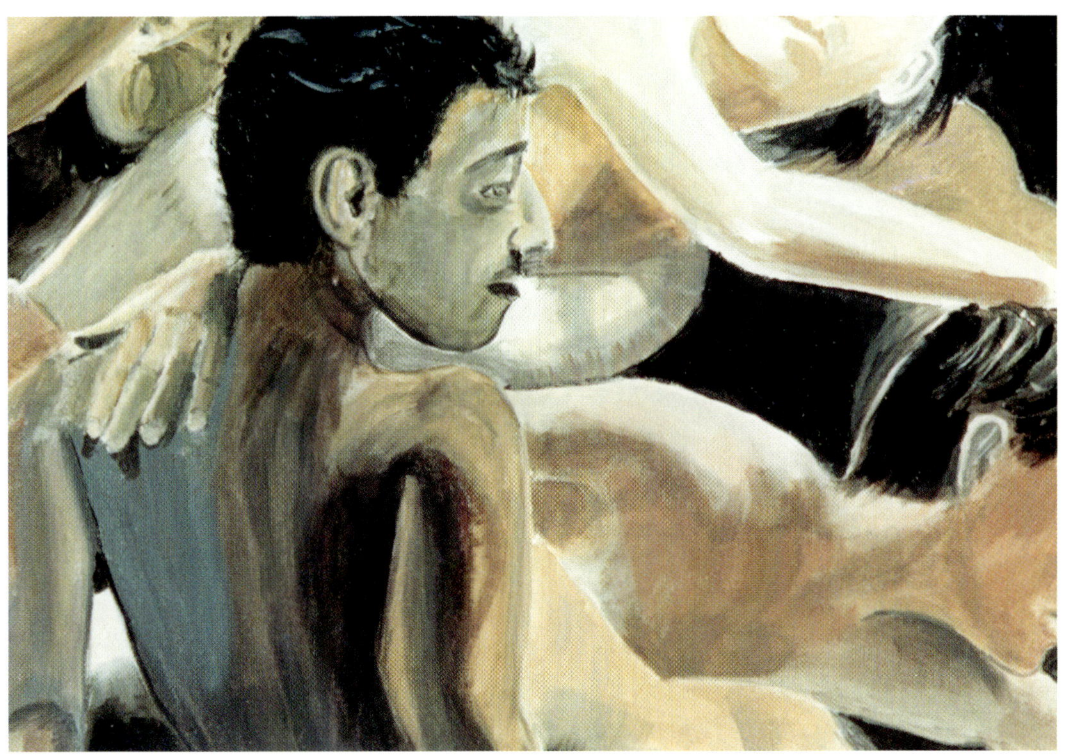

This is a very personal book revealing details of the private lives of real people. Have you ever wanted to talk to someone who had plastic surgery? Not a doctor or an expert, but someone like yourself. Someone who felt like you do. Someone you could talk to honestly. The patients who share the stories here will tell you about their hopes, their dreams, their fears . . . and they will tell you how plastic surgery has changed their lives. They are not movie stars nor celebrities. They are people just like you and me. They are your mother, your father, your sister, your neighbor and your friends, all of whom had the courage to change their appearance. You will see them as they are today and how they appeared before and after their surgery. You'll read about Claudine, who couldn't look at herself in the mirror, and the "Cinderella" story of shy Lillian, who spent her whole life believing she was never as pretty as her sisters. There's Luella, who needed a second facelift, but wanted to keep her natural expressions.

And then there is Maryann, who feels that "youth and beauty" equaled power and success for women in our society. You'll meet 11-year-old Andrew. Today, he is a successful student and a budding model and child actor. Just a few years ago he suffered emotionally, physically and academically because of the cruel taunts of schoolmates who called him "Dumbo" because of his protruding ears.

These are just a few of the patient "portraits" painted here. It is my desire that these stories will help give you very real and personal insights into my patients' lives.

If there is one fault that this book is surely guilty of, it is that these stories depict all the good without the bad. I believe there is a place for such a book, as there is a proper place for other books that should be read. I wanted to create a book of beauty about my work as a plastic surgeon, my "living" art — the people I helped to change and my other art — my painting and sculpture art. A plastic surgeon's ability to change someone's appearance is truly a marvel of modern medicine. Each time I see my patients, I am awed by their remarkable transformations. And I am truly humbled. It is both a burden and a responsibility I accept.

But, with all things that carry a price tag, the label should include a notice "Buyer Beware." Surgery is serious. Educate yourself, ask questions and arm yourself with as much information as possible. Remember, every surgery carries risk. Know what you are buying beforehand.

There are those people who will not opt for the surgeon's knife — aging lines have become old friends, familiar and comfortable. But for others, surgery fulfills their hopes and dreams of having a face or body that brings a smile to their face when they get up in the morning and look in the bathroom mirror. As a surgeon, I try to make each one whole again, whether it be restoring lost youth, rebuilding a breast lost to cancer, or repairing a face deeply scarred by burns. For a society that places so much importance on appearance, the final question that should be asked is what will make you happy?

Millions of people each year have found their answer in the plastic surgeon's office. I do not act as my patients' judge or jury, but try to understand their needs, motives and desires. Today, advanced techniques provide patients more options and more choices, more affordably than was possible even a few years ago.

The patients' stories you will read include photos of patients before and after their surgery and as they appear today. You should be aware that some patients may have had more than one procedure and some may also have had previous procedures by another doctor before becoming my patient. But in every case the patients, photos and procedures depicted are my work.

The before and after photos of the patients have not been retouched. The stories are real, and the experiences are in the patients' own words. While these photos show actual patients, it is important to understand that these photos should not be interpreted as an endorsement of results that you may expect. Every patient is unique and individual, and results may vary. It is also true that no two patients heal in exactly the same way. Only through a consultation with a board-certified plastic surgeon will you know what results you can realistically expect to achieve through plastic surgery, the risks involved, and what procedure may best help you achieve your goals.

I hope this book will answer some of your questions and help to show you the beauty of my work through patients and through my paintings and sculptures. I thank the reader for indulging me this time we share together.

— Daniel Man, M.D.

Boca Raton, Florida

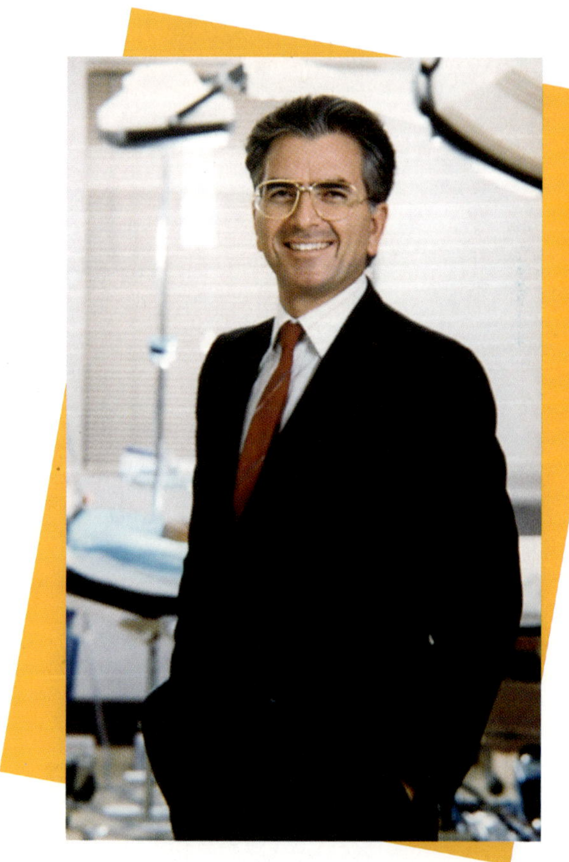

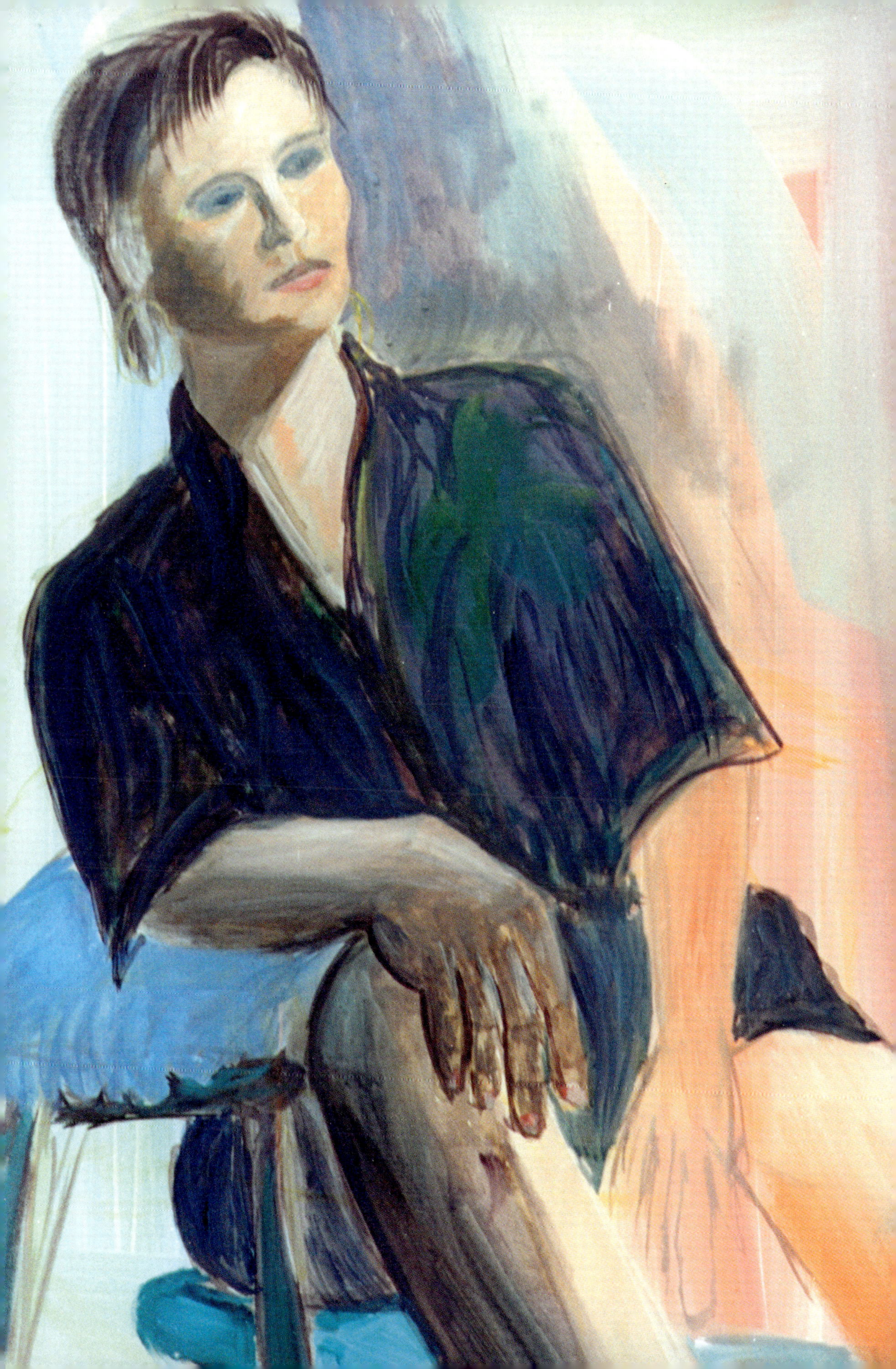

Part 1 Introduction

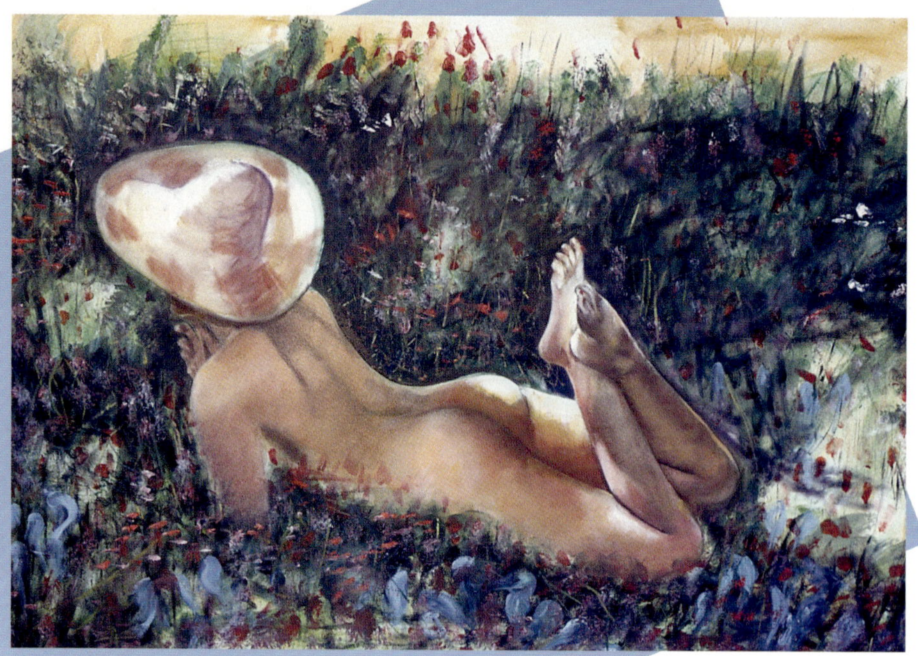

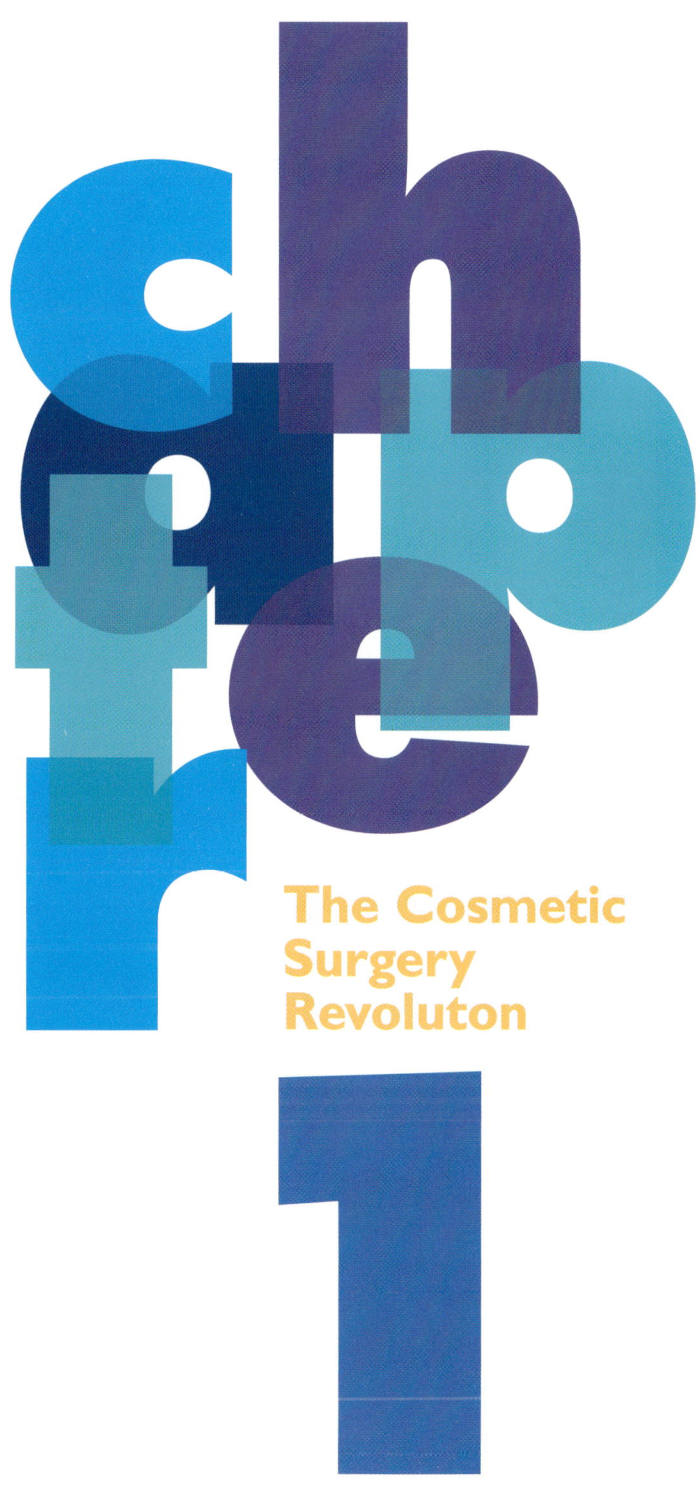

The Cosmetic Surgery Revoluton

THE COSMETIC SURGERY REVOLUTION

There is a new kind of war being waged in America and throughout the world — the war against aging. With our society's constant emphasis on youth and beauty, it's no wonder we (yes, even the authors) find ourselves attracted to the possibilities offered by cosmetic surgery. How often have we looked into the mirror and wished we could change something about our appearance — a prominent nose, bags under the eyelids, wrinkles, frown lines? The endless search for physical perfection is creating a revolution of new anti-aging remedies.

Who Is Doing It?

According to the American Society of Plastic and Reconstructive Surgeons (ASPRS), the professional society that represents board-certified plastic surgeons in the U.S., 1.5 million people undergo elective cosmetic surgery each year. What kinds of things do people want changed? Most cosmetic surgery today is selected by women, though men are joining them with increasing frequency. A few years ago, approximately one in ten cosmetic surgery patients were men. Today, men can account for 20 to 25 percent of a plastic surgeon's practice. And the numbers are growing.

An Ancient Practice

Although we might believe that cosmetic surgery is a product of our modern society, it is not new. Its roots date back many thousands of years. Ancient societies practiced their own form of cosmetic surgery to improve appearance or restore the body after injury or accident. Though their tools were often crude by modern standards, ancient practitioners performed rhinoplasties, reconstructive surgery on ears and even skin rejuvenation. Today we live in an exciting, ever-changing world of medical science and new discoveries that not only help us live longer, but have also improved the quality of those years.

Modern tools include lasers that can remove wrinkles, scars, stretch marks and discolorations as well as endoscopic procedures that allow surgeons to perform intricate surgeries through very tiny incisions. For a society obsessed with appearance and youth, the modern age of plastic surgery is a welcome refuge offering more options, more affordably than at any other time in our history. And the future promises to be even brighter.

What Is Beauty?

Our concepts of beauty and attractiveness continue to change from one society to another and even from one generation to the next. We know from history that what one culture holds as beautiful, another may not. Our modern-day versions are most closely tied to the ancient Greeks who strove for graceful lines, balance and proportion. We even have a mathematical definition, called "the golden proportions," to achieve balance and harmony. As surgeons, we mark and measure millimeters and distances between each feature, turning the face and body into a road map to beauty.

The importance of being attractive has become universally accepted, whether we admit it or not. It is also true that, whether we intend to or not, we treat attractive people differently based on their appearance. Often we derive our first impressions of people within the first 30 seconds of meeting them! One study suggested that cute babies get more attention, even from their own mothers. (Ritter and Langlois, *Developmental Psychology* May 1995). The research also showed the reverse — infants, it seems, also prefer to look at attractive faces.

People often judge our abilities by our appearance. Attractive people are often considered brighter and more successful. One study reported in the *Wall Street Journal* suggested that, appearance can even make or break a career. (*Wall Street Journal*, August 28, 1991).

Self-esteem and confidence are also tied to our physical appearance. If we look better, we feel better about ourselves and those positive attitudes are reflected in our actions and how others

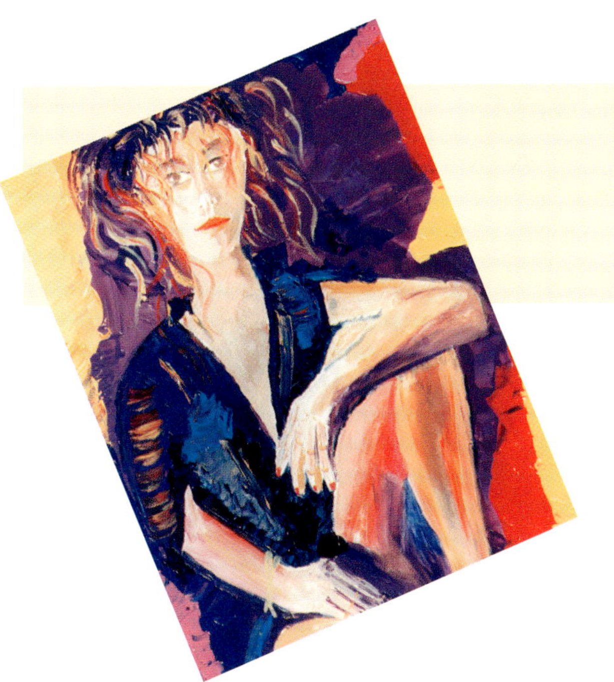

relate to us.

In the past, society seemed to place less emphasis on how a man looked, or at least we seemed to be a lot more forgiving when it came to men. But, this attitude is changing, too. Men care as much about their appearance as women do. Men often seek surgical alternatives in order to be more competitive on the job (*USA Today*, March 21, 1995). Fortunately today, plastic surgery can change what we don't like.

A Modern Solution

Once plastic surgery was a subject kept behind closed doors and talked about in whispers. It was considered a luxury for the very rich and the famous. We wanted celebrities and movie stars to stay

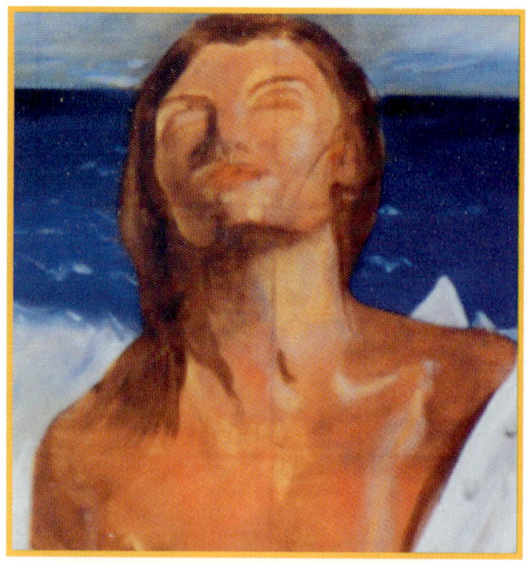

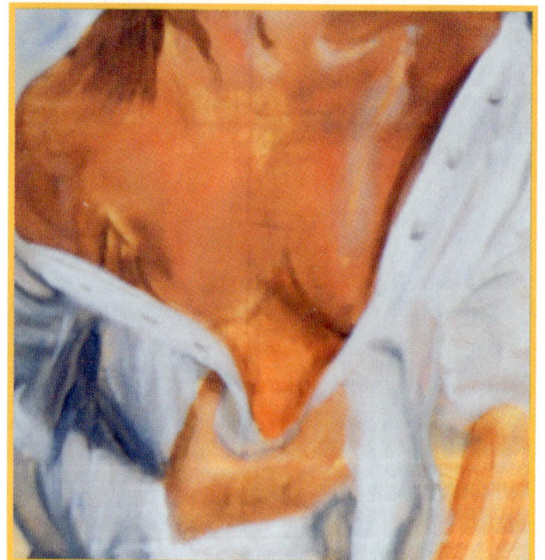

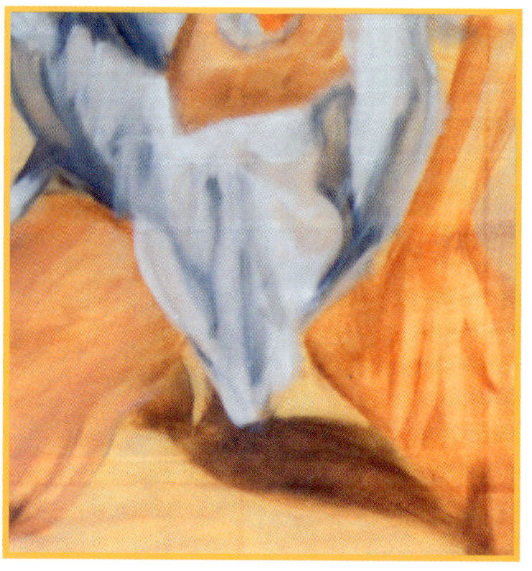

attractive, beautiful and young looking, so we could share vicariously in their glamorous lifestyles portrayed on television and in celebrity and glamour magazines. Fortunately, times change and with it our opinions and values. Today, plastic surgery is much more readily accepted than even a few years ago. It is considered a valuable service for those who want to improve their appearance. As one patient in her 60s confessed, "When I was younger, I always said plastic surgery was not for me. Wrinkles and lines meant character. The only problem was that, when I got older, I had more 'character' than I wanted."

Top Five Procedures

What are the things that people want to change most? As we age, the face is often the first place we notice changes. According to ASPRS, of the top five cosmetic procedures performed in the U.S., most involve the face. They include eyelid surgery, nose reshaping, liposuction, collagen injections and facelifts.

Top States To Have Plastic Surgery

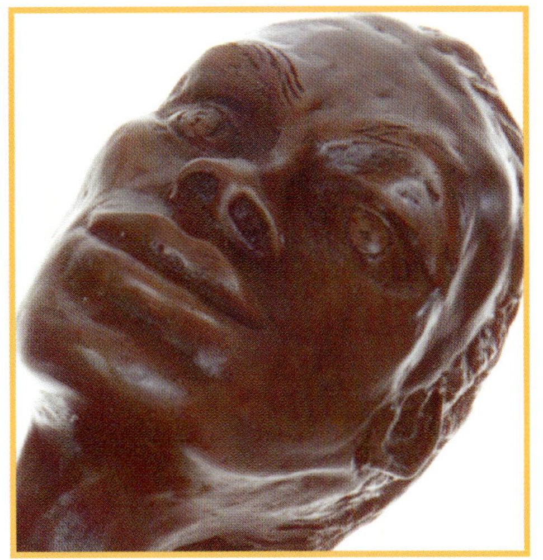

You might wonder where most cosmetic surgery is performed. If you guessed California, you're right. You may be surprised to learn that Florida is second in the number of cosmetic procedures performed by plastic surgeons, outranking New York and Texas which have larger populations.

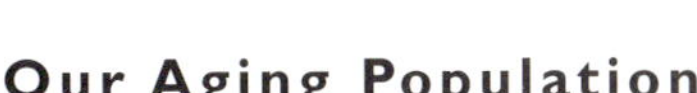

Our Aging Population

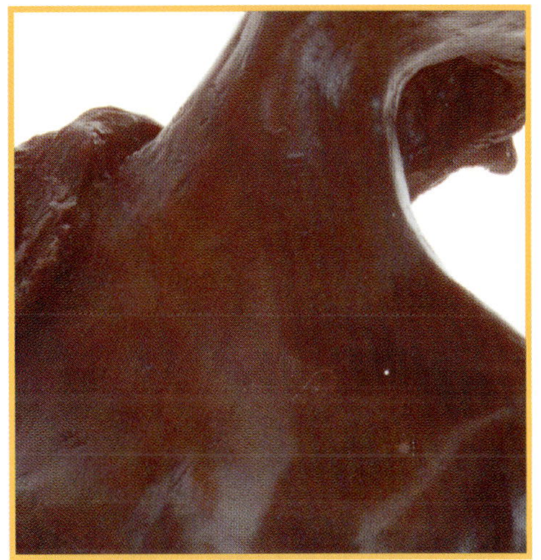

Why all the interest in plastic surgery? The shocking truth is we are no longer a society of the young. Our population as a whole is getting older, as evidenced by baby boomers who have now reached the "unfashionable" age of 50. This means the median age is now 40, and by the 21st century there will be a new senior boom to fuel the anti-aging industry. People over the age of 65 will outnumber teenagers in the year 2025, and experts predict the median age will reach 50 sometime after the year 2000. (Source: *Age Wave* by Ken Dychtwald, Ph.D., 1990). Whatever the age, our society still thinks young and it will do anything to hold on to past youth.

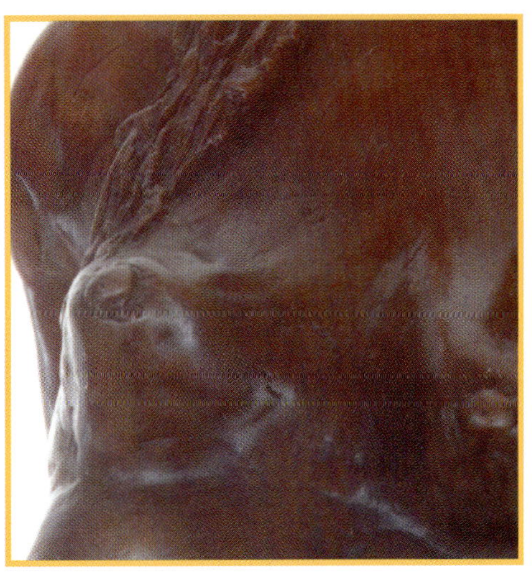

Why Have Surgery?

Most people will opt for cosmetic surgery simply because it makes them look better. Looking good has social and psychological benefits as well; when you look good, you feel good and your self-esteem and confidence improve. Cosmetic surgery is also practical for business executives caught up in corporate downsizing who find they have to compete in a younger market. For some, it helps to know that cosmetic surgery has never been more affordable. Advances in surgical techniques and skills mean that most elective cosmetic procedures are now being done on an outpatient basis in the doctor's office, cutting the high cost of hospital surgery, in many cases by half or more.

Cosmetic surgery is also less invasive. This means patients heal faster, with minimal discomfort, and they recover in days and weeks, instead of months. Though medical science has made tremendous advances, those seeking alternatives to aging should remember that plastic surgery is still surgery. Every surgical procedure carries risks which should be considered carefully and only after consultation with a board-certified plastic surgeon.

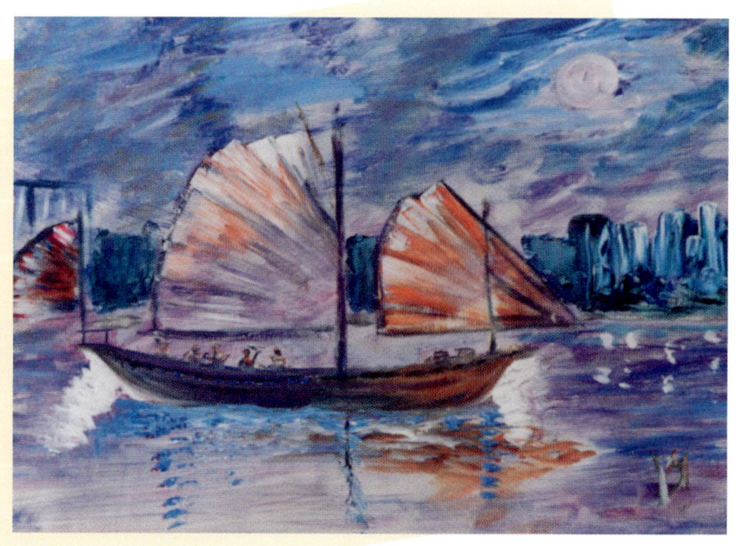

Most-Asked Questions

Most people want to know three things about plastic surgery: 1) How much will it cost? 2) Is it painful? 3) When can I resume my normal activities? If you are thinking of having cosmetic surgery, get as much information as you can beforehand. Ask questions. Lots of them. Hopefully, the following chapters will help provide some answers.

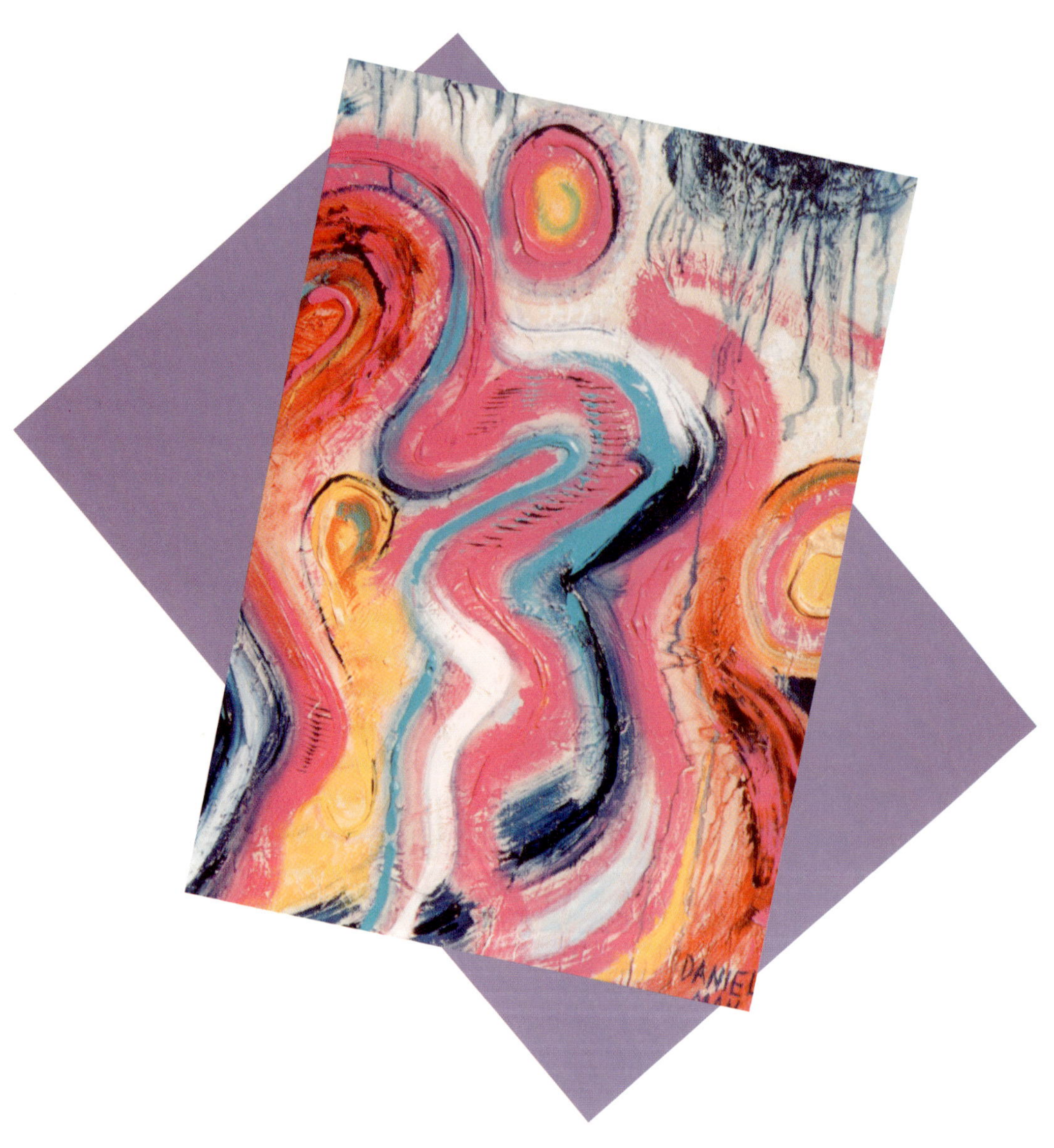

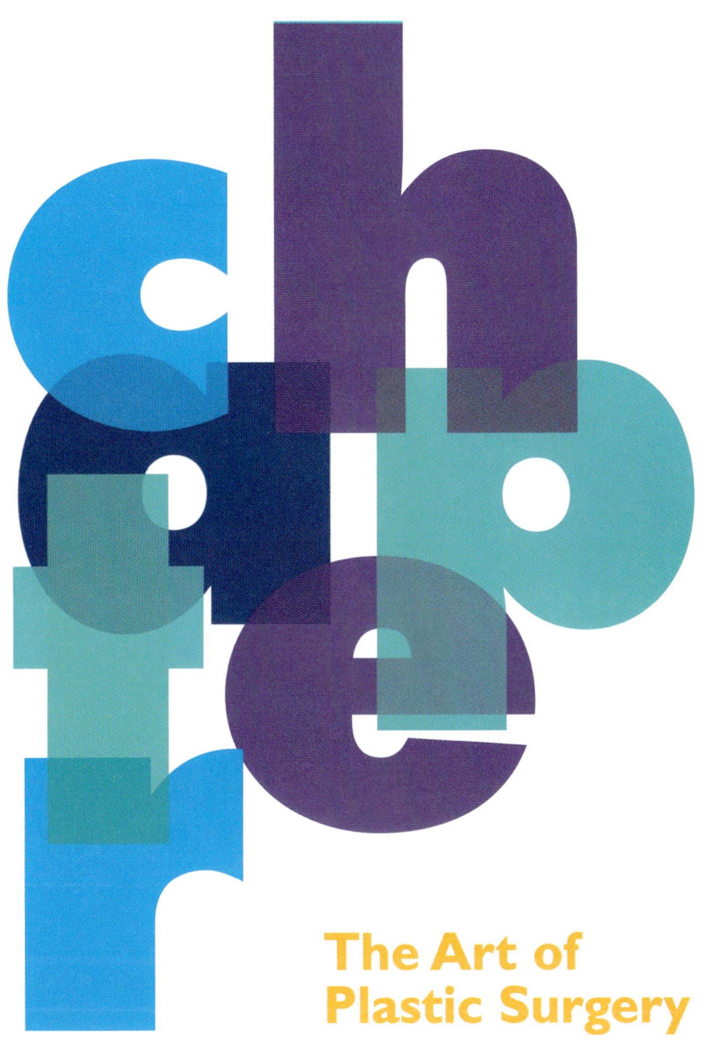

The Art of Plastic Surgery

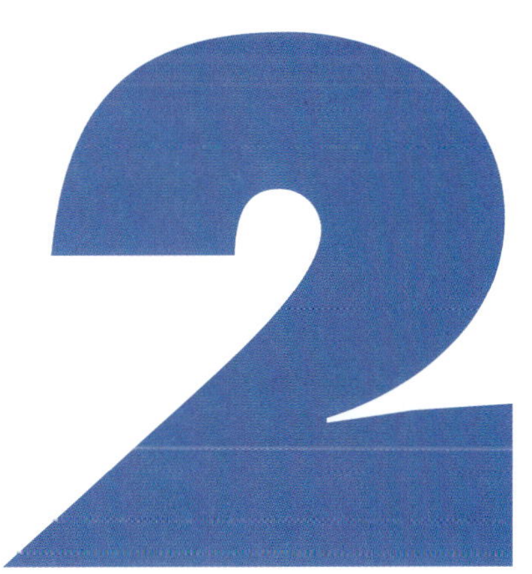

THE ART OF PLASTIC SURGERY

I was born the son of a surgeon in Afula, a small city located in northern Israel about 60 miles outside of Tel Aviv. I knew at a very early age I would be a doctor like my father, and by age 16, I knew I would be a plastic surgeon. As a young boy, I was always interested in how things were shaped. Some of my earliest childhood memories involve sitting on my family's porch carving wooden statues. I would walk through the nearby woods and see a rough tree root that would catch my eye. I would pick it up and run home excited with my new find. I couldn't wait to change its shape. I especially liked carving old olive tree branches, the feel of the wood in my hands, and the patterns that the grain made with its yellow, black and brown rings. I also enjoyed its fragrant wood aroma. When I finally finished my carving, the shape was very pleasing to me and I would immediately present it to my mother as a gift. She was very proud of my little wood carvings, which she hung on the kitchen wall for everyone to see.

A Young Man Dreams

During my university years, I had several opportunities to tour Europe. I traveled to Paris and visited the Louvre museum. I was awed by the works of the great masters, including Michaelangelo, Matisse and Rodin. I was thrilled by what I saw, and I yearned to be an artist too. In school I read that Michelangelo would examine a piece of marble for days, sometimes months, before he could envision the work of art that was inside. I felt this too. I believe there is art in every object. Sometimes its beauty is hidden, lying just beneath the surface. One only has to look deep enough to find it.

Seeking Perfection

I remember another story — this one about the famous artist Matisse, who often visited the museums where his paintings hung. His visits would strike horror in the face of the museum curator, who watched helplessly as Matisse set up his paints and brushes and continued to work on his paintings as they hung on the museum wall! It seems the world considered his works completed masterpieces, but Matisse considered them works in progress and continued seeking perfection, never feeling his work was done.

Sculpting a face or body out of clay, it is easy to make changes. Soon forgotten is the old shape as it takes on a new form. As an artist, I begin with one dimension, then I add a second, then a third. For me, the picture is complete when the pieces talk to each other. The nose fits the face and the mouth fits the nose, and so on — everything in balance and proportion. Then it is beautiful. Working with clay, I immediately have an added dimension, which I can mold and bend into a new shape. Its shape begins to speak as it takes on a new form. It moves and is full of life.

Molding the Human Form

An artist has many opportunities to correct his work. He can remold or paint over what he doesn't like. He can go out and take a walk and think about how he would like the finished work to look. This is not true in plastic surgery. A surgeon basically has one chance to get it right. With the human body, the surgeon works with muscle, skin, bone and fat. Though human flesh has the ability to be molded into a new shape and form, it is very different — it is life held in the surgeon's hands, a sacred trust of one human being to another.

Plastic surgery is the combination of applied art and science. Surgeons must be familiar with the sense of aesthetics and science — how they can be combined, and the limitations of each. Years of medical training have given me the knowledge of the underlying anatomy and the technical skills to create the face or body a patient desires.

Every patient is unique. When I meet patients for the first time, I watch the way they enter the consultation room. I notice how they look and how they carry themselves. I listen to how they speak. I talk with them and feel their skin and examine their bone structure. But, most of all, I listen to what they tell me about their lives, their hopes, their fears and what they want their surgery to achieve. A patient may bring in a picture of herself that was taken 20 or 30 years ago and say, "Can you make me look like this again?" I nod my head, understanding this desire which has been shared by many patients before. I attempt to understand her body image. Sometimes, she projects what she thinks others see in her. Or, she projects the ideals placed on her by a culture obsessed with youth and beauty and constantly reflected in the news media and the popular cinema. I use all this information, combined with my experience in surgery and in art to understand what she is looking

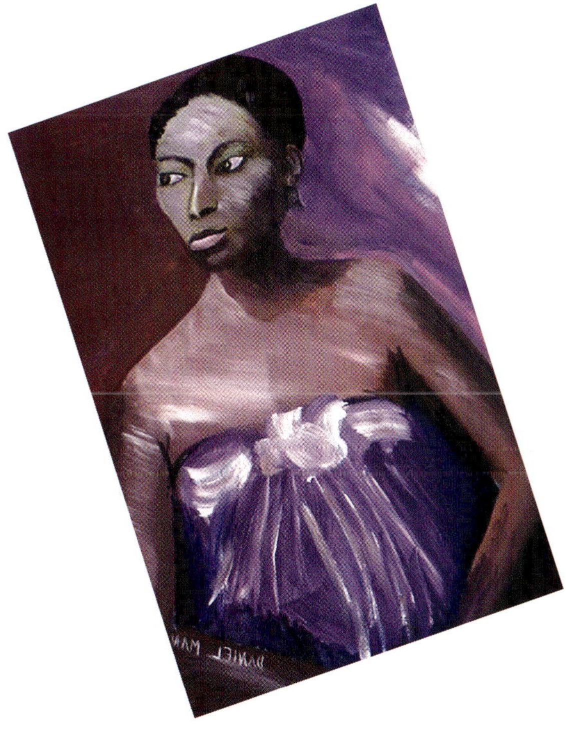

for to improve her body image. Finally, I try to envision the inner person, the inner beauty, and the potential that are lying so close to the surface. When I look at her, I visualize a finished work of art that truly expresses how she feels inside.

Youth & Body Image

Usually, our body image is tied to our youth. I will see a young girl who wants her breasts enlarged. I ask, " Why now?" She will give a host of reasons, "I did not have the money until now," or, "My boyfriend was not sure." I may see another woman who is older. At 56, this woman shows signs of frown lines, deep furrows on her brow and heavy eyelids. The fine jaw others admired in her youth is sagging now and has taken on a jowled look. I ask her, "Do you think about this every day?" If she answers "yes," then it is probably time for a change.

Turning Back the Clock

Cosmetic surgery is not a panacea. It won't improve your love life or guarantee a big job promotion. But it can make you look better and feel better about yourself. The rest is up to you. Aging is an inevitable consequence with which we must all live. But, we don't have to live with an aging appearance. Our youthful appearance has been altered by the aging process. As we age, our bones shrink and we add more fat. These changes leave many people unhappy. They don't like what they see in the mirror. There is a conflict between their age and their body image, which is reflected whenever they see a picture of themselves. Some people are attached to the body image of their youth. Inside they feel much younger and they would like the outside to correspond to their feelings. They would do anything to stay with the body image of their youth.

In my practice, I see many patients who truly suffer from an aging appearance. As a plastic surgeon it is my job to help people who want to change look better, so they feel better about themselves. Fortunately, medical science has given us that ability.

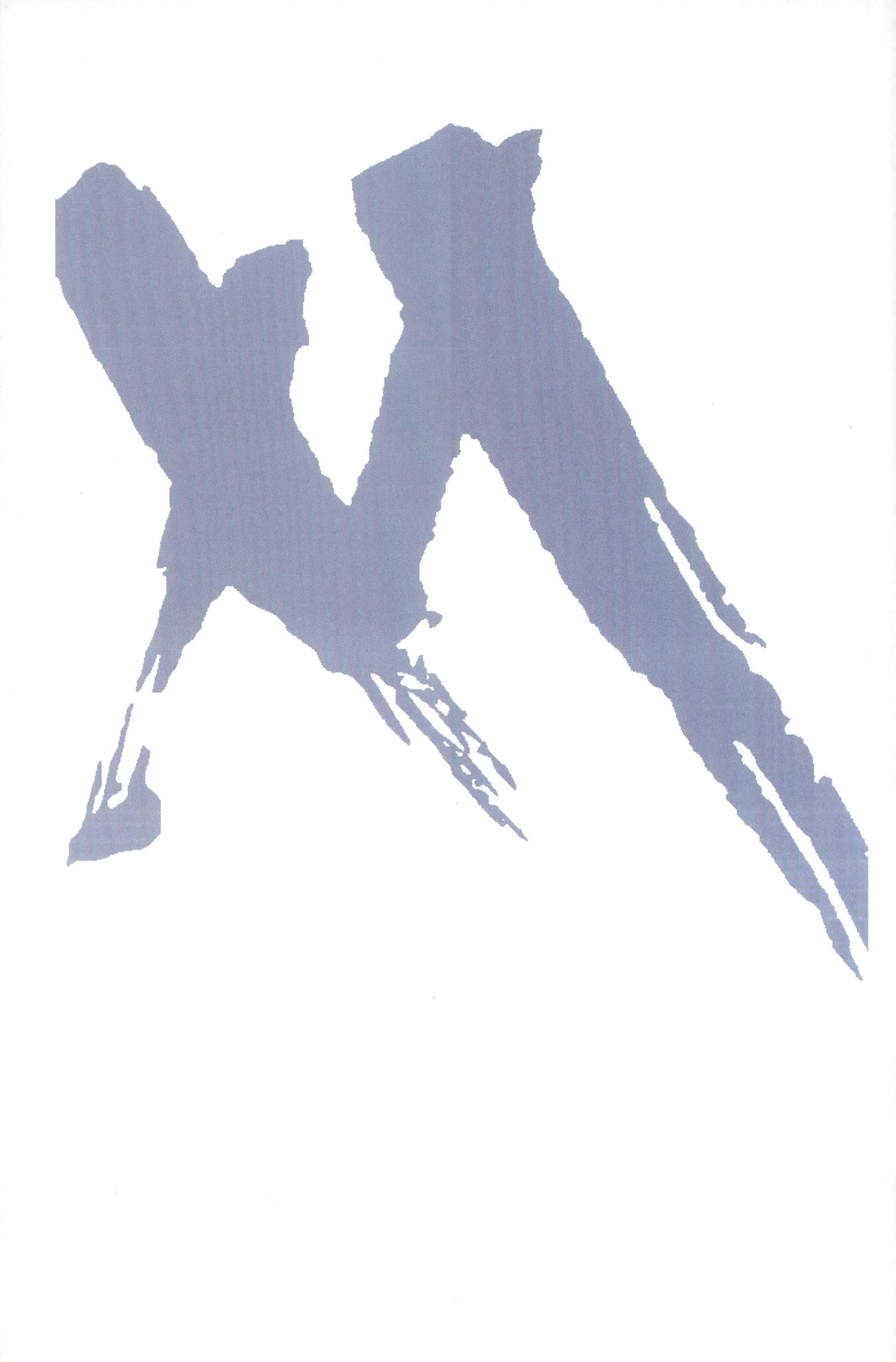

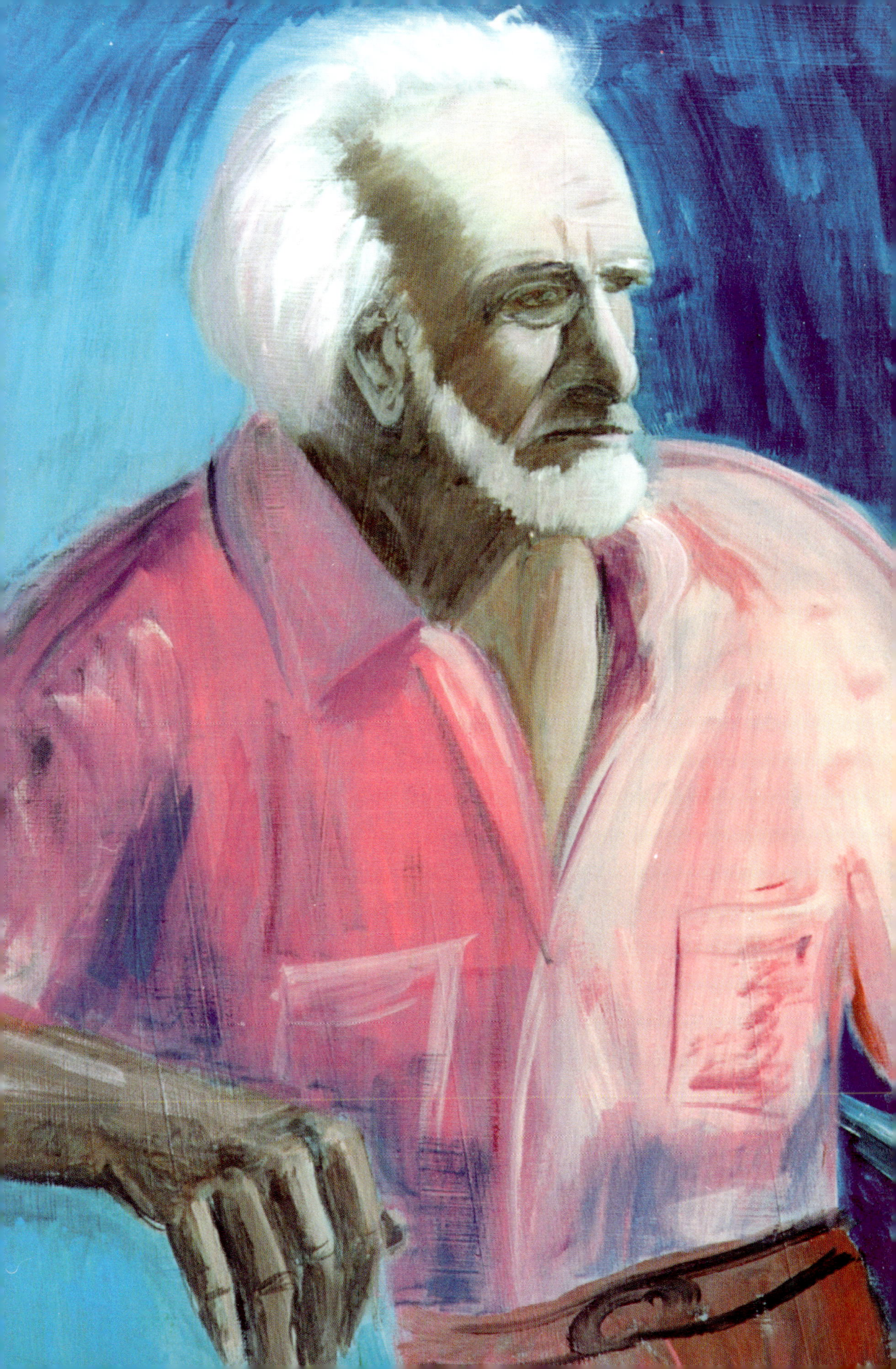

Part 2

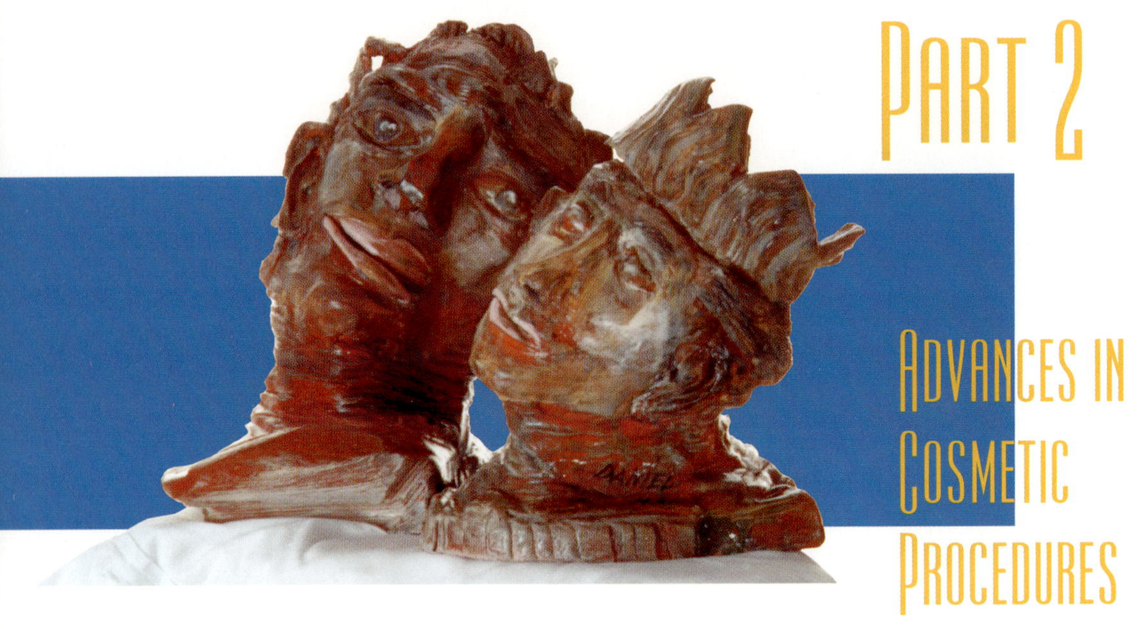

Advances in Cosmetic Procedures

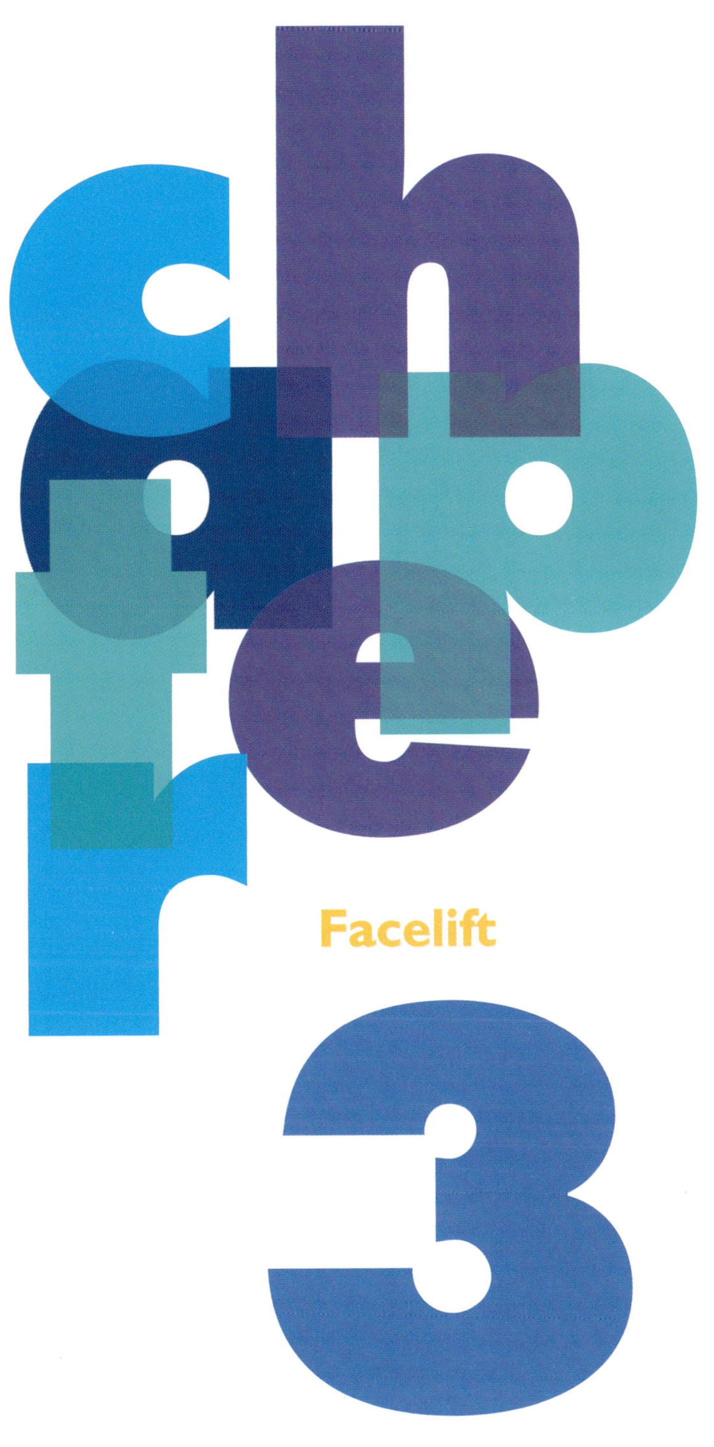

Facelift

3

FACELIFT

A facelift is the surgical procedure used to correct the aging face. As we age, the muscles of the face and neck sag, jowls form as the jaw line becomes less defined and thickens with layers of excess fat. Smile lines, the creases from the nose to the mouth, become deeper. The eyelids become fleshy and heavy as fat deposits form on the upper and lower eyelids. Fat pads make our cheeks plump and round in youth, but diminish and fall with age.

Everything seems to sag as gravity takes its toll. No longer firm and taut, the skin loses its elasticity, becoming loose and lax. Sun damage and age cause wrinkles, lines and brown spots to form, giving the skin a rough texture and uneven appearance.

Is Younger Better?

Who is the best candidate? It is not surprising to see patients in their late 30s and early 40s considering a facelift. At this age, there is very good skin elasticity and muscle tone that allow for excellent results. A good candidate for a facelift is one who has skin that still retains some elasticity and has a strong, well-defined bone structure.

FACELIFT

Rhytidectomy

Purpose: *Tightens sagging skin and muscles of the face, removes jowls and gives a more pleasing contour, giving the face a more youthful appearance. May be combined with a neck, eye or forehead lift and laser surgery.*

Surgery: *Length is 2 – 4 hours, or more depending on the extent. Outpatient surgery, often with an overnight stay.*

Anesthesia: *General or I.V. sedation.*

Recovery: *Patients experience postoperative tightness, swelling and bruising for several weeks. Numbness may last up to several months. Back to work: 1 – 2 weeks. Avoid strenuous activities for 2 – 3 weeks. Makeup: 1 – 2 weeks.*

Risks: *Nerve injury, poor healing, infections, scarring, bleeding, change in hairline.*

Cost: *$6,700 – $20,000.*

**(Note: Prices may vary based on physician fees, anesthesia, surgical setting and number of procedures. Data is based on a compilation of sources including Dr. Man.)*

Of course, this is the ideal. More often, the rule is the patient who does not possess perfect proportions, has loss of muscle tone, severe wrinkling and lax tissue. In many cases, the patient may also have had a previous facelift. These patients can still expect excellent results.

Advances in surgical and anesthetic techniques allow patients to undergo surgery with less discomfort, scarring, bruising and down time — time lost from work or activities. Patients have surgery in the morning, stay overnight, and usually return home the next day.

How Long Does It Last?

The life span of a facelift is also improving; facelifts are now lasting longer (seven to ten years) thanks to new and improved methods being used by plastic surgeons. These advances are particularly good news for patients who have had previous facelifts and for smokers whose skin has little or no elasticity, and often heal slowly.

More "Natural Looking"

Prior to the 1970s, facelift surgery was pretty much a nip and tuck process that basically required the surgeon to separate the outer skin (facial tissue) from the underlying muscle, pull the skin up and back, and trim off the excess. If the surgeon pulled the skin too tight by overcorrecting, it could result in a "wind-blown" or "pulled" look, especially if the skin had little elasticity left.

Advances /New Tools

Modern facelift techniques, however, go much deeper and are more complex. New uses of video magnification, endoscopy and laser tools are also available today. Excess fat and skin are removed with laser assistance, while the underlying layers of connective tissue and muscles called the platysma and SMAS are tightened. SMAS stands for superficial musculoaponeurotic system, which attaches the layers of sagging, connective tissue to the underlying facial muscles and bones.

The Total Picture

In addition, plastic surgeons today take a much more artistic approach. They look at the face as a total picture, not just parts of it. Anatomically, the face is a complex structure of fat, cartilage, bone, connective tissue, muscles and nerves. The underlying structure of our face is what gives it its shape and expression. When facial structures fall or become lax, they usually do so as a unit. Fixing only parts of the face may not complete the total picture or achieve the patient's desires.

Every facelift is different and individually planned for each patient. I always ask patients what they don't like about their appearance. Sometimes it is necessary to combine several techniques in order for patients to achieve their desired results. Depending on the patient's needs, I may

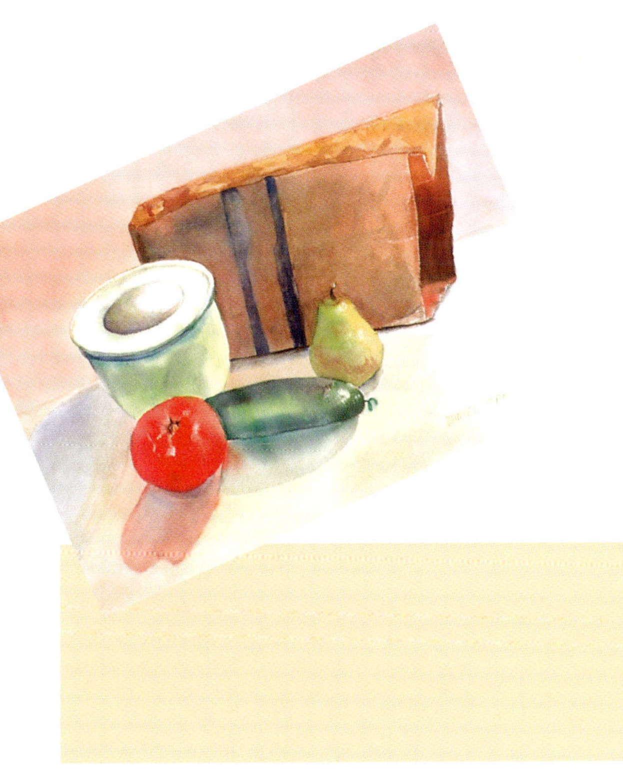

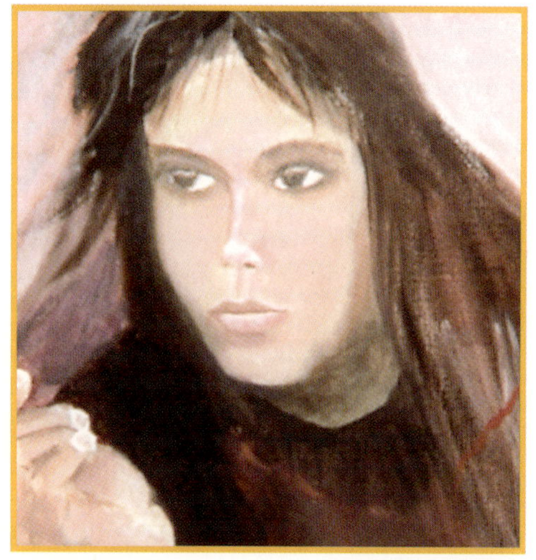

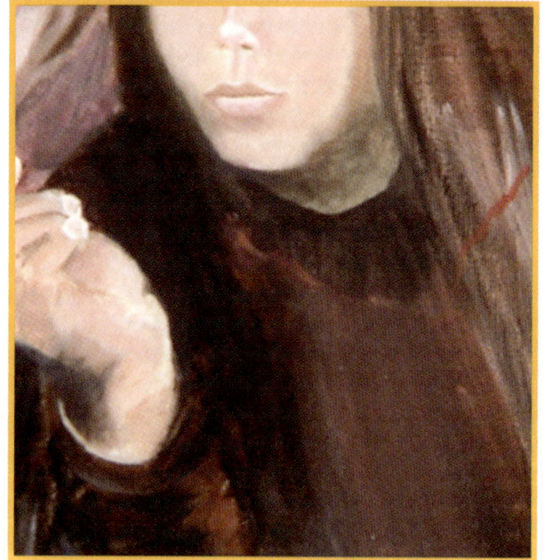

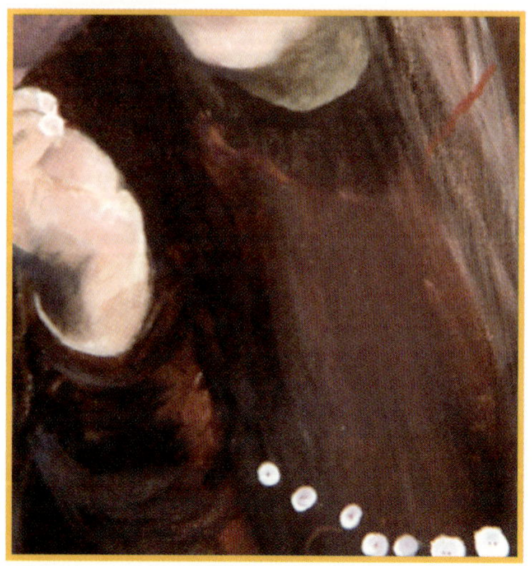

recommend that a facelift be combined or followed by laser resurfacing, an endoscopic forehead lift, eyelift, chin implant, cheek augmentation or nasal contouring.

Patients often ask about their skin. As one of my patients reasoned, "Why drape old, sun-damaged skin over a newly restructured face?" A facelift will eliminate many wrinkles, but fine lines, blemishes, acne scars and sun-damaged skin will remain. In this case, I would recommend that the patient also have laser skin resurfacing or the Skin Rejuvenation Peel® to remove sun damage, brown spots and pigmentation irregularities. (More details about lasers and peels are covered in Chapters 4 and 5).

More Innovations & Advancements

In the late 1980s and early 1990s I originated a new facelift technique to reduce the "pulled," or "wind-blown" look, sometimes associated with traditional facelift surgery. This technique utilizes a crescent-shaped, balloon device called the "Man Facelift Expander", (Reported in

Plastic and Reconstructive Surgery, October 1989), which is placed temporarily under the skin and inflated for several minutes and then removed. The surgeon, instead of pulling the skin in only one direction, as is performed in the traditional facelift, is able to stretch the skin circumferentially in all directions at once, similar to the way the skin is stretched naturally. This helps prevent a tight, "pulled look" since it allows additional skin and wrinkles to be removed while giving a more "natural" looking appearance. Looking natural is the key. "Natural" facelifts are also tailored to a patient's particular expressions which are unique to each patient and are left intact. When performing a facelift on men, the surgeon will also take into account the patient's natural hairline, sideburns and beard growth.

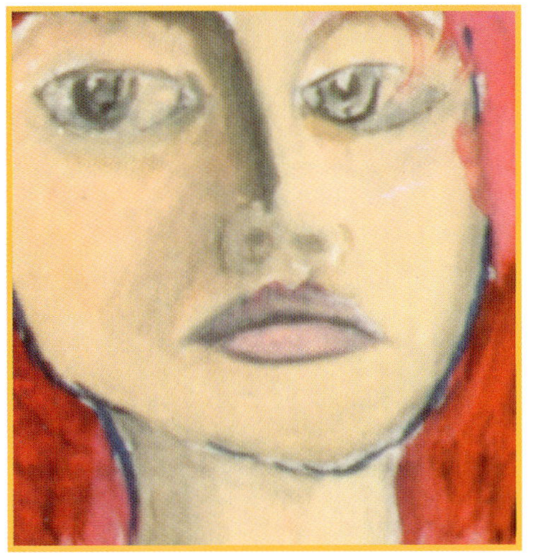

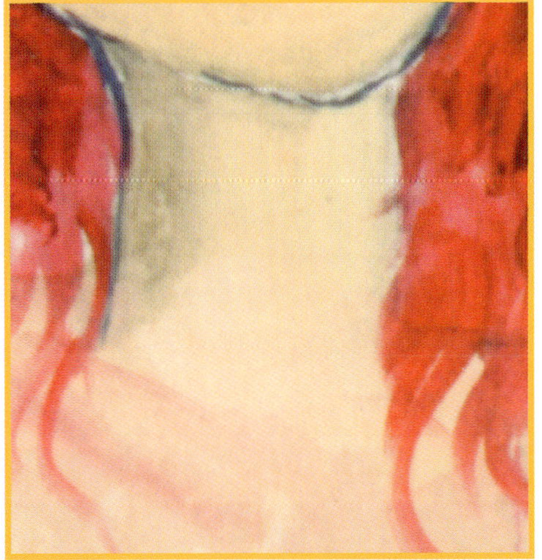

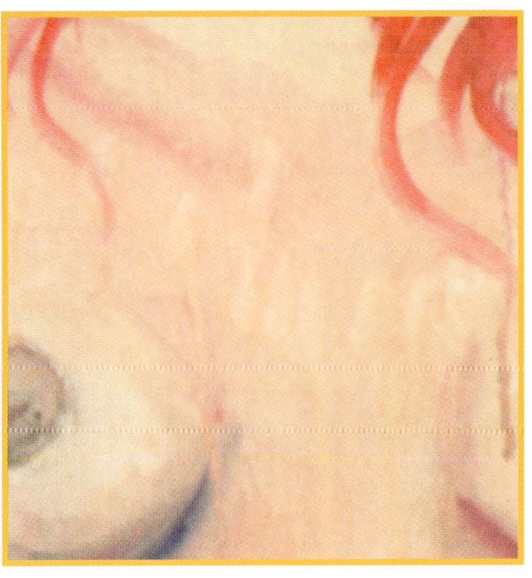

This process also reduces tension on the suture sites during closure, which is important for good healing to occur, and achieves less hair loss in front of the ears.

Endoscopic Facelift

Another innovation is the endoscope. The endoscope is a small, telescope-like instrument that allows the surgeon to see inside the human body. The endoscope has been adopted for nearly every surgical procedure from joint surgery to hernia repair. Using the endoscope, the surgeon can see the structures under video magnification in order to tighten muscles, remove fat and perform a number of intricate procedures. The plastic surgeon no longer has to create an ear-to-ear scar, for example, in the case of a forehead lift. This is especially beneficial to patients who have thinning hair or receding hairlines.

Less scarring means less pain, less bleeding and faster recovery.

Laser Assistance

Lasers, too, have become a valuable tool for the plastic surgeon. A marvel of medical science, lasers help to cut, cauterize and vaporize tissue and blood vessels.

A facelift alone will not remove all wrinkles. Modern lasers, such as the erbium and carbon dioxide laser, can be used at the same time to help smooth out wrinkles, resurfacing the skin and removing fine line wrinkles, such as crow's feet around the eyes, lines over the upper lip and acne scarring. (More about lasers is discussed in Chapter 4).

I believe that the endoscope and the laser will find more and more applications in cosmetic surgery, as plastic surgeons continue improving results and speeding recovery for patients.

Risks & Complications

Though facelift surgery is generally safe, side effects and complications can occur. These should be discussed candidly with your surgeon.

Thousands of women and men undergo successful facelift surgery each year. But, there is no guarantee. Any doctor may perform cosmetic surgery, but would it make sense to go to a gynecologist to have cataracts removed? It is important to check your doctor's credentials. Get to know the doctor and talk to several patients. Ask how many procedures of the kind you are considering the doctor has performed. Make sure your doctor is board-certified in the practice of plastic surgery and that he or she serves on the staff at local hospitals and has privileges to perform plastic surgery at those hospitals. Your surgeon should also be in good standing with the American Society of Plastic and Reconstructive Surgeons and local medical societies. (See Chapter 18, The Consultation: Finding a Doctor.)

Surgery Length

A facelift usually takes from two to four hours, longer if additional procedures are being performed at the same time. It may be performed under general anesthesia, or with intravenous sedation in an outpatient surgical facility. Before surgery, patients are asked to stop smoking, stop taking aspirin, have blood tests and an EKG, and have a medical clearance from their family physician.

In my practice, patients have surgery and stay overnight. They may choose to go home the next day or several days afterwards. Sutures are usually removed between four to ten days after surgery, and many patients are able to go about their everyday activities and return to work in two to three weeks.

Patients should review the risks with their doctor prior to surgery. Most patients develop temporary swelling and bruising. Possible complications include, but are not limited to, bleeding, swelling and bruising, nerve injury and loss of sensation (which usually returns), infection, reaction to anesthesia, hair loss, scarring and problems in healing. Some patients may experience transient depression soon after surgery, which should pass.

FACELIFTS

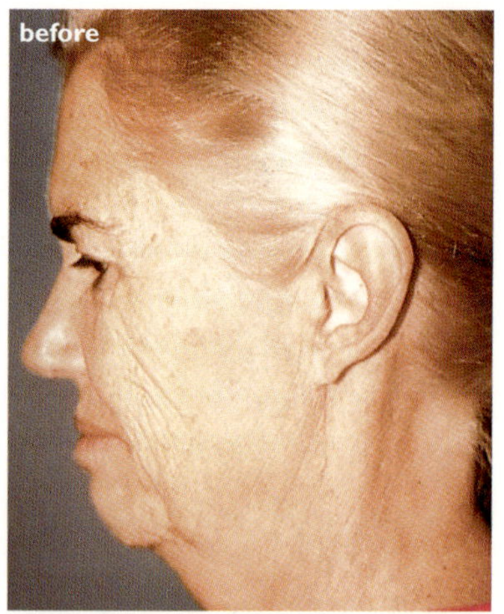

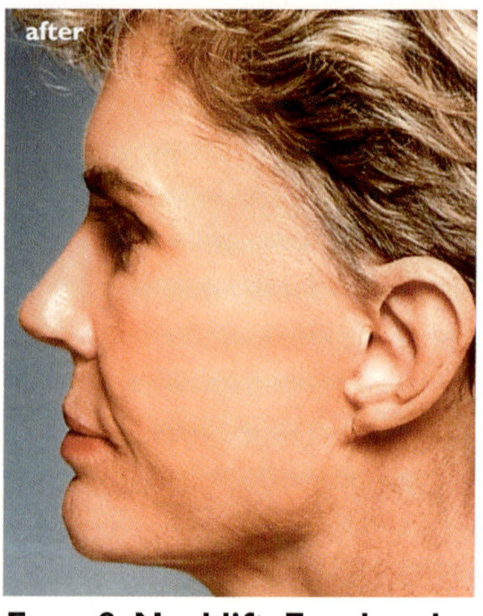

Face & Necklift; Forehead Lift; Lower & Upper Eyelids; Chin Implant and Skin Rejuvenation Peel.

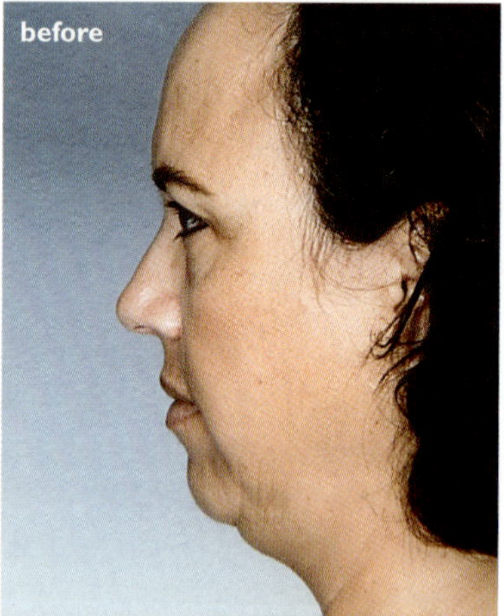

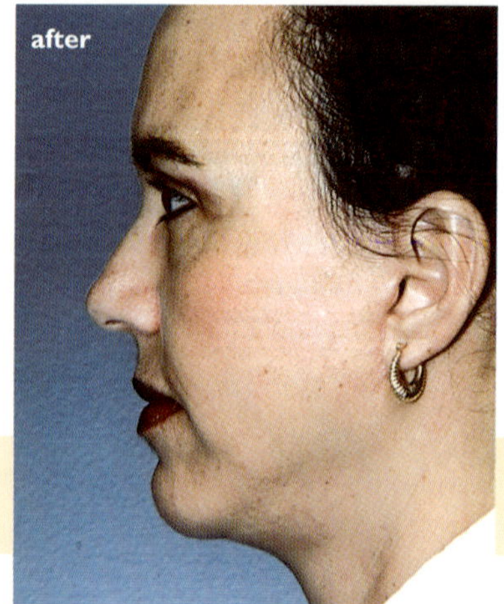

Face & Necklift; Chin Implant; Liposculpture Upper & Lower Eyelids, Earlobe.

FACELIFTS

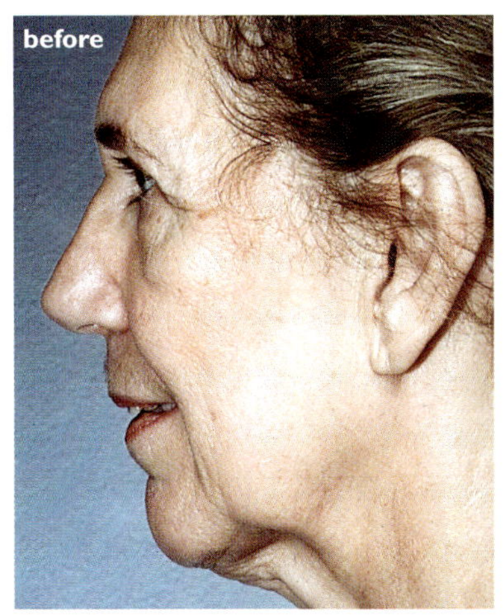

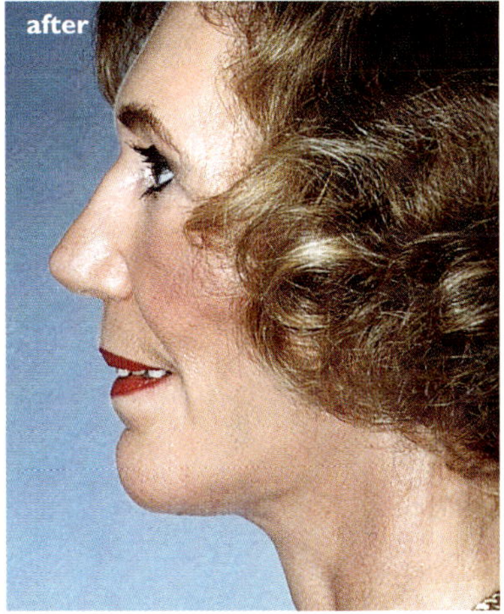

Face & Necklift;
Endoscopic Forehead Lift;
Upper and Lower Eyes;
Full facc Laser

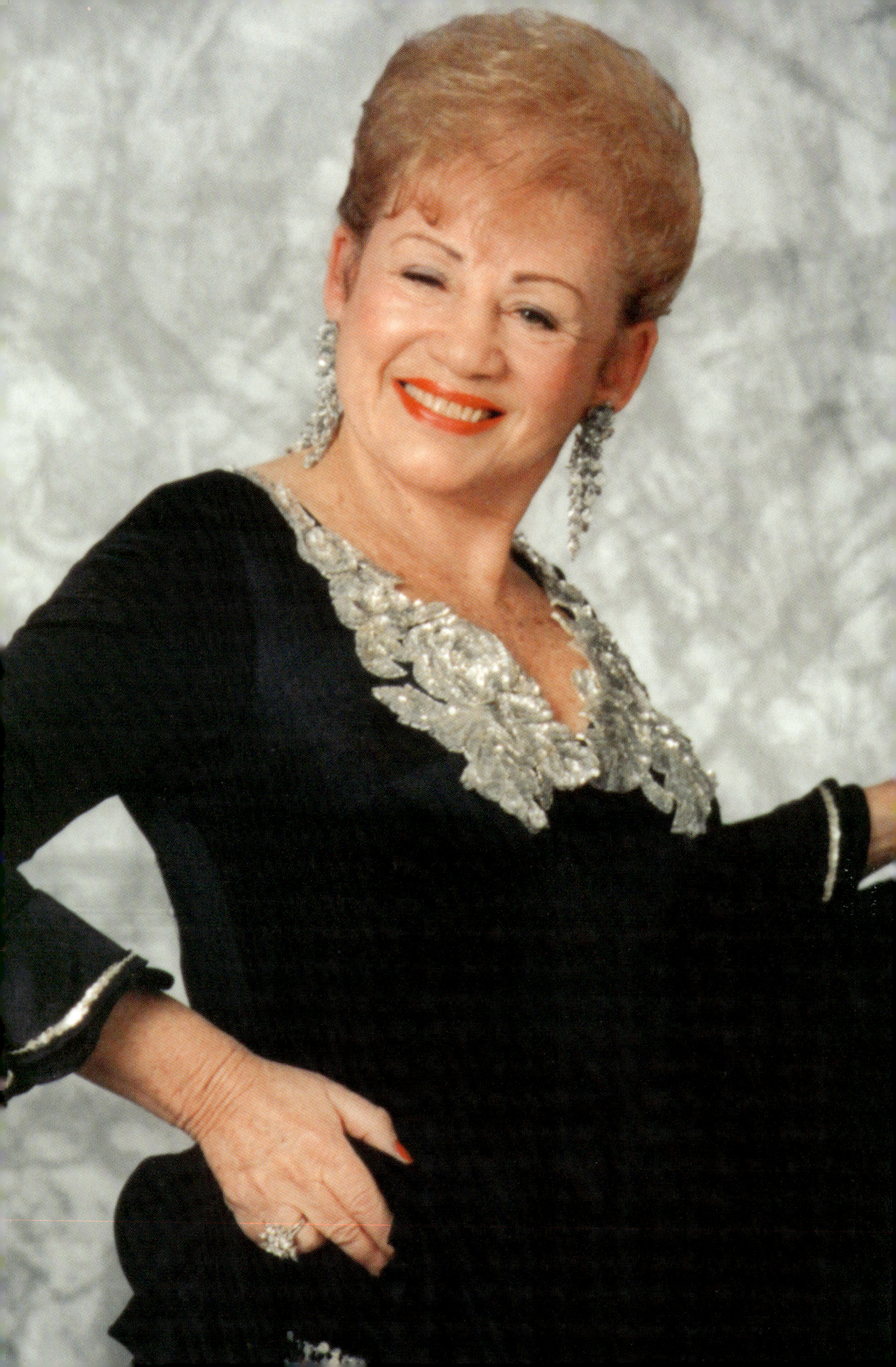

PATIENT PORTRAIT

SYLVIA SHEAR
FACE & NECK LIFT, FOREHEAD LIFT, CHIN IMPLANT, UPPER EYELID
AGE: 72

I was 65 years old when I realized my face and neck were sagging. I wanted to look good, so when I won $5,000 in the Florida Lottery, I knew exactly what I wanted to do with it.

My husband and I have been married for 53 years. He thinks I am as young and beautiful as the day we first met, when mutual friends introduced us. I remember how he accompanied me to the shoe store one day shortly after we were introduced. At the shoe store I tried on a pair of shoes. The radio was playing and he said let's test them. So we started dancing right there in the store. It was wonderful. That's when I fell in love with Sol and I knew I wanted to marry him. We've been dancing ever since. We danced in the dance studios in Brooklyn. When we retired to Florida, we kept dancing. Now, we go to Luigi's Ballroom at the Italian-American Club. We've been going there for over 16 years. We do the tango and the disco, and we love Latin rhythm and waltzes, too.

Dancing keeps us young. It's great for staying fit and it's a great way to meet people. You meet the nicest people dancing. I stayed very active and felt young. What I felt inside didn't match the outside. So I had the facelift. My husband was very supportive. Anything I wanted to do was okay with him.

Two and a half weeks after my facelift I went to have my hair done. My hairdresser said she couldn't get over how good I looked. The scars were so fine you hardly saw anything.

Now when I'm dancing I know I look as good on the outside as I feel inside.

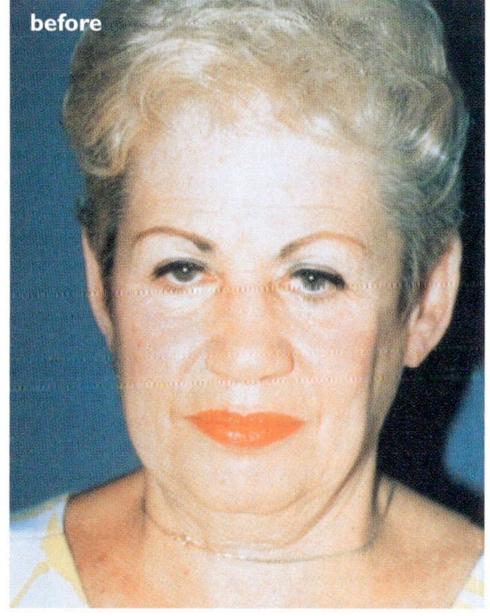

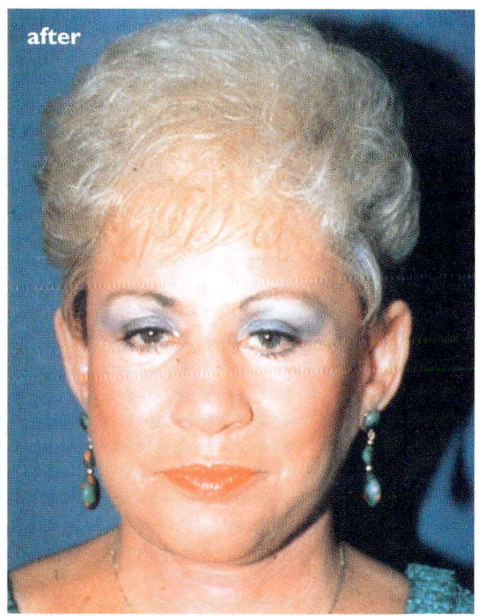

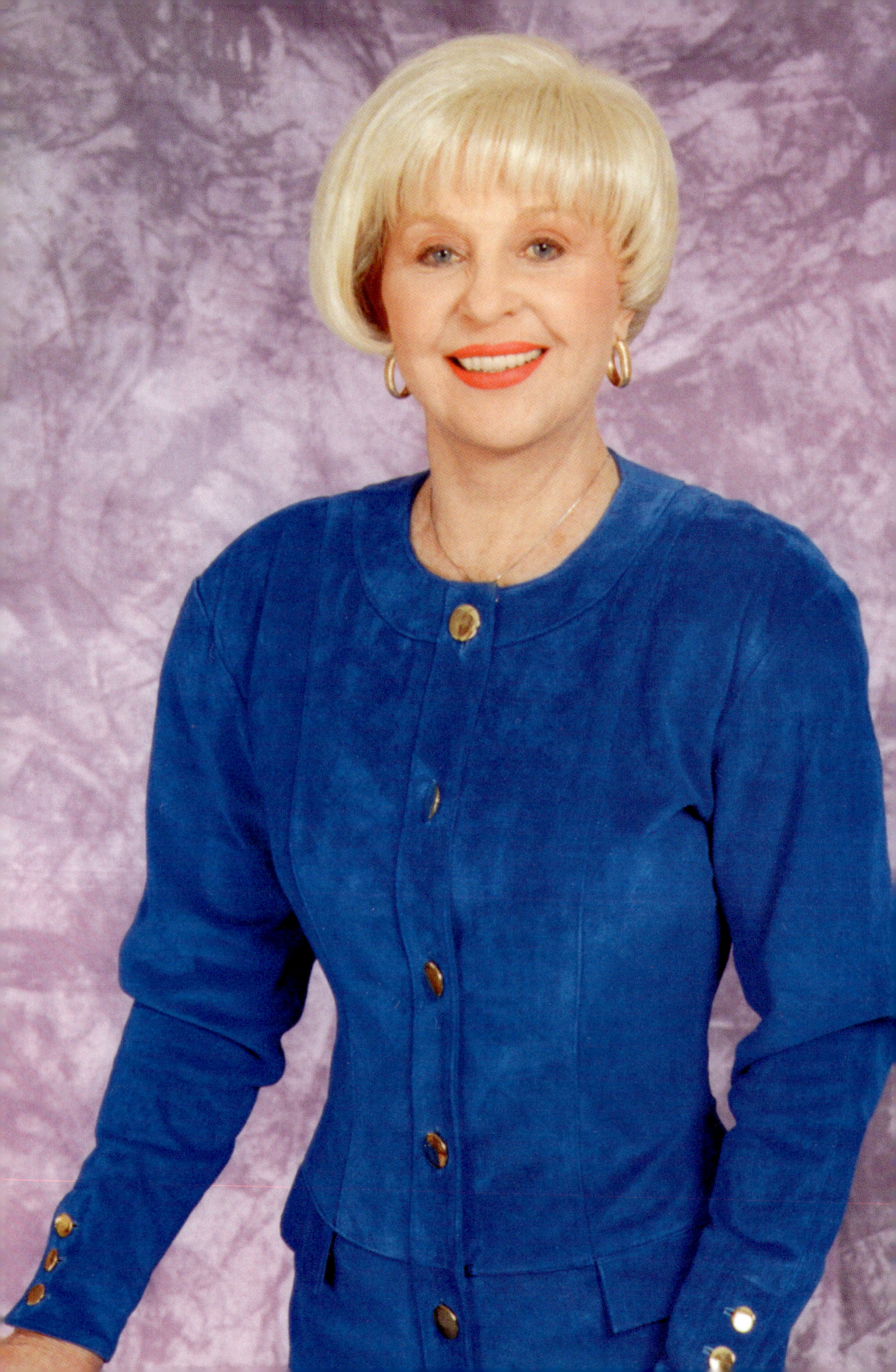

PATIENT PORTRAIT

LILLIAN PRIMPAS
FACE & NECK LIFT, FOREHEAD LIFT, CHIN IMPLANT, EYE LIFT, SKIN REJUVENATION PEEL
AGE: 66

When I was a child my family would gather every Saturday night in the kitchen. The men would play cards and the women would talk. I wasn't shy; I would sing and dance like a dimpled Shirley Temple and they would all laugh and applaud. It was a happy time. When I was 5, my cousin and her boyfriend came to the house. They looked at my 3-year-old sister Virginia exclaiming, "Isn't she cute?" And they took her with them when they went out, while I was left at home. I didn't understand why. But I thought that they left me because she was cute and I was ugly. Oh, the things children think! That cut into my heart like a knife. I never forgot it. I think that experience colored my whole life and made me withdrawn. I didn't dance or sing anymore. I grew up feeling that I wasn't pretty. I would always try to hide my face whenever anyone paid me a compliment because it always made me feel self-conscious. I never really heard the compliment. I just felt exposed and uncomfortable. It was so bad that whenever I walked into a room, I would sit in the back and hide because I didn't want people to look at me. Now I can stand in front of a room full of people and speak.

I had always promised myself a facelift when I got older. I knew it was time when George, my husband, would sit and stare at me. Before, he always gave me compliments. Now, he just looked. When I said, "What are you looking at?" He said, "It's time." When we went out one night I really tried to put my make-up on with care. In the elevator, George looked at me and said, "It's really time."

My facelift has made me a new person. It is miraculous what this has done for me. I even got my dimples back. Before my surgery, I had spent my whole life being shy and withdrawn. I had this terrible feeling of inferiority.

I was in the grocery store and I noticed a woman who followed me up one aisle and down the next. Everytime I stopped, she stopped. But, she wasn't putting anything in her cart. She was staring at me. I mean really staring. This kept happening for several aisles. So, I finally turned to her and asked if I could help her find something. "I'm sorry," she said, "but, your skin looks so beautiful, I can't help staring at it. Do you mind if I keep walking with you?" I said okay. I didn't tell her I had anything done, and she didn't ask. That was one of the first times I realized how good I looked. What a great feeling that was.

George loves my new looks too. Now, when we're at the breakfast table, I stare at him. "What?" he asks. I smile and say, "It's time."

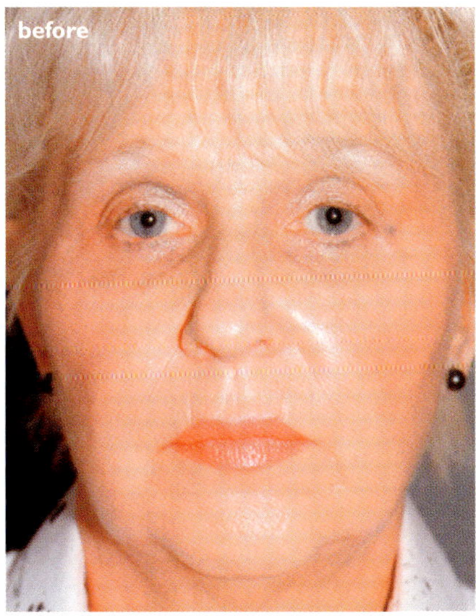
before

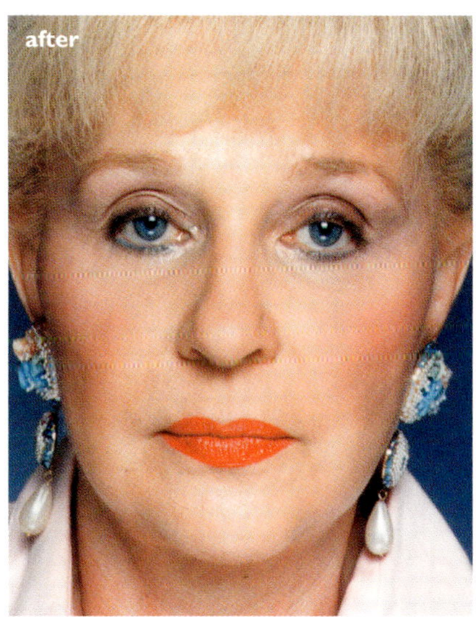
after

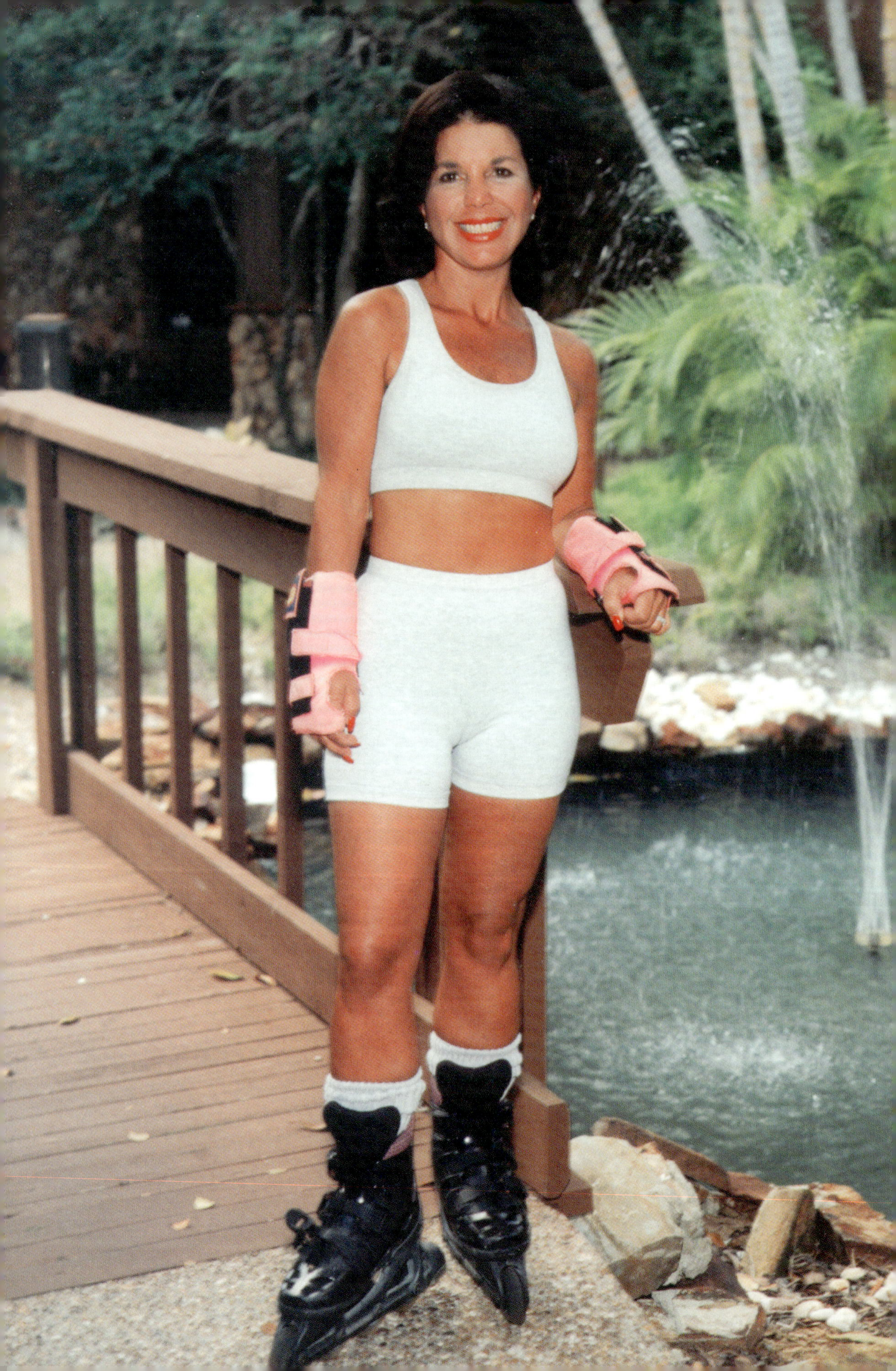

PATIENT PORTRAIT

RISE WEST
FACE & NECK LIFT, FOREHEAD LIFT, NOSE SURGERY, LIPOSUCTION, FAT INJECTIONS, UPPER & LOWER EYELIFT, BREAST SURGERY, MEDIUM PEEL
AGE: 48

This all began when my 76-year-old father expressed interest in having a facelift. His interest surprised me, so I researched plastic surgery for my father and began to look into the subject. I wanted to find the right doctor for him. I must say I was very thorough, because I wanted my father to be satisfied.

When my father and I went for his consultation, I asked a few questions about my own appearance. I wanted to have my eyes done. We do a lot of entertaining because my husband is in the commercial investment real estate business and I think it is important that I look good. My husband has to look at me all the time, and, although he tells me I'm beautiful, I realized that I wasn't looking so great.

I didn't realize how bad I really looked until I saw my results. Before my facelift, I looked frumpy — and tired. When you are in your 40s you can look tired even when you're not. But now, I look like a kid again! You can tell how pleased I am with my facelift because that really got me started on self-improvement. I was so thrilled about the results that I just couldn't wait to look even better. Now, I've had my eyes, my nose and my breasts done. I've had liposuction on my knees, my inner thighs, my saddlebags — and I'm not done yet! I watch my diet, I'm dedicated to my exercise routine. I like to Roller Blade. It makes me feel better, healthier and more self-directed. I look at other people and I look to see if they had anything done. I see people who are walking around looking like a mess — and I can't believe it. They have their hair colored and their nails manicured, but they look bad. Their faces are sagging, they have wrinkles all over, and they have bags under their eyes. I wonder about peoples' priorities. I see people driving $100,000 cars, but they look terrible. I want to tell them, "Go have your face done, or get a nose job."

I'm so excited about the way I look. My doctor contoured my face to look much prettier, and he gave me the breasts of a 16-year-old. My husband said I should attach a mirror to my arm so I could keep it with me. I promised myself that I was never going to look old and frumpy again. There is no stigma anymore to plastic surgery. Everybody goes to the dentist routinely so they will be able to keep their teeth. This is the same thing, it's just another kind of maintenance. I plan on maintaining my face and body so I can keep getting better and better.

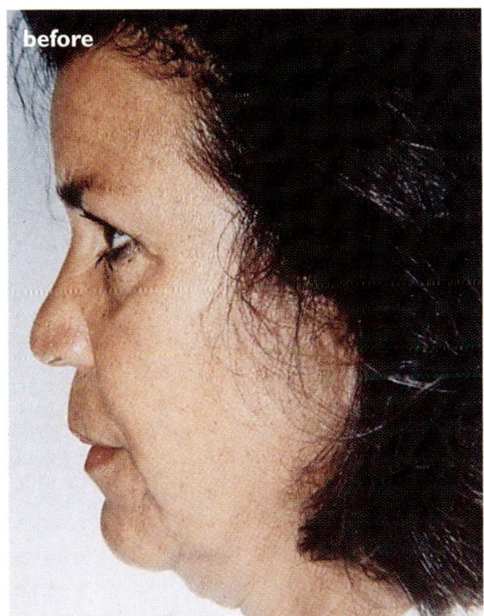
before

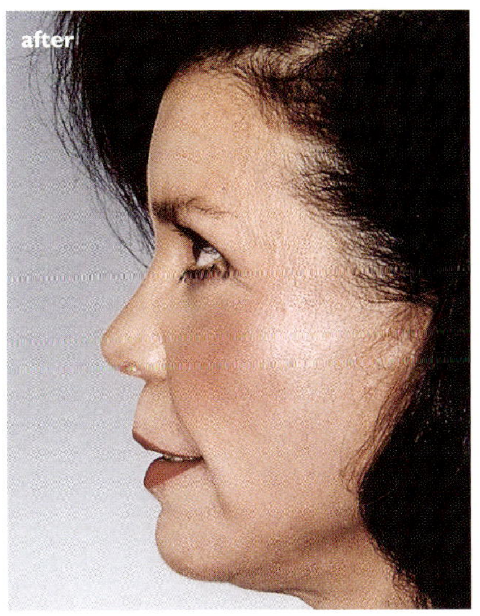
after

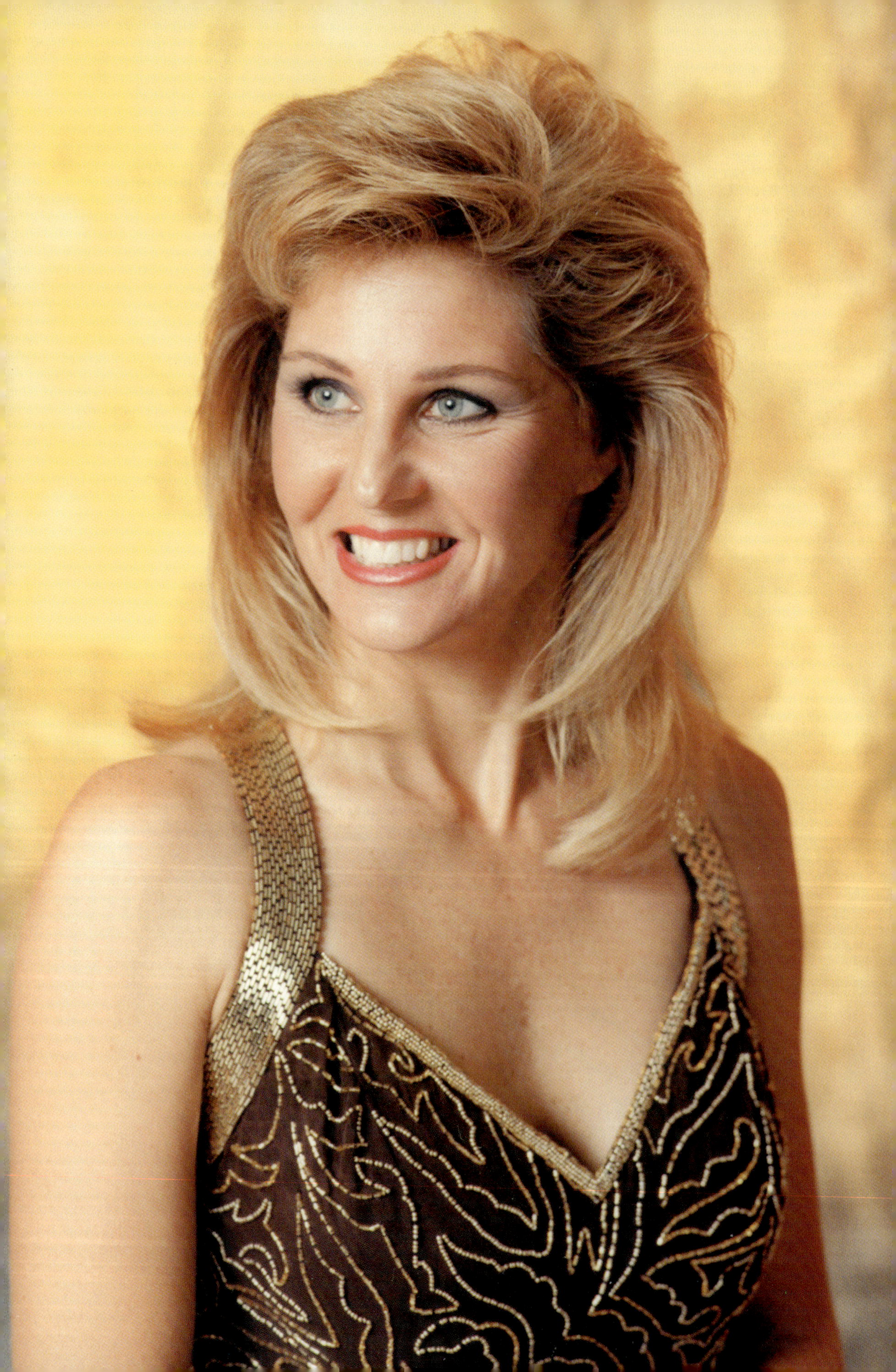

PATIENT PORTRAIT

SHARON MAIN
FACE & NECK LIFT, UPPER & LOWER EYELIFT, BREAST SURGERY
AGE: 38

Having plastic surgery was a family decision. I was concerned about the money because I don't contribute to the household income. I'm staying at home to raise my 4-year-old twins. It keeps me very busy. A year ago I noticed my skin beginning to sag. My face had absolutely no elasticity. Everything about it was dropping. My jaw was sagging, so was my neck. I think it runs in my family because I've got my Dad's jaw. I had heard that the younger you go for a facelift, the better the results. Why wait till you're 50 and sagging and then have it done? I was 38 when I had my facelift.

I plan on going back to work when the kids go to school. I know it's very competitive out there. But I'll be ready when that time comes. In the meantime, I'm very happy. I do mom stuff all day. My husband is an airline pilot, so he travels a lot. We like to spend our time with the kids.

After my kids were born, my breasts began to sag. So I also had my breasts lifted. I believe surgery is safer and a lot more advanced than it was even a few years ago. The majority of people in a few years will think nothing about going to their plastic surgeon. It's like going to the dentist. Having your eyes done today is nothing. Nobody keeps it a secret anymore. I think women doing it are liberating men. After one of my last visits to the doctor, my husband plopped down in the chair and said, "I think maybe I'll get rid of this," grabbing his middle. Everybody thinks about it. Men too.

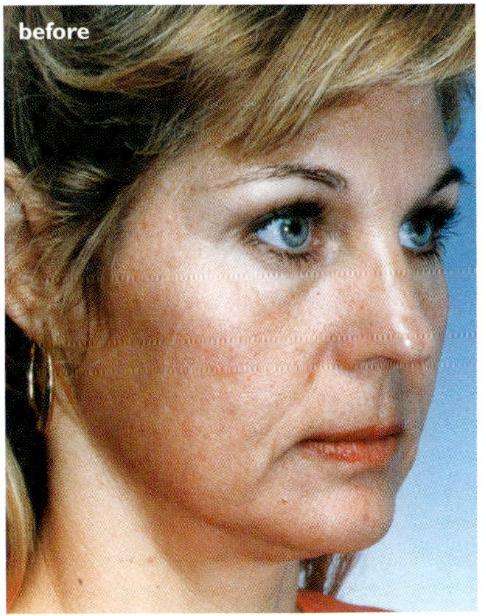
before

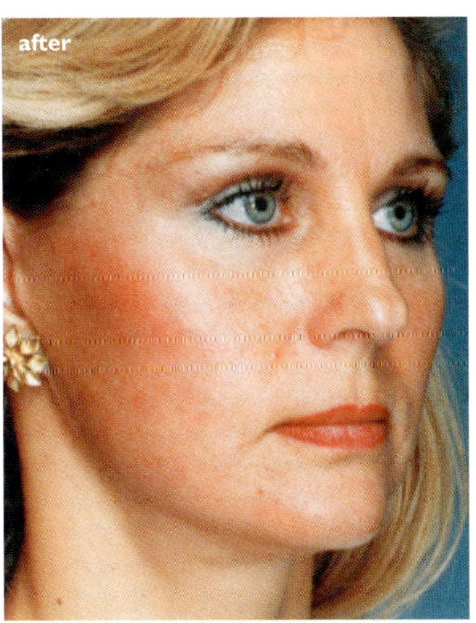
after

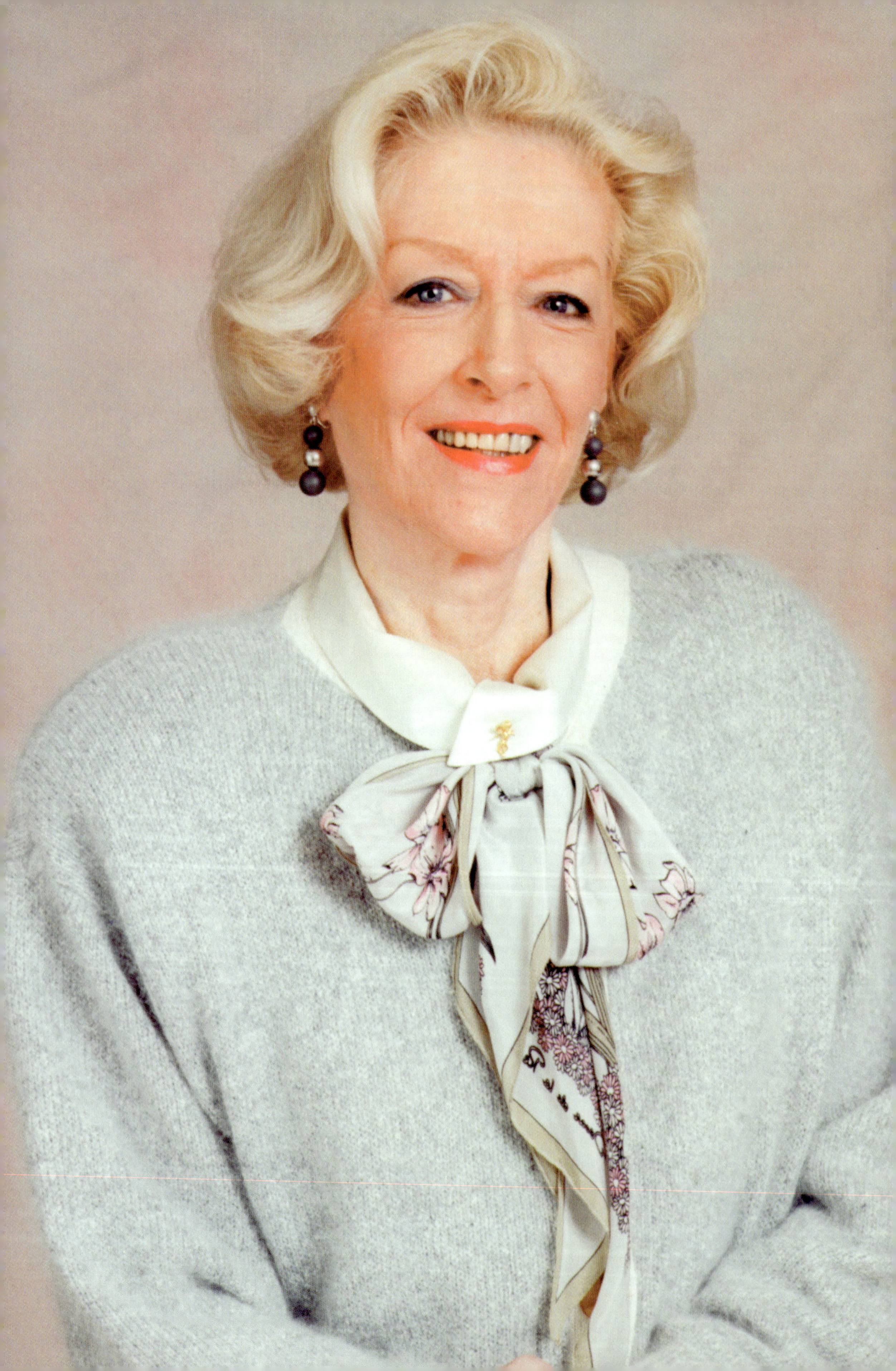

PATIENT PORTRAIT

LUELLA BAILEY
FACE & NECK LIFT, CHIN IMPLANT, GLYCOLIC PEEL
AGE: 77

God gave me my natural expressions, and I wanted to keep them. I had a previous facelift years ago, which felt artificial, like something was holding me up,. I am a former model and beauty and skin care consultant. My husband, Porter, and I started the first esthetician school in Florida.

When you had a facelift twenty years ago, you were hospitalized for ten days. There was bruising. I had to wear a heavy dressing like a helmet on my head for two weeks. I even went home with it!

Today, a facelift is a lot different: There are no heavy dressings, and recovery doesn't take weeks and weeks. When I had my second facelift, I stayed overnight and I went home the next day. I had very little discoloration, no bruising and no pain. I went back to work and I was lecturing in front of a large audience at our esthetician conference the very next week.

Before I had my surgery, I went for consultations to quite a few doctors. When they told me they would show me how I would look on a computer, I politely declined. A computer is just a program, with only so many choices that the doctor can put together. It's not real flesh. It can't tell you that the face on the computer screen is how you are going to look — and it sure can't tell you if the doctor can give you the result that the computer shows.

I wanted my new facelift done by someone who understands skin like I do. When the facelift heals, it is the skin that people see. The doctor has to understand how to drape flesh over the underlying bone, and if he doesn't understand that, if he is just pulling skin up and cutting it off, then he is only a technician and not an artist.

I know that the results depend a lot on the condition of the skin before surgery. It has to be in good condition. It has to be toned and supple, well hydrated and nourished so that it won't dry out and become sensitive from all the anesthesia. If skin is functioning at its maximum before surgery, then recovery will be that much faster. I looked until I found a surgeon who understood all of this and even more.

It's been five years since I had my facelift, and it is still very natural looking. My sagging neck is gone, my lips are relaxed and natural and so are my eyelids. I don't have that awful "pulled tight" look that you see today on some people, even celebrities. The scars from my old facelift were very wide. The doctor fixed that, too, with this facelift. He went into the same areas and now they are very narrow and have faded so that they are barely visible.

Since, my surgery I have also changed my make-up. I've stopped wearing high neck shirts, which I wore to cover the neck wrinkles, and I've added more exciting jewelry. I don't think anyone would guess that I'm 77 years old. Porter, my husband, says I look just like the girl he married half a century ago.

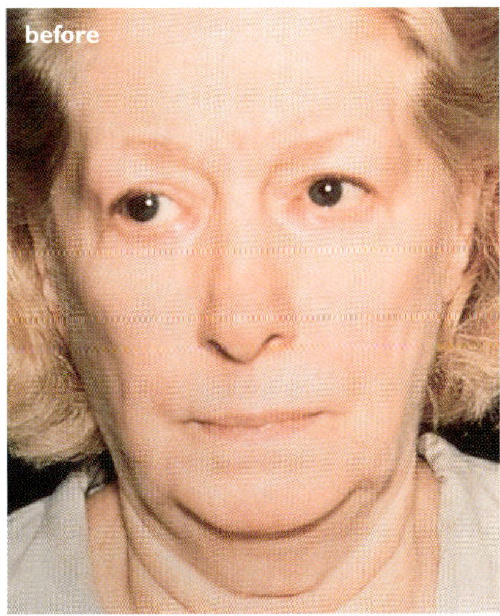

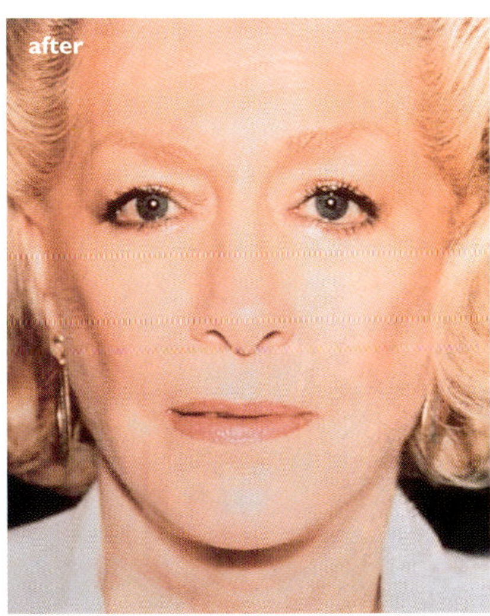

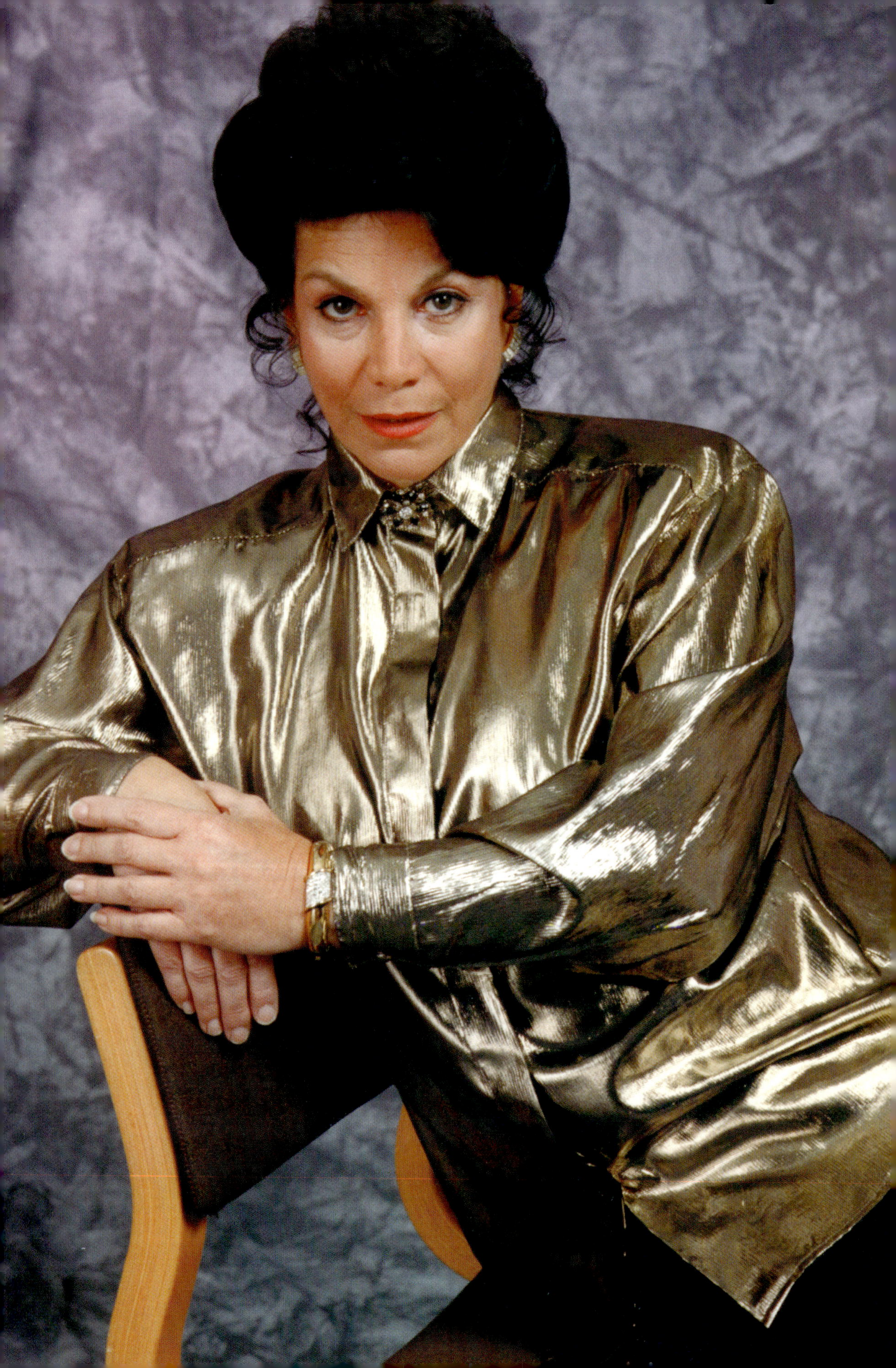

PATIENT PORTRAIT

MARYANN PENNINGTON
FACE & NECK LIFT, FOREHEAD LIFT, UPPER EYE LIFT
AGE: 50

I always knew I would have a facelift when I needed it. I remember talking about it with my father when I was young. My dad was a tall, handsome man. My family is Italian and we have very thick skin. I literally lost all definition to my face just like him! I guess it's hereditary.

One morning I was blow-drying my hair I was leaning from one side to the other, and I noticed that my face was leaning with me. Everyone has a chin line and a neck line, but my face was one big round ball of flesh that wobbled back and forth. I had no chin line and no neck line and I knew that all the makeup tricks in the world — all the special skin products and everything I had learned from years in the beauty business would not solve my problem. So I decided when I had my next birthday I would have a facelift.

I believe that youth and beauty are the equivalent of power for women. Today, women are very much an important part of the work force. It's very competitive. You have to sell yourself every day and be able to go out and represent a company in a professional manner and look good while you're doing it. It isn't a matter of choice. To be successful you have to look good.

Hairdressers know a lot about cosmetic surgery because we see it every day, and our clients tell us about it, too. I have talked to hundreds of clients who have had cosmetic surgery. Once I put someone in the shampoo bowl and hit the hair with water I can see the scars. So, I would tell them I was going to have a facelift. Some would say, 'Honey, you're too young and pretty, you don't need a facelift.' I don't think having a facelift is a question of your age. It's how you feel inside. I also think you should have a facelift when you're younger and still have some elasticity left in your skin. Why look old when you don't have to?

My facelift is the best thing I ever did for myself. I'm so thrilled that I still get choked up about it. I had my surgery on a Tuesday and the next Monday I was sitting at a bar, telling the whole world what I had done. Other than some swelling, I had no pain, no discoloration. I looked great in just a few days.

My doctor let me see photographs of other patients. And, I was given phone numbers of patients. I called one patient and we met. She let me examine her face and she even pulled her hair back and let me feel her scars. She answered every question I asked. Boy, did I ask a lot of questions. It is amazing how many of us spend more time looking for the right hairdresser than for the right doctor.

Years ago women had to wear spit curls in front of their ears because of the scars but with my facelift there were hardly any scars. After my surgery, my husband Byron, who is also a hairdresser, said, "You can hardly see the scars, it's the best work I have ever seen."

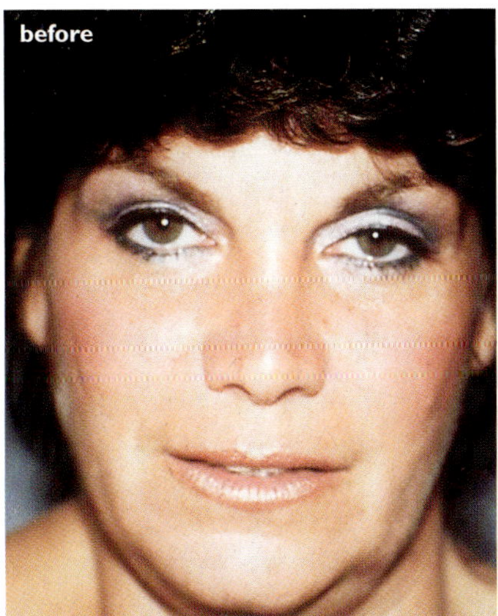
before

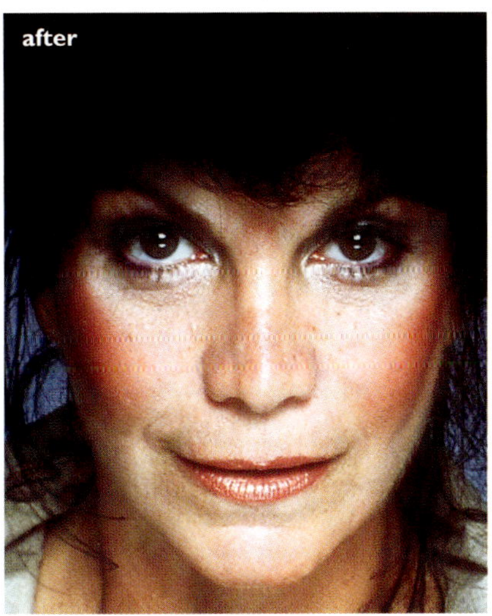
after

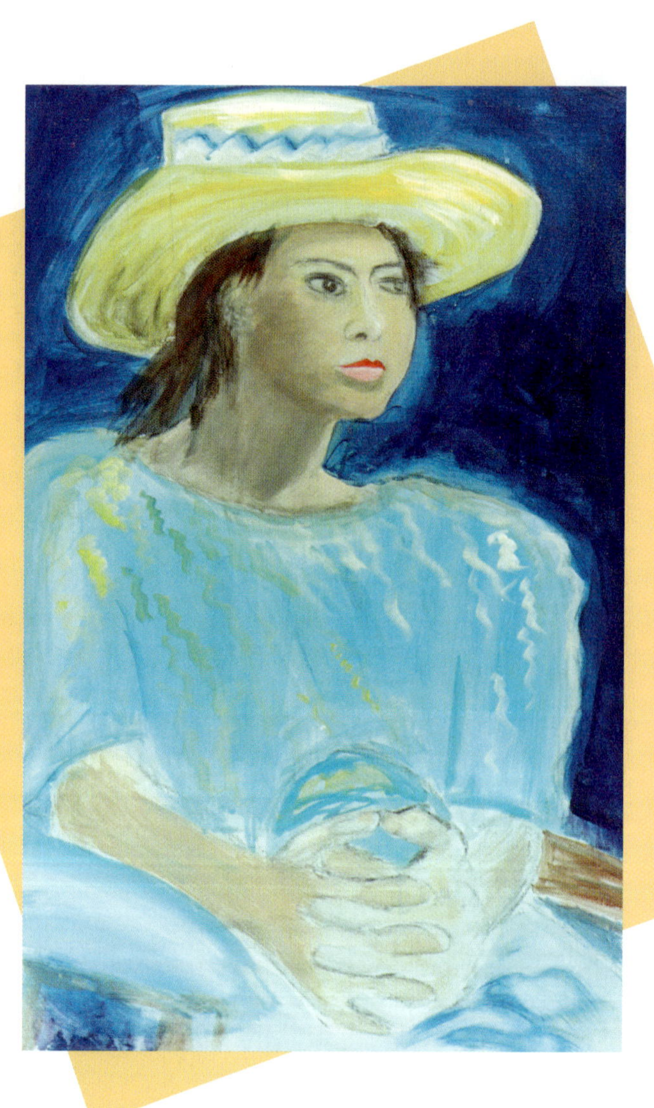

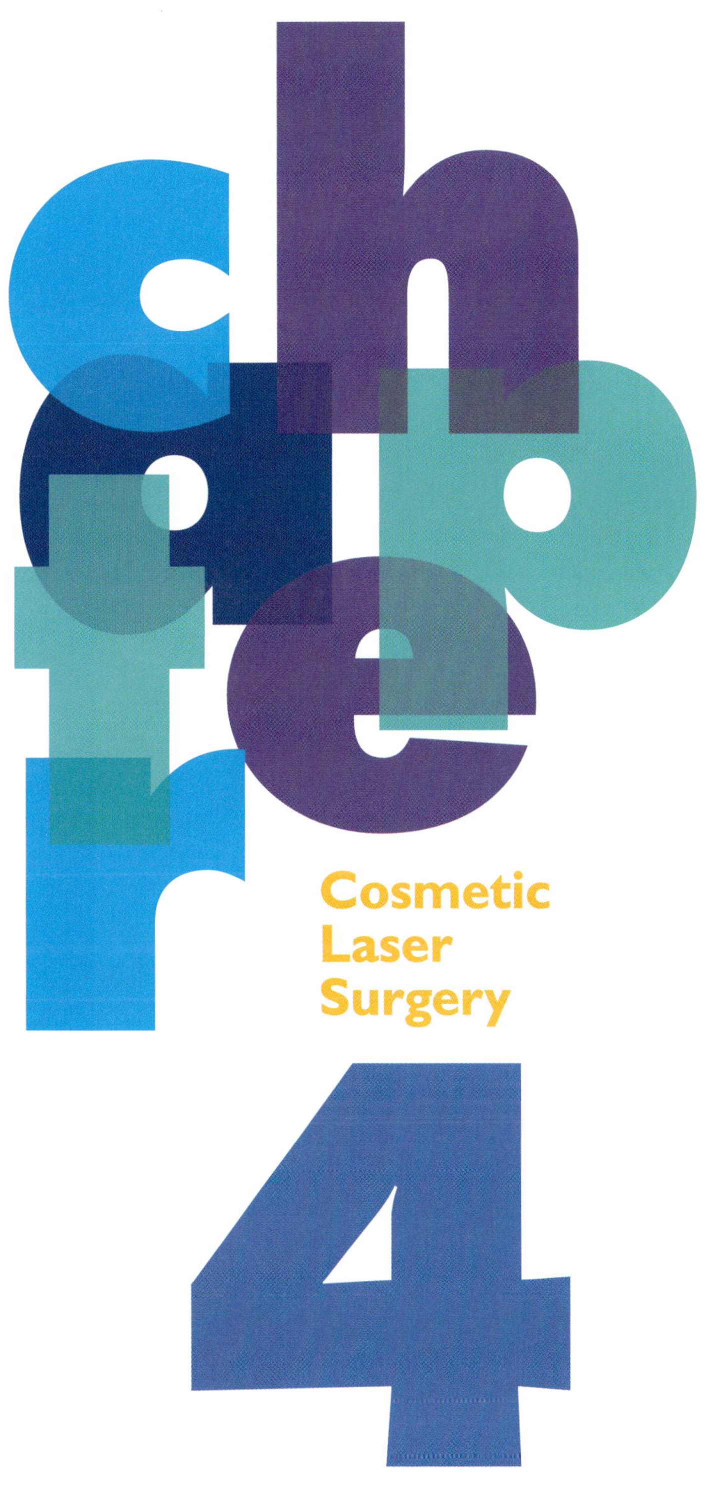
chapter
Cosmetic
Laser
Surgery
4

Cosmetic Laser Surgery

Welcome to the modern age of cosmetic surgery and lasers. Lasers are an important and valuable tool in the plastic surgeon's arsenal against aging and are revolutionizing the treatment for many cosmetic procedures including wrinkles, sun-damaged skin, acne scars, spider veins and tattoos. They are also used to assist plastic surgeons during many surgical procedures including facelifts, endoscopic forehead lifts, blepharoplasty (eyelifts), neck lifts and cheek lifts. They can help remove stubborn lip lines, repair scars and lesions, smooth out stretch marks, and remove warts, moles, birth marks and unwanted hair.

As a surgical instrument, lasers can even replace the scalpel because of their ability to cut and cauterize at the same time, sealing blood vessels and vaporizing tissues with less bleeding and scarring. Their unique ability to target specific tissues with minimal thermal damage to surrounding tissues helps account for their widespread applications and almost universal appeal to patients and surgeons. Less damage to tissues offer many post-operative advantages for

Cosmetic Laser Surgery

Procedure: *Laser Skin Resurfacing. Purpose: Removes wrinkles, lines, sun damage, acne scars, blemishes and uneven pigmentations in order to give the skin a smoother, younger appearance.*

Treatment: *15 minutes for small areas, 1 – 1 1/2 hours for full face laser.*

Anesthesia: *Local anesthesia, intravenous sedation.*

Where: Outpatient surgery.

Recovery: *Redness 7–10 days, to several months. Can be covered with makeup. Back to work: 7–10 days,*

Risks: *Burns, lightening of the skin, infection, scarring.*

Cost: *$1,900–$6,000.*

**(Note: Prices may vary based on physician fees, anesthesia, surgical setting and number of procedures. Data is based on a compilation of sources including Dr. Man.)*

patients, including less bleeding, bruising, swelling and pain. The result is that patients heal faster and return to everyday activities much sooner. Studies indicate that after laser treatment there is an increase in elasticity and smoothness, as well as improvement to the skin's texture. (*Journal of Dermatologic Surgery,* "Resurfacing of Atrophic Facial Acne Scars With A High Energy, Pulsed Carbon Dioxide Laser," by Tina Alster, M.D. and Tina West, M.D., March, 1996:22:151–155.)

Types of Lasers

Though Albert Einstein originated the concept for the laser in 1917, the world waited nearly half a century before it first became a reality in the 1960s. Developed for industrial and military uses, its applications in medicine would soon follow, and today there are as many uses for lasers as there are types of lasers on the market.

The word laser is an acronym for light amplification by stimulated emission of radiation. Basically, a laser is an extremely high-energy, intense beam of light. Some lasers are visible to the eye, while others appear only in the infrared light spectrum. Lasers usually are named for the mediums in which the laser light is conducted. Some use gas mediums like carbon dioxide, erbium, argon and krypton, while others use liquid dyes, or solids such as crystals and precious gemstones. Future lasers will use new crystals and will be developed by scientists to aid mankind in cancer research and new antiaging discoveries.

Lasers In Medicine

The first medical laser had a solid ruby tip and was used to treat skin lesions and to perform surgery of the larynx and ear. Today, lasers are utilized by nearly every medical discipline including plastic surgery, ophthalmology, neurosurgery, dermatology, gynecology, cardiology, oncology, otolaryngology and others.

The laser is a very sophisticated and precise medical instrument. All lasers are not alike. Each laser has its own unique properties and tissue interaction capabilities. The effect of the laser on tissues varies depending on the water, melanin (pigment) and hemoglobin content of the different tissues. Some lasers are selectively absorbed by pigmented tissues without affecting other tissues, while other lasers are absorbed by water and are indifferent to color and pigment.

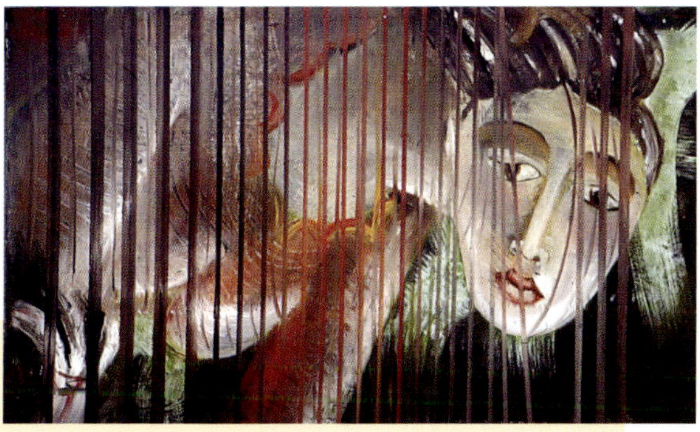

There are many types of surgical lasers used today and many more are being developed. Here are a few examples of lasers used in plastic surgery:

Carbon Dioxide Lasers (CO_2) are the most widely used of all surgical lasers. Sometimes referred to as the "workhorse" of lasers, this laser is an example of a gas laser. It is invisible to the human eye and requires a special aiming beam in order to direct the light. This laser penetrates all tissues because of its ability to be easily absorbed by water which comprises 80 to 90 percent of all human cells. In its *continuous* wave form, the carbon dioxide laser can be used to cut and cauterize tissues and assist in a variety of surgical procedures including face, neck, eye and forehead lifts.

Pulsed Carbon Dioxide Lasers use short bursts of high energy to penetrate thin layers of tissues. The pulsed carbon dioxide laser has the ability to vaporize tissues instantaneously with minimal thermal or heat damage to surrounding cells. In this form, it offers an excellent way to instantly vaporize the top thin layers of epidermis and upper dermis, removing wrinkles, sun damage, problem lip lines, brown spots, crow's feet around the eyes, and uneven pigmentation. It is also an excellent tool to smooth out acne scars and pits, moles and other blemishes.

YAG Lasers: Q-switch Ruby, Alexandrite, and Nd:YAG are color-specific, targeting pigmented tissues and red blood vessels. The Q-switch Ruby and Alexandrite lasers have a propensity for black and blue pigments, such as those found in tattoos. The Nd: YAG laser is absorbed by red pigments and is very effective at eliminating pigmented lesions such as "strawberry patch" or "port wine stain" birthmarks, tattoos, abnormal blood vessels, hemangiomas, and "liver" spots or brown age spots. Tattoo removal may require a combination of these lasers and several treatment sessions.

Argon Lasers emit a blue-green light and have a preference for the color red where they are heavily absorbed. This makes it a very effective means for treating spider veins and vascular abnormalties.

Erbium (ER-YAG) is a new type of laser that is being used for skin resurfacing and wrinkle removal. It causes less heat damage than CO_2 lasers and allows quicker recovery, and can often be performed with little or no anesthesia. The erbium laser is absorbed by the top layers of skin and works by vaporizing the top layer to eliminate wrinkles, lines and sun damage.

Pulsed Dye Lasers use a liquid laser system and emit a yellowish light. This laser has a unique ability to pass through other tissues without thermal damage or scarring while targeting red pigmented tissue and red blood cells. This

laser is an effective treatment for vascular lesions, hemangiomas and birthmarks. It is used to vaporize abnormal blood vessels, spider veins and port wine stain birthmarks. It also helps reduce scars. This laser is very useful for treating infants and children with these conditions.

The Copper Vapor Laser is a yellow light that can also be used for treating pigmented areas.

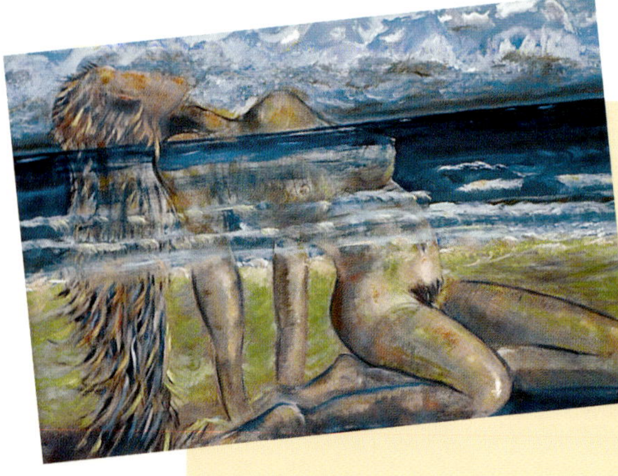

Types of Procedures

Cosmetic surgery will continue to benefit from lasers and the rapid advances in the field of laser surgery. The laser has many advantages both for the surgeon and the patient. Laser surgery has no systemic risks, and it can be performed on many more patients of all ages, including those with heart and kidney problems. Treatments are brief, usually 1 to 1 1/2 hours, and are performed in the doctor's office or outpatient surgical center under local anesthesia and sedation. Small areas can be done in even less time.

Lasers are considered a nearly bloodless procedure because of their ability to cut and seal blood vessels and nerve endings simultaneously. This characteristic speeds patient recovery since blood vessels and tiny capillaries do not have to coagulate on their own, and nerve endings are not left frayed. This contributes to less swelling, bruising and post-operative pain.

The following is an overview of types of cosmetic laser procedures.

Laser Skin Resurfacing

Laser skin resurfacing is one of the most exciting advancements in the field of anti-aging medicine. Using an advanced, high energy carbon dioxide or erbium laser, the surgeon is able to remove wrinkles, sun damage and blemishes from the skin. Total facial skin resurfacing or smaller areas such as crow's feet around the eyes and "smoker's" lines around the mouth can be treated. Laser resurfacing can also be used to smooth out acne scars and irregular pigmentation and has the advantage that it may be performed in combination with other surgical procedures including facelifts and eyelifts.

While a facelift or eyelift may remove excess skin and wrinkles, these procedures do little to improve the skin's texture. Laser surgery offers some advantages over traditional forms of wrinkle reduction including chemical peeling and dermabrasion. Laser skin resurfacing gives the surgeon precise depth control and instant visual verification. The surgeon can immediately see the degree of skin tightness and uniform consistency. For some patients who do not want to undergo facelift surgery, total facial resurfacing can offer substantial skin improvement by removing wrinkles, fine lines, crow's feet, lip lines, sun damage, brown spots, acne scars, forehead and frown lines, irregular pigmentation and discoloration, as well as yielding some degree of "tightening" skin.

How Does It Work?

The laser beam vaporizes the water in the top layers of skin causing a constriction of the tissues. The surgeon regulates the amount of laser energy and precisely controls the removal of each layer. After treatment, patients experience some discomfort and redness, which looks similar to a bad sunburn. Makeup can usually be applied in seven to ten days. The skin continues to improve in texture as the laser appears to benefit the cells by causing tissues to form new collagen and elastin fibers.

Laser Blepharoplasty (Eyelid Surgery)

Laser-assisted blepharoplasty is a procedure that removes excess skin in order to tighten baggy, droopy eyelids, remove fat pads from under the eyes, resurface the skin of the eyelids to improve its texture and remove lines around the eyes including crow's feet, squint lines and discolored skin. The laser decreases the need for an external incision on the lower eyelid.

Lip Lines

Smoker's lip lines and creases around the mouth are often the most stubborn lines to remove. While a facelift will tighten the skin, these wrinkles often remain after surgery, requiring laser treatment to this specific area.

Tattoo Removal

Tattoos consist of permanent colored dyes, injected into the skin to form patterns and messages. Often these tattoos lose their appeal and their owners decide to have them removed. Tattoos usually contain more than one color. Dyes usually vary in color and consistency. Because no one laser is effective at treating all pigments, a combination of lasers may be used, requiring several treatment sessions.

Acne Pits, Scars, Stretch Marks

The carbon dioxide laser appears to be a promising tool to smooth out acne pits and scars left from chicken pox. The pulse dye laser can improve stretch marks and hypertrophic scars by reducing the redness, bumpiness and irregularity of scars that may have resulted from surgery. It also shows promise for reducing stretch marks caused by pregnancy.

New Trends

A new trend in cosmetic surgery is the development of non-invasive laser centers that offer a wide range of cosmetic face and body treatments using the most advanced laser and light procedures to beautify and rejuvenate the face and body. New centers, including Nova Laser Light Cosmetic Centers, provide such services as non-invasive facial rejuvenation using the latest lasers and light machines, varicose vein treatments, hair removal, and body contouring with cellulite reduction.

Other types of laser-like treatments include hair and spider vein removal. Hair removal is performed with the use of laser-like, intense light devices such as the EpiLight®. These devices now offer a new high-tech way for men and women to remove unwanted hair from the face, legs, back, arms and other areas. This procedure promises to replace often painful traditional salon and over-the-counter treatments including electrolysis, plucking, hair removal creams and waxing kits. The process comprises a laser-like, high-intensity light that penetrates large numbers of hair follicles and their roots, without damage to surrounding tissues.

PhotoDerm™ is a laser-like device that emits an intense pulse of light to treat unsightly pigmented vascular lesions and discolorations of the face, legs and body such as sclerosis of leg veins (spider veins), stretch marks and birthmarks such as port wine stains, hemangiomas, age spots and some tattoos. Treatment comprises administering an intense pulse of light, similar to the flash of a camara, to the skin. Patients report feeling a slight pinch. No anesthesia or pain medication is required. Several treatments are usually needed.

Cellulite Reduction

One of the newest European body contouring treatments helps smooth skin and reduce the "orange peel" look caused by cellulite. Called Endermologie®, this treatment uses a special electrical massage device to smooth cellulite and smooth the dimpling look of the skin.

COSMETIC LASER SURGERY

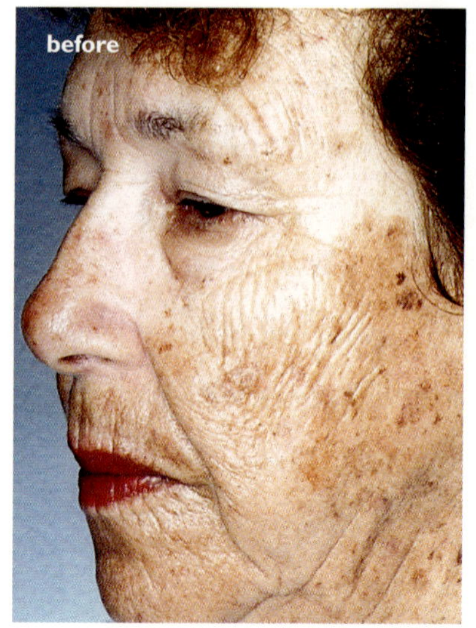

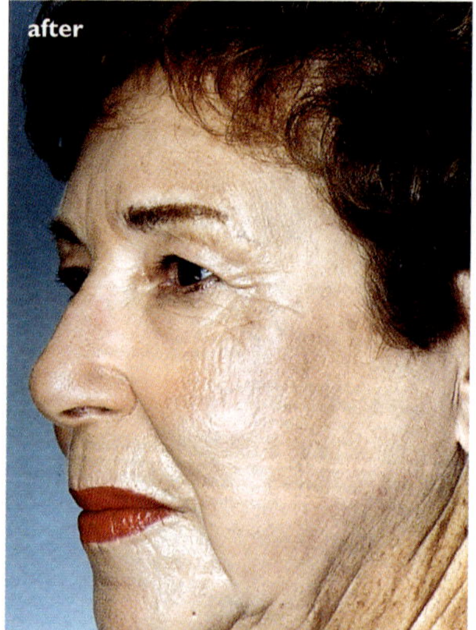

Full Face Laser

COSMETIC LASER SURGERY

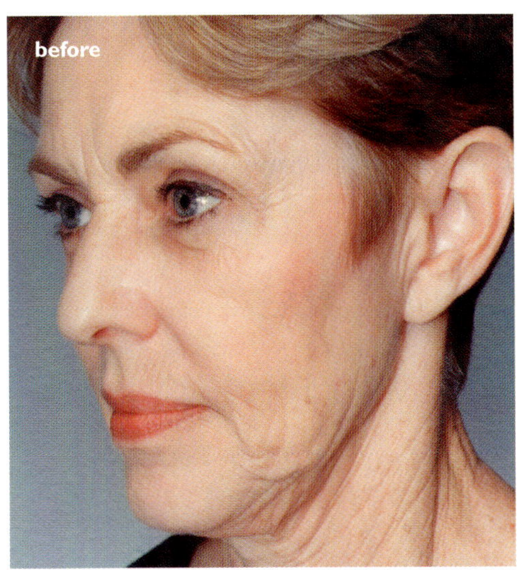

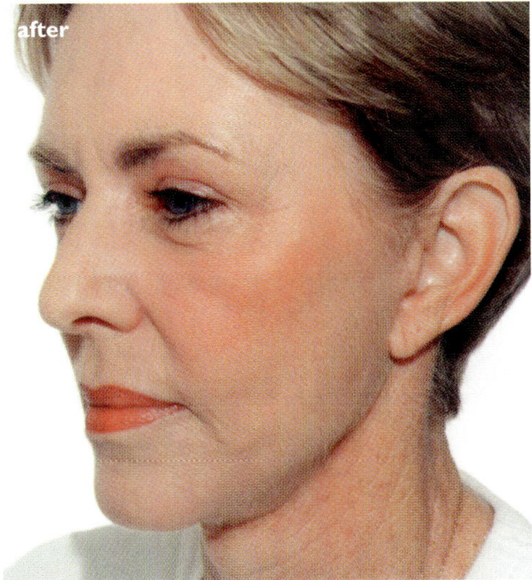

Face and Necklift; Endoscopic Forehead Lift; Upper and Lower Eyes; Full Face Laser

PATIENT PORTRAIT

ISABEL BRAUT
FULL FACE LASER
AGE: 69

My face looked like a map of the United States. I had lines and wrinkles everywhere. Every time I looked in the mirror, I got a chill up and down my spine, and cringed. Now I can look in the mirror without crying. Laser surgery has made a big difference in my life. I feel very attractive. I'm amazed at what it did for my eyes. Now they're very attractive and quite lively looking. I think my whole attitude has changed.

I'm originally from New York and I moved to Florida nine years ago. I was a sun worshiper, and I used to go to the cabana club and the beach. My family practically lived at the beach. I guess the sun began to take its toll on my face. I'd been thinking about having surgery for about five years. I was thinking about it, but not really seriously because I was afraid to have a facelift. I heard about the laser and felt it was the thing for me. Thankfully, the doctor agreed.

The procedure went very well. I had no pain. I didn't even feel the injection he gave me to put me to sleep. The redness was gone in eight to nine days and I looked great. I even went to the beauty parlor the tenth day. Nobody knew I had it done except my hairdresser, and he knew because I told him beforehand. He was really excited about the results and wanted my doctor's name.

My family was really excited, too. I went to the Orient to visit my son. He couldn't get over my face. My son is 50. Now he says he wants to do something. I also have a younger son who is an attorney, and he said, 'Mother you look beautiful.' That really made me feel great. Everyone who sees me can't get over the way I look. People stare at me and whisper to one another. They all point to me and say, 'she's the lady who had her face done with the laser.' I think that's quite flattering.

Laser surgery has changed my whole outlook on life. I think my surgery has enhanced my lifestyle. I'm dating a very nice man. He didn't think I needed surgery, but he's thrilled now that I did it. I notice him looking at me in different ways than previously. He likes it when his friends tell him how wonderful I look. 'What's happened to Isabel?' they ask, 'she looks great.' But they can't seem to put their finger on why. I think it's wonderful.

Since my laser surgery, I try to stay out of the sun and when I am in the sun, I wear sunscreen and maybe a hat. Other than that, I just try to take care of my skin with a facial once in a while.

I'm retired and at the age when it is important to take care of yourself and do the things you've always wanted to do. Maybe, in my case, it was good that I waited, because now I could have the laser surgery I always wanted.

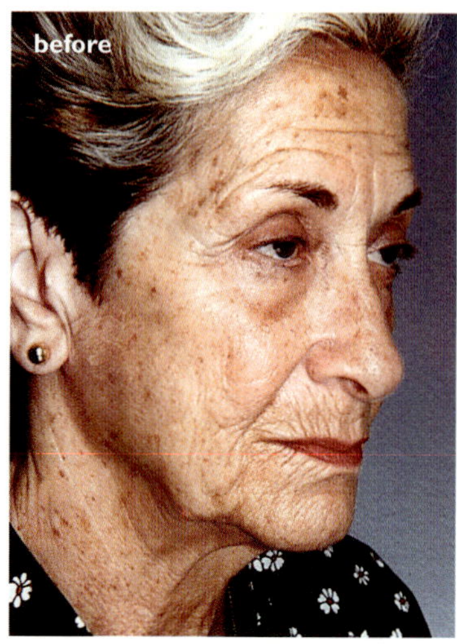
before

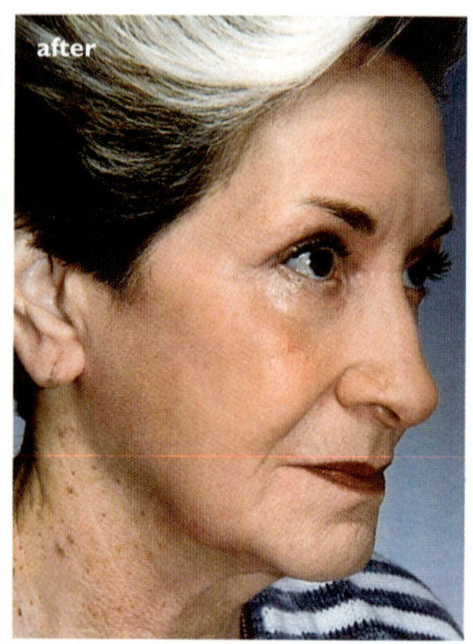
after

PATIENT PORTRAIT

JOHN DE PASQUALE
FULL FACE LASER, ENDOSCOPIC FOREHEAD LIFT; LOWER EYES
AGE: 52

I had a lot of wrinkles on my face, probably because I've lived my whole life on the beach. I love to fish, swim and scuba dive. Being out in the sun all the time caused me to have severe sun damage. My face had lots of lines and wrinkles and brown spots. I also had a problem with my heavy eyelids, which caused the skin to push down over my eyelashes. Every morning when I woke up , I would feel like I was seeing the world through spider webs. My eyes looked tired all the time, whether I got eight hours sleep or was out dancing all night.

I originally went to the doctor to have my eyes done. The doctor said I should do the whole thing and get rid of the wrinkles. He said because my eyelids were so heavy, he couldn't do it all in one shot. I thought that was a good idea. I didn't know anything about laser surgery, but he explained it all to me. I'm very happy, and I was really surprised at the results. It looks very natural.

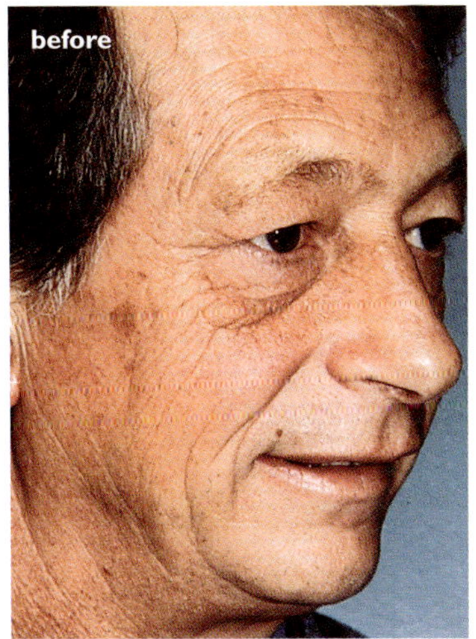

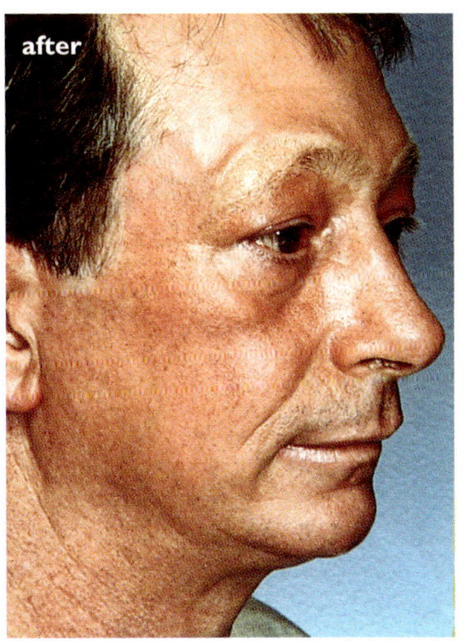

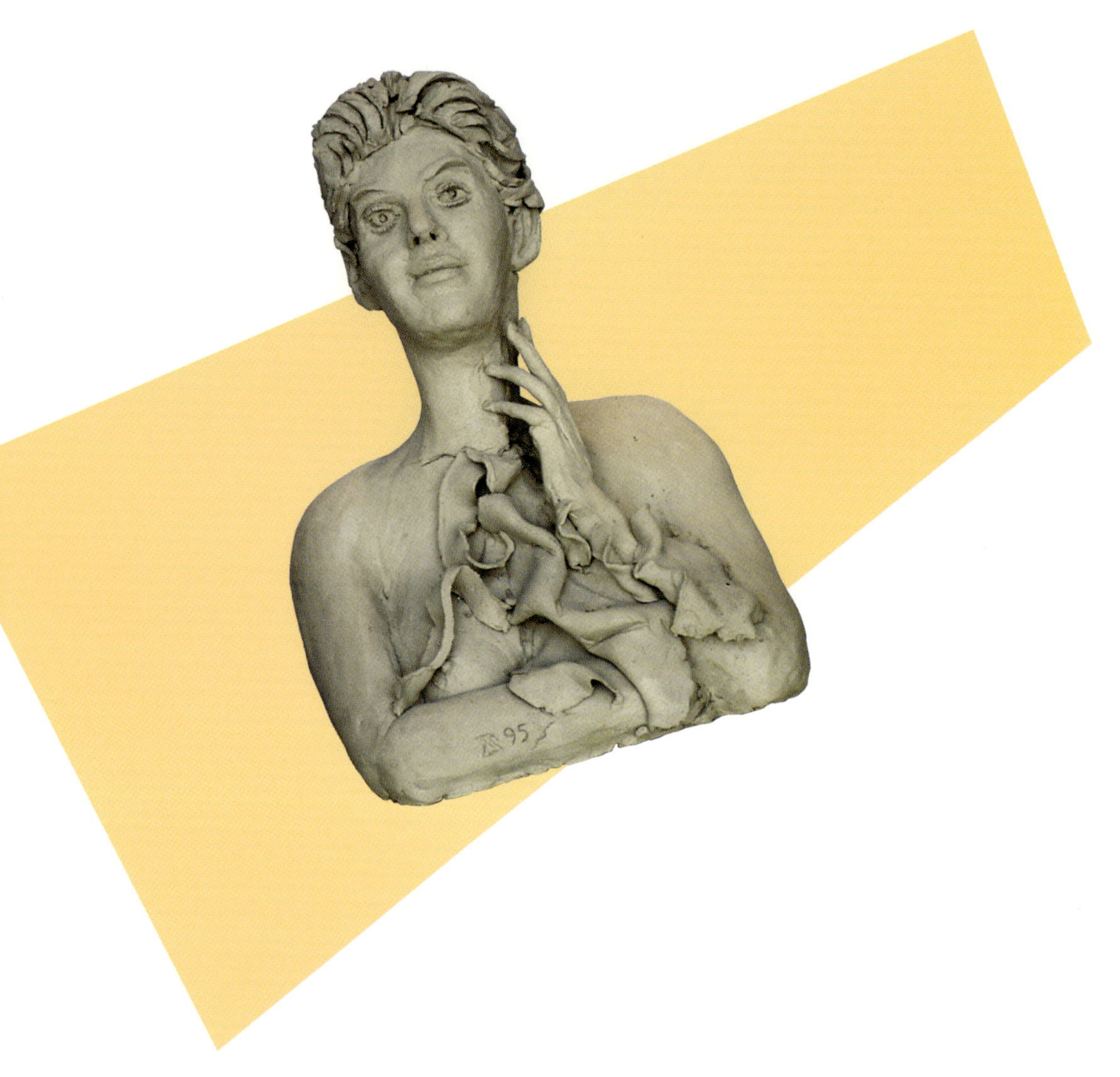

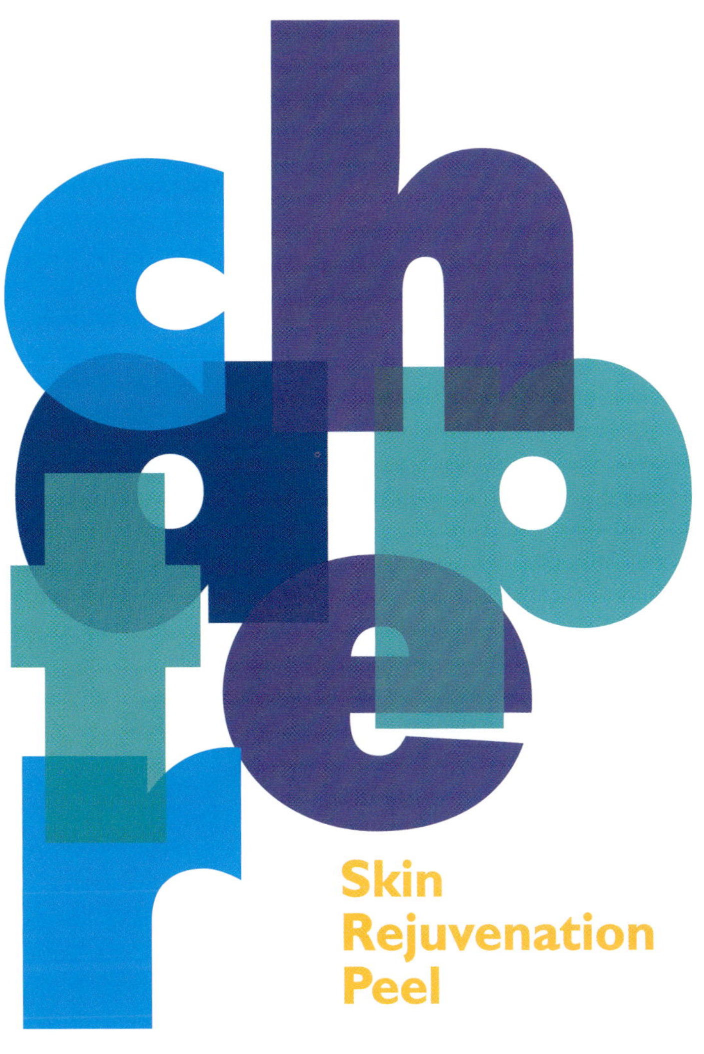

Skin Rejuvenation Peel

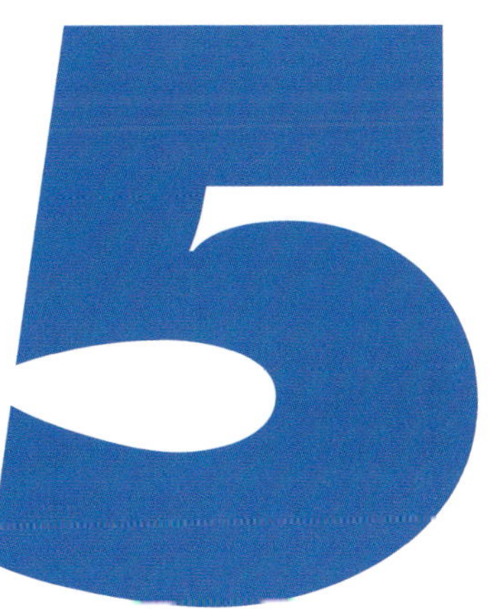

Skin Rejuvenation Peel

The concept of a youth-enhancing "magic potion" or "magic wand" to improve the skin's appearance has intrigued mankind for thousands of years, beginning with the Egyptians 4,000 years ago and followed by the Greeks. One of the earliest examples of an attempt to restore a patient's youth was recorded 1,600 years before the birth of

Christ by an Egyptian physician in his instructions to a patient. This recording described the preparation and application of a special "potion" or ointment and was found in an ancient papyrus writing entitled: "The Beginning of the Book of Transforming An Old Man Into A Youth." An addendum to a surgical treatise, it states:

"Anoint a man therewith. It is a remover of wrinkles from the head. When the flesh is smeared therewith it becomes a beautifier of the skin, a remover of blemishes, of all disfigurements, of all signs of age, of all weakness which are in the flesh. Found effective myriads of times."

- From An Anthology of Plastic Surgery *by Harry Hayes, Jr., M.D*

General Overview

Light Peel

(Alpha Hydroxy Acid)

Purpose: *Improves skin's texture and very fine lines. Removes top layer of dead skin cells.*
Length of procedure: *1/2 – 1 hour.*
Anesthesia: None. **Where:** *Outpatient*
Recovery: *Patients experience tingling of skin and slight redness.*
Back to work: Immediate.
Cost: *$90–$120*

Medium Peel

(Trichloracetic Acid)

Purpose: *To remove wrinkles, lines and smooth out uneven pigmentation and blemishes. Improves skin texture.*
Length of Procedure: *1/2 – 1 hour.*
Anesthesia: *Local or I.V. Sedation*
Where: *Outpatient* **Recovery:** *Patients experience temporary redness, swelling, itching and sun sensitivity. Redness may persist for several months. Back to work: 5 – 10 days; Makeup: 1 – 2 weeks.*
Risks: Infection, scarring, whiteheads, hypopigmentation.
Cost: *Medium peel $1,100 – $1,400*

Deep Peel

(Phenol Peel)

Purpose: *To remove deep lines and wrinkles, rough, sun-damaged skin, remove discolorations and uneven pigmentations.*
Length: *30 minutes – 2 hours.*
Anesthesia: *I.V. Sedation*
Recovery: *Tingling, itching, tightness, discomfort, boredom, as patient may stay in facility for 7 days.*
Back to Work: *1 – 2 weeks*
Risks: *Infection, scarring, prolonged redness, loss of pigment.* **Cost:** *$6,475 – $7,500*

Throughout the centuries, people have looked to "magic potions" and youth-enhancing drinks to turn back the aging clock and restore youthful skin. Cleopatra bathed each day in sour milk to keep her skin soft and smooth. It was said that the 15th century Spanish explorer Ponce de León drank from every body of water he encountered, searching for a youth elixir and the "Fountain of Youth." Today our multi-billion dollar cosmetics industry is a testimonial this search continues. So is plastic surgery.

How to remove wrinkles is a question that has fascinated and plagued the world for many centuries. It is still a question that plastic surgeons continue to ask and search fervently for answers.

Skin Rejuvenation Peel: A Magic Potion?

A truly remarkable feat of modern-day medicine is the plastic surgeon's ability to reverse the effects of aging skin through lasers and chemical restoration. Surgery alone does not make aging skin look younger. A facelift can tighten sagging muscles and remove excess tissue, but it will not restore the skin to its former youthful glow and vibrant appearance. For this, one requires laser skin resurfacing or chemical restoration through peeling.

If there is such a thing as a youth-restoring "potion" or "lotion," then the chemical peel could be called its modern-day version. Peeling is a very popular means of improving the skin's appearance. There are many types of peels in use today. They range from the mild enzyme peels used to exfoliate the skin and control open pores, dehydration, excessive oiliness, acne, blackheads and comedones; to the light peels such as the glycolic acids and alpha hydroxy acids; and finally to the medium peels, such as trichloracetic acid, and the deep phenol peels.

Light Peels (Alpha Hydroxy Acid)

The light peels include the alpha hydroxy acids (AHAs), which are derived from food products including vegetables and fruits. Alpha hydroxy acid is applied to the surface of the skin and it helps to loosen the "glue" that binds the dead skin cells together, providing rapid exfoliation. The most common types of AHA are *glycolic acid,* the acid found in sugar cane; *lactic acid,* the acid found in sour milk; *citric acid* found in fruits; and *tartaric acid* which is in grapes. *Salicylic acid,* also a common exfolliant, is derived from aspirin. These products are commercially available in very mild concentrations, ranging from 3 percent to 10 percent at department store cosmetic counters, drug stores and salons. Physicians offer stronger concentrations, which can give even better results, in addition to better control.

Retin- A, short for retinoic acid, a vitamin A derivative, has been successfully used as an acne treatment and has also demonstrated its ability to smooth the skin and remove fine lines. As a light peel, it helps smooth a dry complexion by removing the dead cell layer.

As we age, our ability to slough off these cells slows. Peels are best used under a doctor's guidance, as they make the skin photosensitive and can cause skin irritations and redness.

Light peels help make the skin look smoother and fresher by removing the dead cell layer and promoting new cell growth, but they do little to remove deeper lines and wrinkles. For this, a medium peel such as trichloracetic acid (TCA) or the deeper phenol peel is needed.

Medium Peels

Medium peels most commonly utilize trichloracetic acid (TCA) to help reduce the effects of fine lines, blemishes and pigmentation irregularities. TCA will make the skin tighter and smoother looking, giving it a fresher appearance.

Deep Peels (Phenol)

According to the American Society of Plastic and Reconstructive Surgeons, chemical peels are very popular. Though chemical peeling is not a surgical process — there is no cutting with a scalpel — it is invasive, meaning it penetrates the body, in this case, the outer layers of the skin. Therefore, it should be performed by a qualified surgeon.

Phenol is the deepest peel and gives the most dramatic results. The "mother" of all peels, phenol, or Skin Rejuvenation Peel® has the capability to remove deep lines and wrinkles, sun damage, rough and dry skin, pigmentations, acne scars, lines, blemishes, under-eye circles, lip lines, forehead and frown lines, pregnancy masking, discolorations, surface acne scars, brown

spots and even some pre-cancerous lesions.

Phenol has been used since 1903. For the patient with many wrinkles and sun damage, a phenol peel is one of the most effective means of achieving younger-looking skin. Matching the right peel to the right patient is critical to its success. The peel is customized to the patient's skin type and needs. Someone who has a lot of sun damage, rough skin, deep lines and wrinkles, and pigmentation irregularities will require a stronger peel than someone with mild sun damage and fine lines. For many patients, the Skin Rejuvenation Peel® can have excellent results. It can also be used after a facelift to enhance the overall appearance, while improving the texture and look of the skin.

Peels also work to "tighten" the skin, shortening the earlobes which grow longer as we age, and refining the tip of the nose. The neck and chest areas, pre-cancerous areas and even the hands have shown marked improvements using various peels. In some cases, repeated treatments may be necessary, as brown spots on the hands can reappear.

How Long Does The Procedure Take?

TCA and phenol peels can be applied to the whole face, or to specific areas. With the TCA peel, the process takes about 30 minutes to 1 hour for a full facial peel. The phenol peel takes about one to two hours. Medium peels require a shorter recovery time, and usually can be repeated, as the results are less dramatic than the phenol. Phenol peels have a longer lasting effect and the results continue to get better with time, as the skin forms new collagen and elastin. There are very few procedures in plastic surgery that have the longevity of the phenol peel. The end results have been reported in the medical literature to last as long as 20 years.

Protecting The Skin

Even though there is more education about the hazards of over exposure to the sun, the medical literature reports significant increases in the number and severity of skin cancers (melanomas) including basal cell and squamous cell carcinomas. A depletion of the ozone layer, a protective shield in the atmosphere, is allowing stronger concentrations of ultraviolet rays to reach the earth.

Despite being aware of the harmful effects of sun exposure, most people continue their habits of bathing on the beach and engaging in outdoor sports without protection. I see many patients who show signs of excessive sun exposure, and I encourage them to take preventive measures to protect the skin, such as wearing protective clothing, hats, sunglasses and using sunscreens with a minimum sun protection factor (SPF) of 15.

Prior to the peel, patients will follow instructions regarding facials, cleansing, exfoliation, massage of the skin, and diet and exercise. This may include the use of Retin-A and other agents which are reviewed with the patient by the esthetician.

Facials prior to the Skin Rejuvenation Peel® are recommended, including hydrating masks, deep pore cleansing, lymphatic drainage and pressure point therapy.

Peels are performed as outpatient procedures in the doctor's office or outpatient surgery center, under I.V. sedation and monitoring in the operating room. The neck is treated with a milder peel. Discomfort is managed by using medications at the time of the peel and for several hours thereafter. In my practice, I prefer to have patients remain under my supervision for a week before they go home. The skin will remain pink or red, similar to a bad sunburn, for several weeks to several months afterwards. Make-up can be worn as a cover-up beginning about 14 days later. Sunscreens are recommended to protect the new skin. After a week or two, most patients return to work and gradually resume normal activities.

Most Common Questions

The most common questions patients ask about peels are: Can I go out in the sun after a peel? Yes, as long as you use a sunscreen. How long does the peel last? The results of the peel will last for many years. However, the clock continues to tick and it is possible you will need more improvements down the road. Patients are advised to stop smoking for two weeks prior to treatment to improve healing, and they are asked to refrain from using chemicals and coloring of hair, including tinting, bleaching, perms and hair straightening. These can be used six weeks after the peel. Possible complications from the procedure many include heart irregularities, infection, numbness, bleaching and scarring. A well-performed deep peel may leave the skin only one tone lighter in color. Patients with dark or black skin should be cautioned when considering chemical peeling or laser skin resurfacing.

Most Common Questions

1) Is the procedure safe? • Yes

2) Is it painful? • No

3) Will my skin look uniform? • Yes

4) Will it get better in time? • Yes

5) Is it long lasting? • Yes

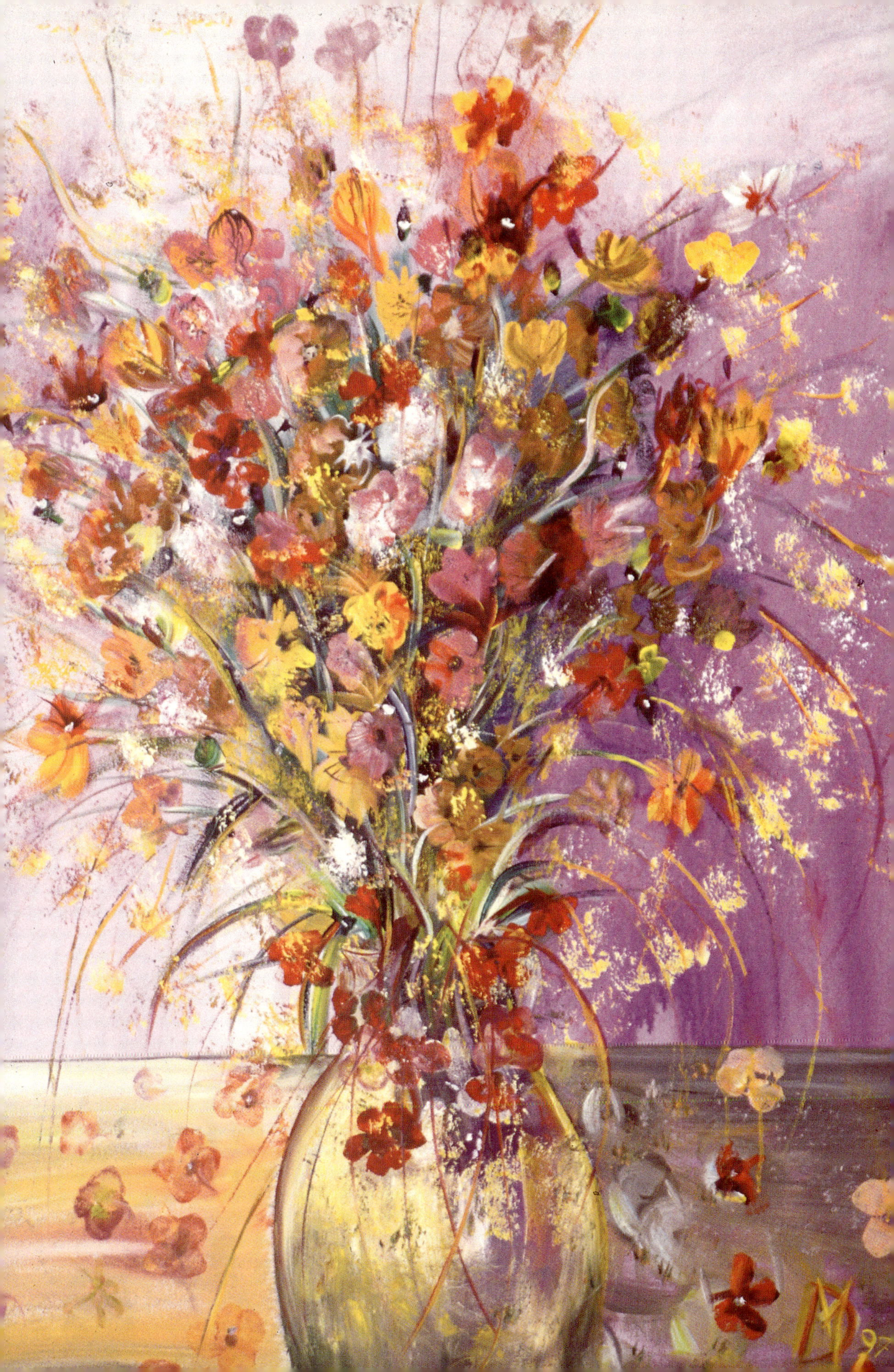

SKIN REJUVENATION PEEL

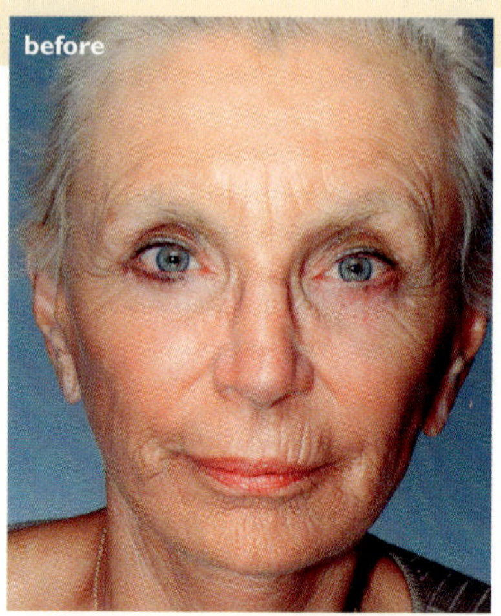

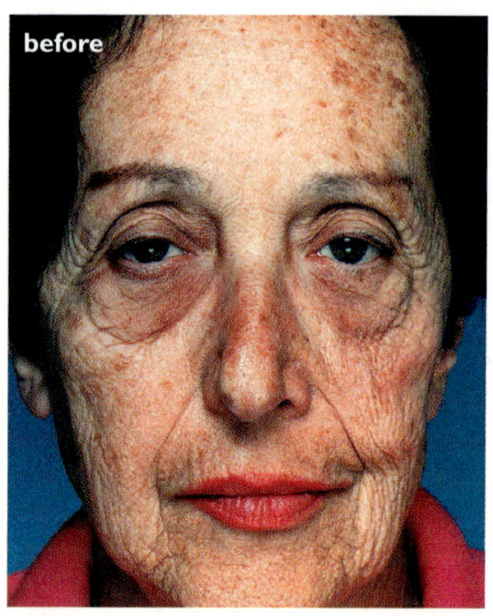

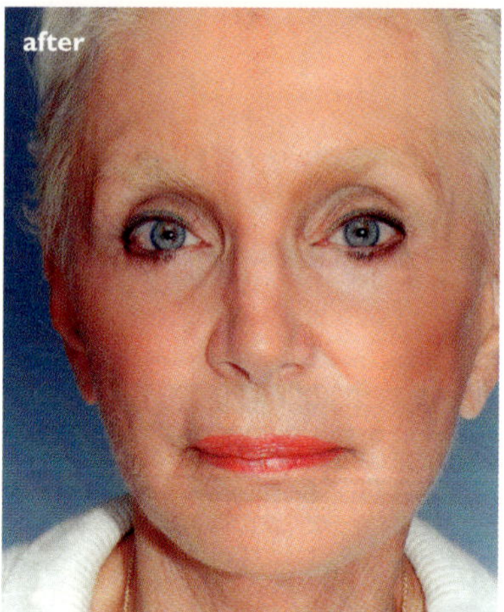

SRP, Upper & Lower Eyes

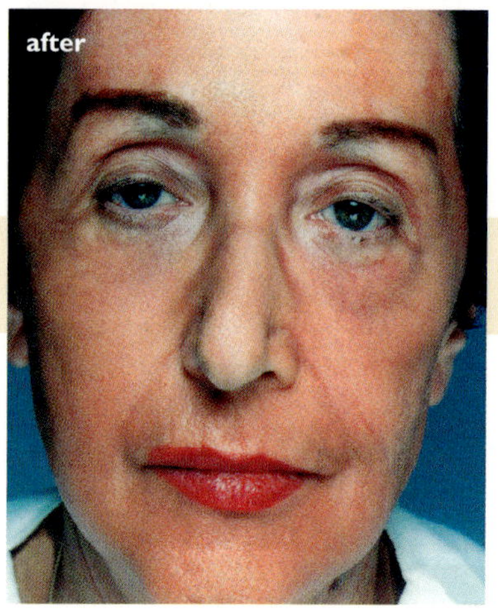

PATIENT PORTRAIT

NATALIE JACOVITZ
SKIN REJUVENATION PEEL
AGE:63

I took my 86-year-old "young" mom to the mall one day. We were in Saks, and it never fails that someone says to my mother, 'Oh I thought this was your sister,' pointing to me. Mom, of course, was always thrilled. While I was crying, she was laughing.

So, I started investigating plastic surgery. There was a lot of damage from all the years of sun exposure. In those days, we didn't think anything about going out in the sun. Before we moved to Florida, we lived in Lido Beach on Long Island. I lived across the street from the ocean, and I remember putting the baby pen up on the beach and spending the whole day there with the kids.

We decided to move to Florida because my youngest son had asthma and we thought it would be better for him. Besides, my husband loved to fish and I told him he could fish 365 days a year if we moved to Florida. I even used to use a sun reflector, that's how much I worshipped the sun. So, you can imagine the wrinkles and sun damage.

One day I remembered the plastic surgeon who was in the emergency room and operated on my son's face. My son had been in a car accident and had almost gone through the windshield. His face and forehead were pretty badly damaged. After surgery my son didn't have a scar or any facial impairment. So I went to see the doctor and he told me he could get rid of my wrinkles with a peel.

That was all I needed to hear. I had the peel. It was great. Now I have no lines on my face and I still go to the beach. The only difference today is that I wear sunscreen and sometimes I wear a hat.

I want my mother to get a peel. But, she says I had more wrinkles than she did. I won't argue with her. When you decide it's something you want to do for yourself, that's when you'll do it. At least now, when we go shopping, people know I'm the daughter and not the sister.

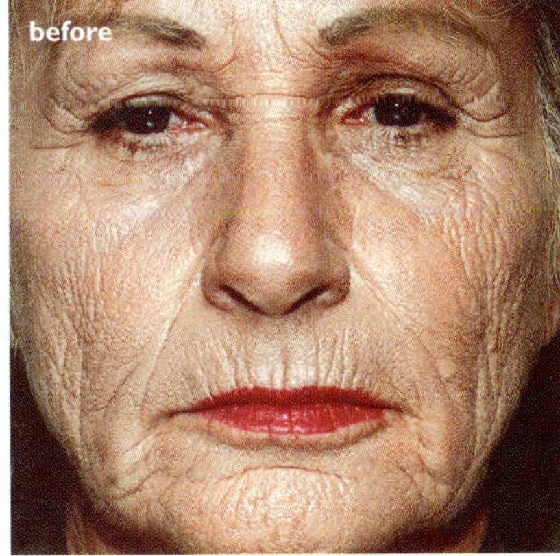

before

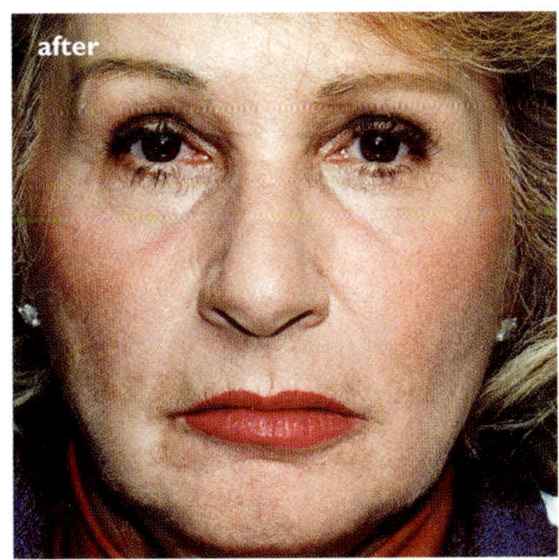

after

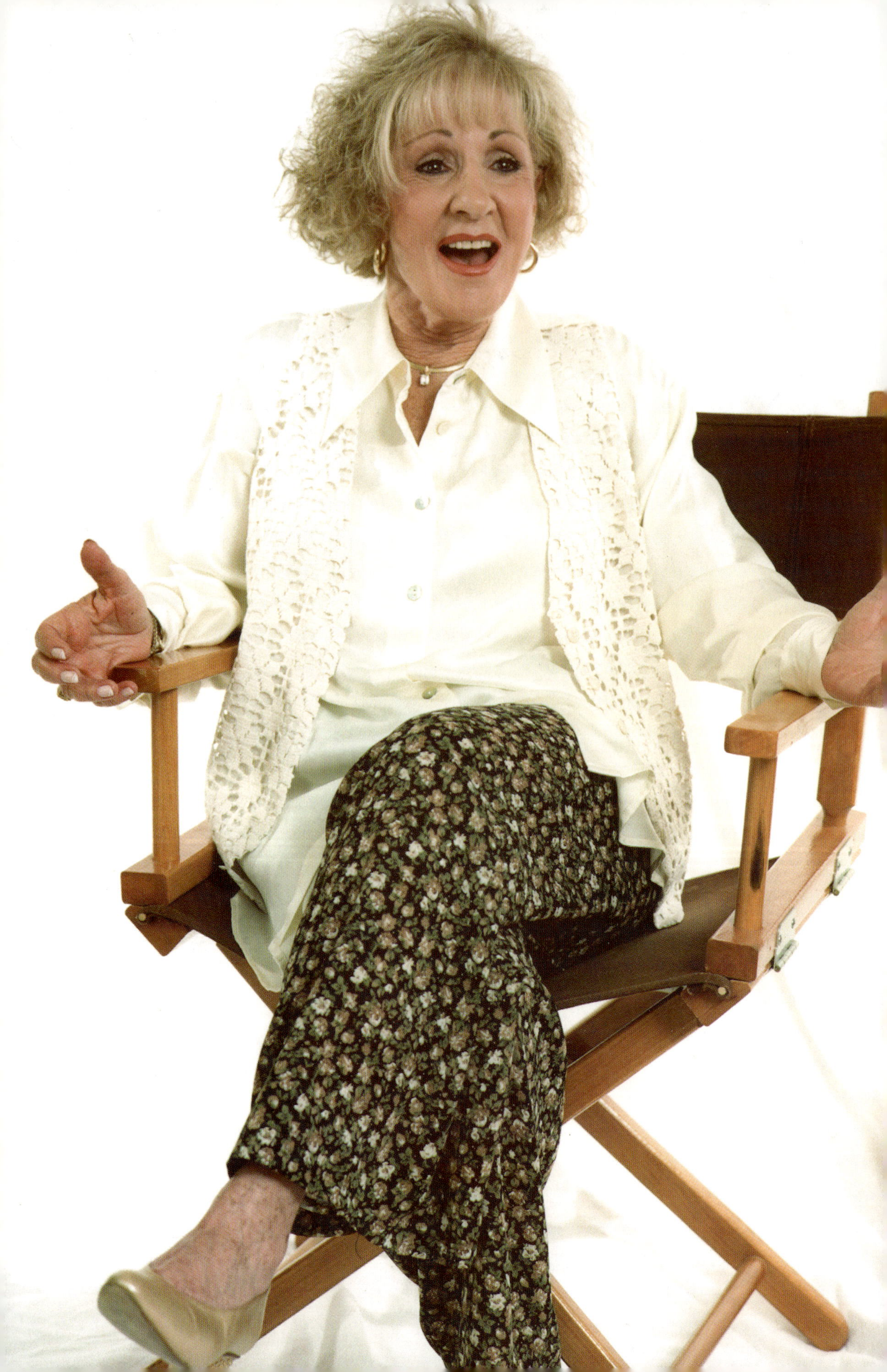

PATIENT PORTRAIT

ZELMA SINGER
SKIN REJUVENATION PEEL
AGE: 66

I've been out in the sun my whole life and I smoked for 33 years. Those are the two things that do such damage to your skin. I was always unhappy with the lines around my lips. Those come from puckering up your mouth to puff on those cigarettes, I guess. I hated the way I looked. But now! I carry my before picture around and show it to people. I can't believe I looked like that.

I was a little nervous about having the peel, but when you want something bad enough, you just take the plunge. If you want something, then you have to accept there might be some risk. You should find out what those risks are by asking questions, and you weigh those risks against the benefits and then decide.

After my peel, I went to California to visit relatives. My sister-in-law had two facelifts, but she still has little lines around her mouth. Now, she says, 'I'm coming to stay with you and have a peel next.' I think that's great because a lot of people always think they do everything better out there in California.

I still go out in the sun a lot. I love to play tennis, but now I wear sunblock. None of the brown spots have come back and I don't have one mark on my face. I have a part time job and when customers come back they often ask for me. They say, 'I want the young lady who waited on me before.' I love it when they say that.

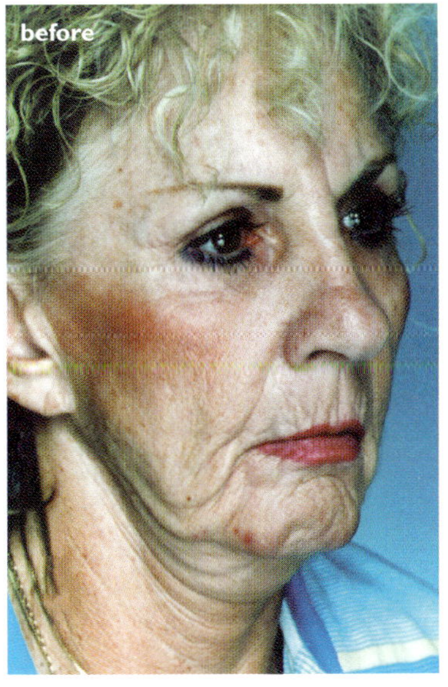

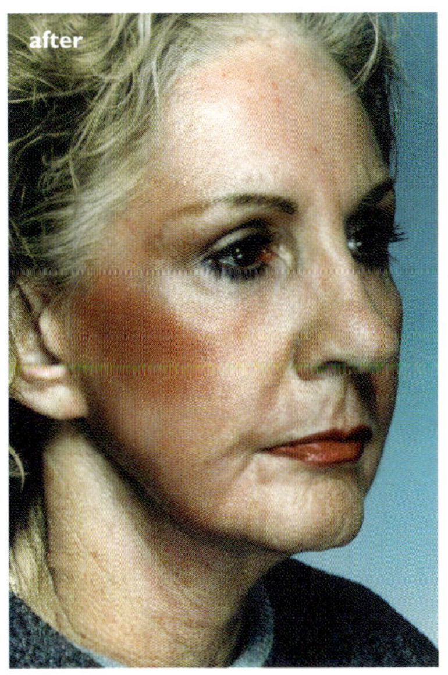

PATIENT PORTRAIT

CLAUDINE GREEN
SKIN REJUVENATION PEEL
AGE: 58

In my home in Zurich, Switzerland, everyone gets a facelift, but nobody talks about it. In America, it's amazing, everyone tells everyone else about their cosmetic surgery. Americans are so open, it's great. I have spent years in the sun skiing, boating and hiking. All that sun has really taken its toll on my skin. I simply couldn't stand looking at myself. I wouldn't look in the mirror because I knew what I would see — freckles, wrinkles and all those age spots — it was just too much to bear. I had to do something. If I would catch a glimpse of myself in a shop window, I would shudder. It was that bad.

So I came to the United States on a holiday and I had my skin rejuvination peel, and then I just went home again. When I went home, I said nothing about having had a peel because that just isn't done in Zurich. I didn't even tell my son. One day he said to me, "You've done something, this isn't the mother I know." I smiled at his quick observation. Then he knew, and he was very pleased to see his mother looking so young and rested.

I plan to retire soon from my work. I am an insurance broker and I'm looking forward to setting up my easel under a beautiful tree and doing the thing I love most, painting. I can look at myself in the mirror now — I am content and look forward to my retirement.

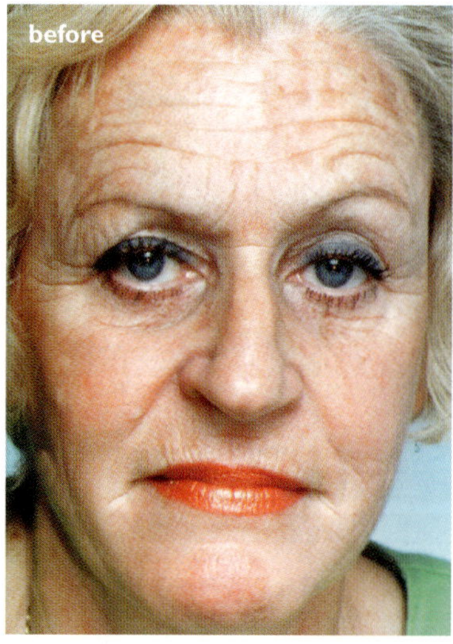

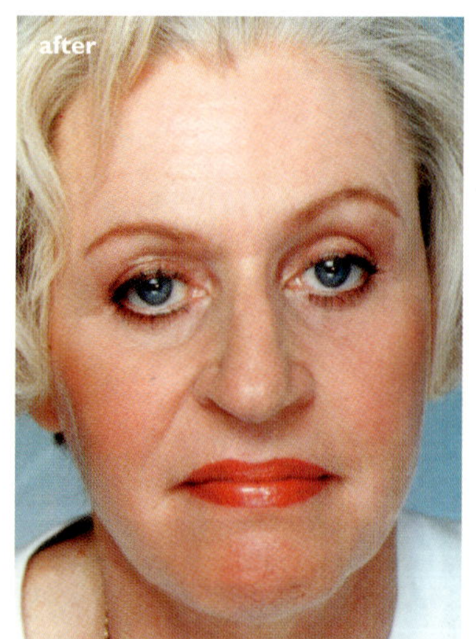

PATIENT PORTRAIT

ANGELA LADESTRO
FACE, NECK, EYE & FOREHEAD LIFTS; SKIN REJUVENATION PEEL; LASER SURGERY
AGE: 74

I had lines everywhere. The lines were so bad I couldn't put any makeup on at all. The makeup would get in between the lines and make me look like a clown. So I quit using makeup. When we would go out I'd complain to my husband and say: "I'm not going to put makeup on to go out." And he would say, "Why don't you get a facelift instead of getting so upset?" My husband wanted me to do this for a long time, but I wasn't ready. It wasn't that I was afraid of the surgery. I had several surgeries including a hysterectomy and I had a tumor removed. But, I thought, I'm getting older, so why not just accept it? My husband continued to encourage me. He was a great supporter of my surgery. So I finally made the decision to do something about the wrinkles instead of just complaining.

It seemed like the deep lines had come all at once. It started with small lines around the eyes, and then I got the deep lines around my mouth, my cheeks, everywhere. I think I inherited my family's genes for wrinkles. I remember when I went to Europe and visited my grandmother. She had deep lines all over her face — the same lines I would inherit many years later. That was when it hit me — I was starting to look just like my grandmother!

I had the facelift surgery first, then I had the skin rejuvenation peel .There was one really deep line right across my face, so deep, I thought the doctor could never get it out. But he did. It was amazing. My eyes look great, and you can see my neckline and chin again. The doctor even did some touch-up with the laser to get out some lines that remained under my chin and around my eyes. I look so different now. It's really incredible.

My husband and I have been married for 54 years, and he thinks he's married to a young girl. I saw my son this summer and he said to me, "Mom you look younger than I do."

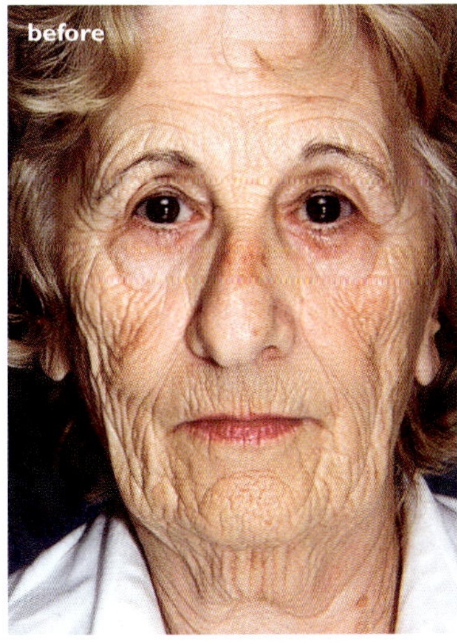

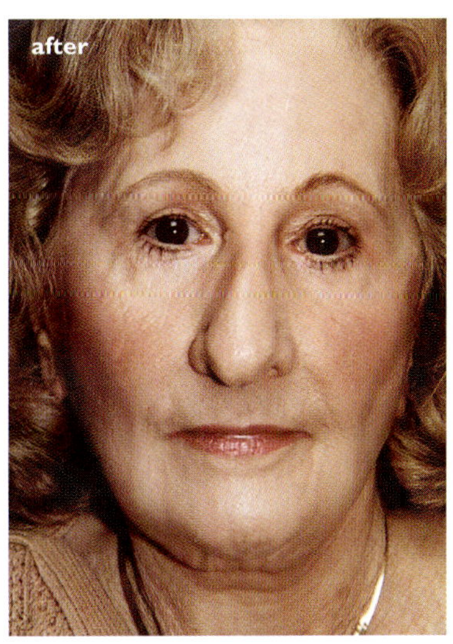

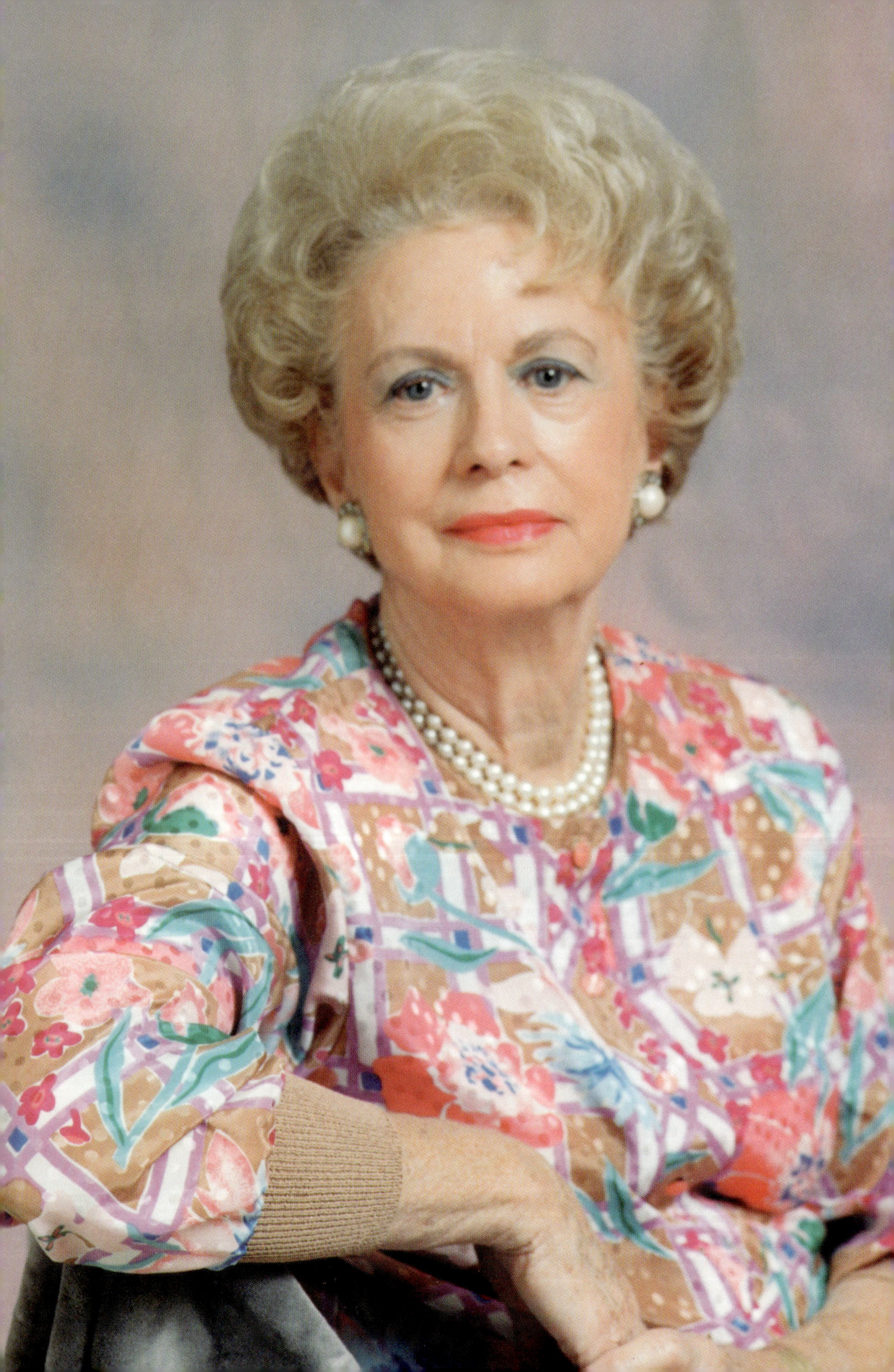

PATIENT PORTRAIT

DOROTHY NEWTON
SKIN REJUVENATION PEEL
AGE: 76

I was an executive with Elizabeth Arden in New York. We had a wonderful building on 54th Street where we sold the most fabulous lingerie and high fashion clothes. Those days were wonderful. It was a great time. We took care of the hair and skin of all the Broadway stars and famous people and celebrities. Everyone came in: Kennedys; Ethel, Pat, Jean, Rose and Jackie; the Rockefellers; Ginger Rogers; Marlene Dietrich; Ethel Merman. Just think of a big name — they all came to Elizabeth Arden's. Of course, we did everything for the skin, and I had all kinds of facial treatments at the salon. But in those days we just didn't know anything about sun damage and nutrition or pollution.

My husband was a vice-president of Chase Manhattan Bank and we were avid fishermen. Fishing is a great release from the pressure of the business world. We would go out to some remote beautiful place and fish for hours up and down the east coast, from Maine to the Florida Keys. The sun damage caused my face to be weathered and lined and I had brown spots and skin cancers. I looked like a dried-up, old prune.

We were fishing in Alaska and I met someone who told me about getting the chemical peel. I really thought I was going to need a facelift. I came to see the doctor and he said he could tell from the lines and the condition of my skin that the peel would take care of it. My friend came along with me for the consultation. Afterward, she said, 'Don't think I'm going to let you go and get beautiful while I look 20 years older, and have to look at you for the rest of my life! I can't stand it!' So she came and we had our peels done at the same time.

We both look great. I'm still out in the sun a lot. I fish and swim and play golf, but now I take care of my face. I wouldn't think of going out without my proper makeup and sunscreen on. All my pals are waiting for my face to collapse, but they are in for a big disappointment. My skin is beautiful, and I get a great big kick out of getting up in the morning and looking at what a peel can do for repairing all those years of being outdoors.

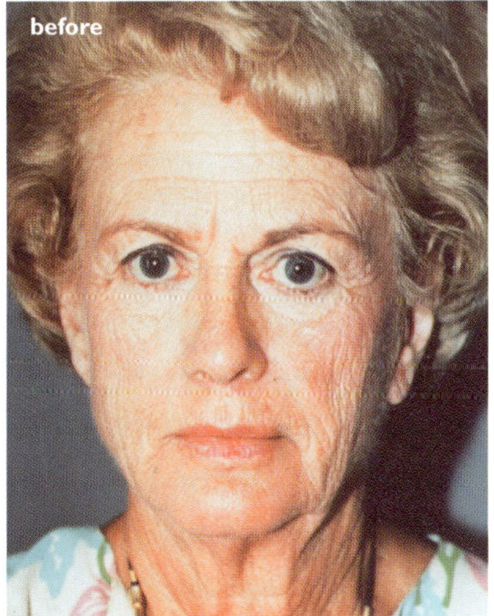
before

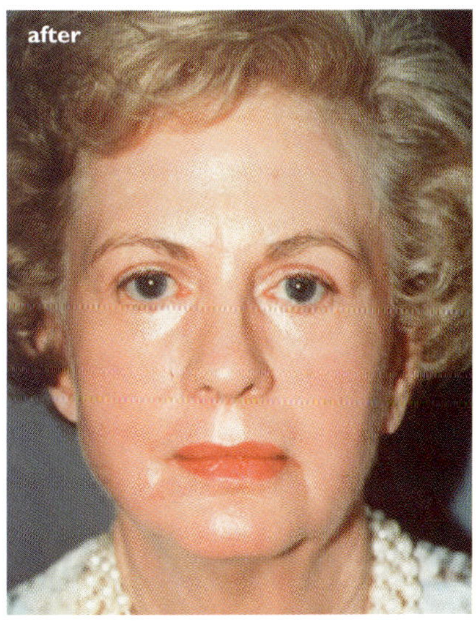
after

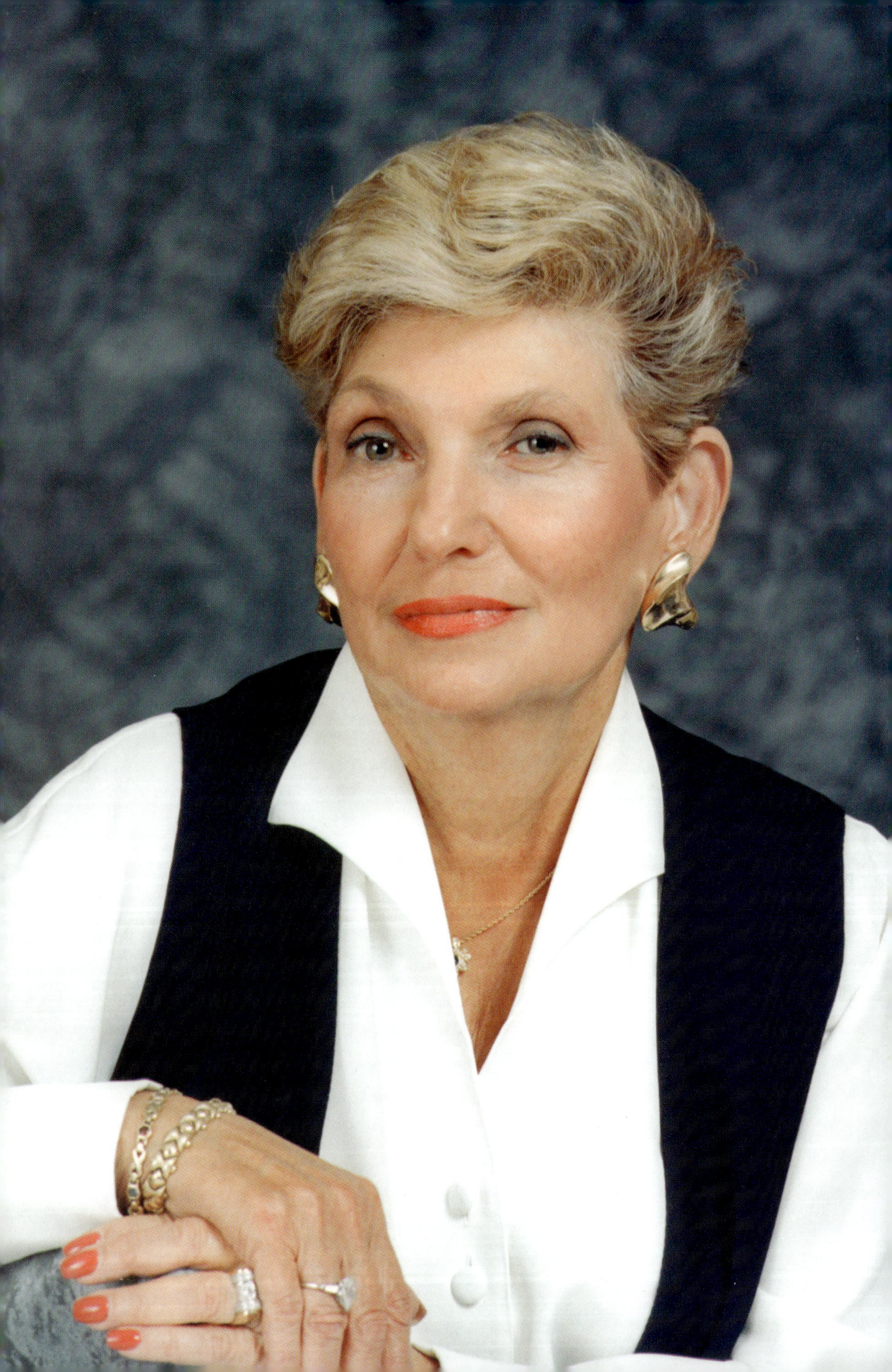

PATIENT PORTRAIT

RHEA HELFAND
SKIN REJUVENATION PEEL
AGE: 65

When I had my consultation, I looked at the doctor's hands. I do sculpture, and I know how important the hands are. They are your most important tool. You have to have the right feeling about the doctor you choose. You have to know that the doctor understands what you want to look like and that he has the skill to give you that result. This is very important. If you can't communicate with the doctor, find another one. For me, I wanted someone that I felt would give me his undivided attention. And I found one. My doctor is a perfectionist, and when he sees me in my follow-up appointments, he is very intent. I can tell he is satisfied with the new face he has given me, and so am I.

I used to do all the things you shouldn't do to your skin. I sat out in the sun all day and I smoked, so I paid the price for all that neglect. I lost my mother, my husband and my father, all in one month — I can tell you that added a few wrinkles to my face. My face wasn't sagging, I was just covered with wrinkles. I didn't give it much thought until my children said, 'Mom, do something!'

Several of my friends had chemical peels. I didn't realize the difference a peel would make for them because when it's your friend, you look past the wrinkles, at the person. But when I saw their before and after pictures, I was astounded. Their faces just seem to glow. They had an attitude-lift. They are all so much more outgoing, confident and happy. I wanted to look and feel the same way.

I had never done much to take care of my skin. I would just wake up, throw some water on my face and get on with my day. That was it. But I have learned so much. I was taught the proper preparation and care of my skin so that it would be right for the peel — and then how to take care of it afterward. All of this is new to me, but I am willing to do it. I'm educated about how to treat my skin now and I don't want to look like I did before my peel — all those age spots and wrinkles, ugh! When I see my "before" pictures, I see an old woman. I didn't feel like one, I just looked like one.

My granddaughter loves my face. She touches it all the time. I was at the swimming pool with her and a stranger said, 'Is that your mother?' She was so proud, she said, 'That's my grandmother!' And she was all smiles.

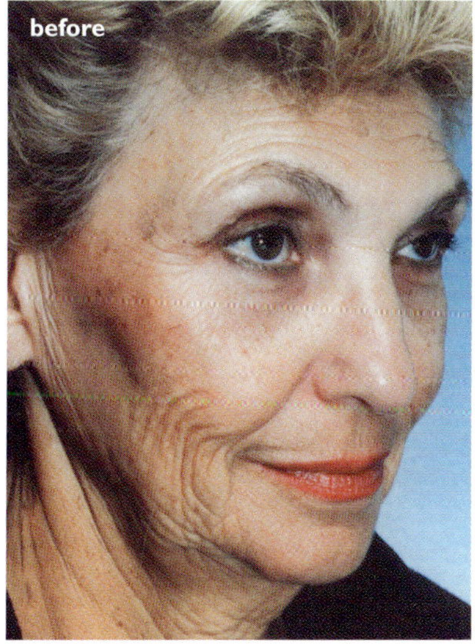
before

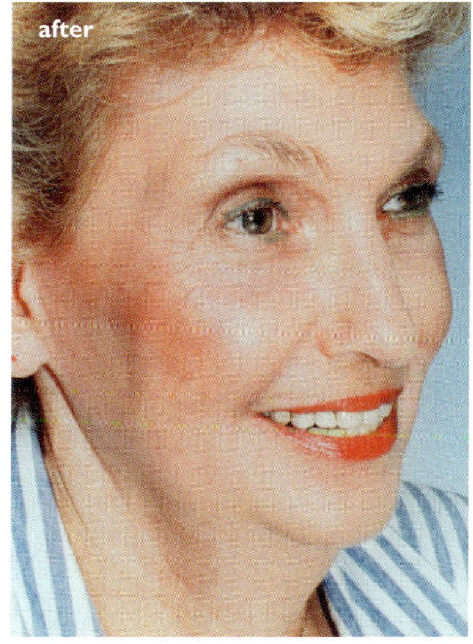
after

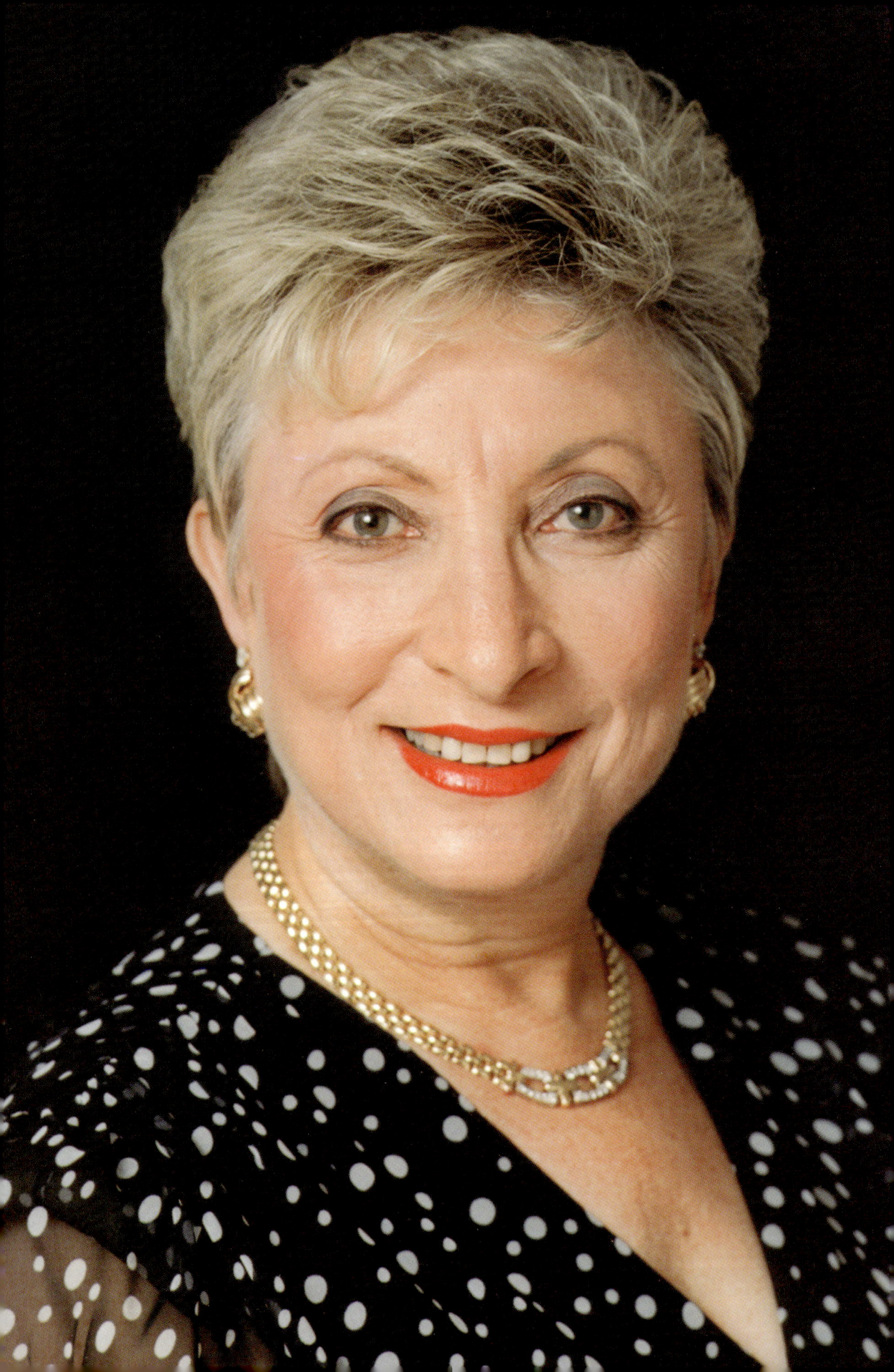

PATIENT PORTRAIT

ROBERTA HERBSTMAN
SKIN REJUVENATION PEEL

I had my nose fixed when I was 16, and I've always known I would have a facelift when it was time. I was surprised when the surgeon said I would look good with just the chemical peel. That was a very nice surprise.

My children thought I shouldn't bother, but it mattered a lot to me how I look, so I made the decision to have something done, no matter what they thought.

I had been to see other plastic surgeons and was given various options. One doctor said he thought the peel would make me look pretty good without surgery.

I admit it. I am very vain. I've always taken good care of myself. When my husband and I travel on our business trips, I don't want to be old-looking. Sometimes it is quite a while before we see some of these people again and I want to look good.

Gratefully, my husband and I have our health. My husband and I discussed everything and agreed that the peel was a good idea. My kids loved me the way I was. It didn't matter to them, but it mattered to me. So I made the decision to do it.

I'm enjoying life. My husband and I have a family business that takes us all over the world. We go to lots of places that most people have probably never heard of, and wherever we go, we have friends.

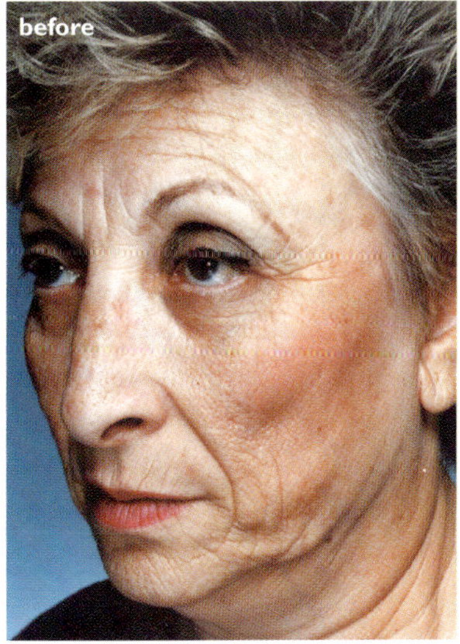

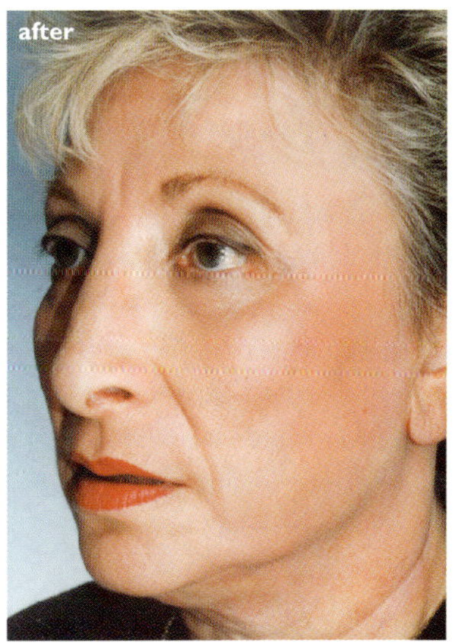

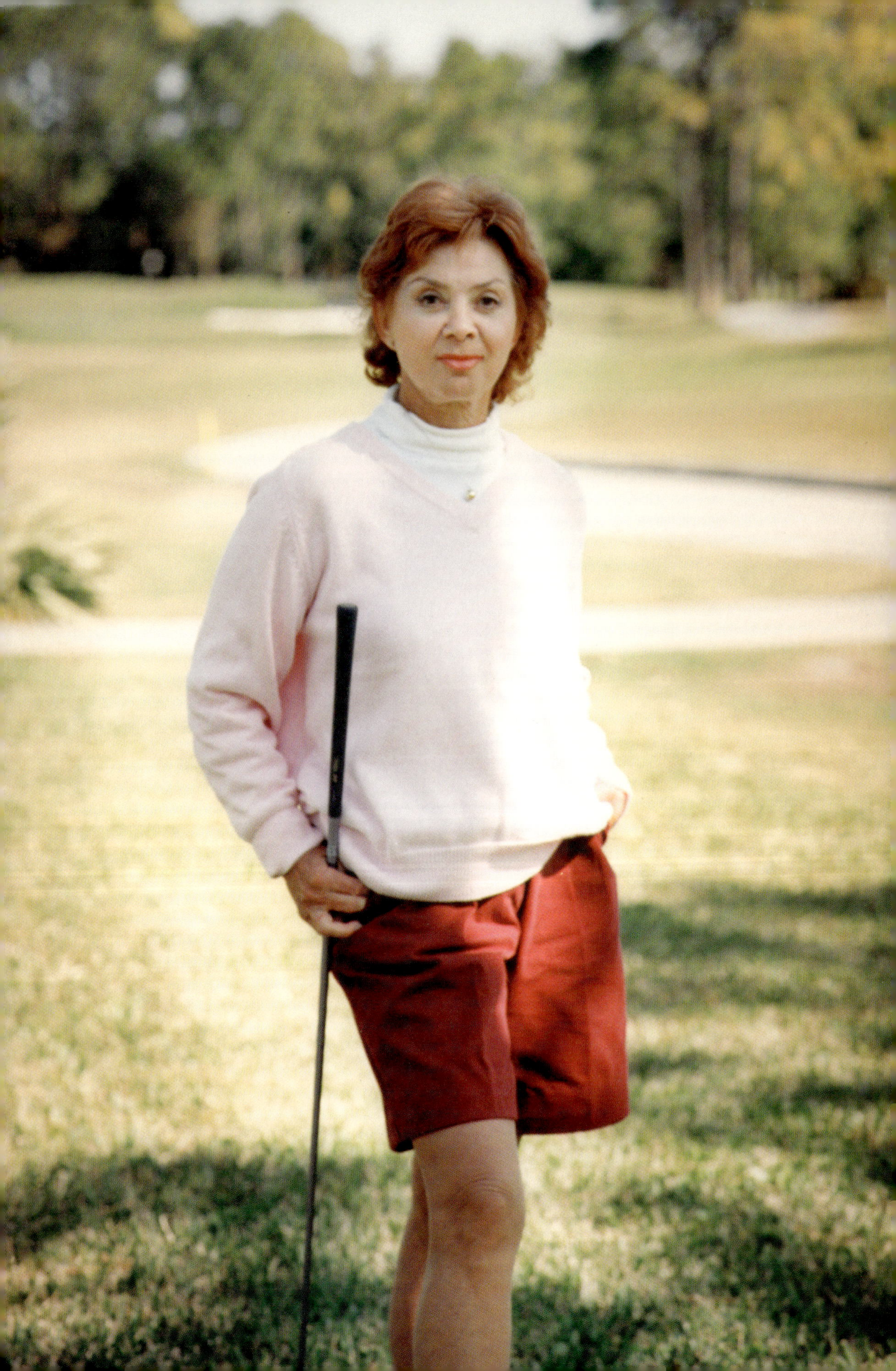

PATIENT PORTRAIT

HILDA GROPPER
SKIN REJUVENATION PEEL

On a trip to visit my brother, I was sitting next to a stranger on a plane and he said, 'Do you mind if I say something personal to you?' I thought he was going to tell me something like, 'You're a nice lady,' because we had been having a friendly chat. Finally he said, 'You are too young and beautiful to have the kind of skin you have.' I couldn't believe it! I was very upset by what he said. For several years I had been going to the dermatologist for a light chemical peel every two or three months. It just sloughs off the dead cells and you look a little fresher, but it doesn't do anything for the wrinkles. Still, it wasn't as if I'd just ignored my skin. When I got to my brother's house, I repeated what the man on the airplane had said to me. My sister, who is 13 years older, said, 'He's right, you look older than me.' That's when I knew I had to do something."

My husband didn't want me to have anything done. I'm 12 years younger than he is and he'd say, 'You're young enough and beautiful enough to suit me. When it's time to find yourself another husband, then you can have it done.' Of course, we'd laugh at that, but he really was not supportive of the idea until he realized just how much I wanted to have something done.

I made several appointments for a peel. Then I'd get scared and cancel. I was letting fear prevent me from doing something I wanted. I finally decided I wanted it enough — and now I recommend it to anybody who wants to listen. The chemical peel actually gives you new young skin. It tightened up my jaw line and the skin on my neck and around my eyes.

I was given a lot of pre-op and post-op instructions. But I've always been one of those people who don't believe in taking pills. At first, I didn't do any of the things you are supposed to do after surgery. I was told to spritz my face with water every few hours, put ointment on every few hours and take pills for the itching. I didn't follow these instructions. I took a shower and got into bed, and then I thought I was going crazy with the itching. I realized I had the top layers of skin burned. Layers were coming off, that is all part of the healing process. I got right up out of bed and took the pills, did the spritzing, put on the ointment, and then I was fine.

I'm the youngest of five and, as a teenager, I tried to look older and sophisticated so I wouldn't be the baby of the family. Now I put a piece of black tape on my driver's license to cover the year I was born.

When people see me they say, "You look wonderful. Your skin looks gorgeous. You look terrific, but it must have been so painful?" It wasn't.

When I see my 'before' pictures, I can't believe it's me. Why didn't someone tell me that I looked that ugly before some stranger did?

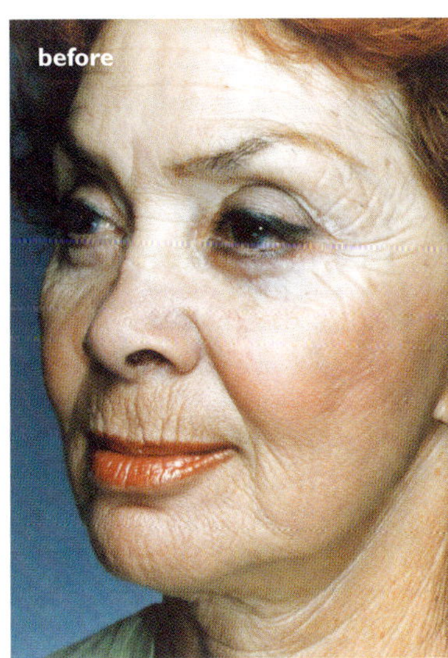

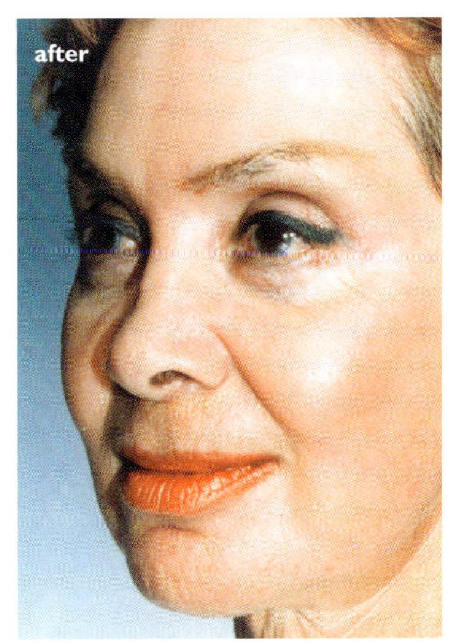

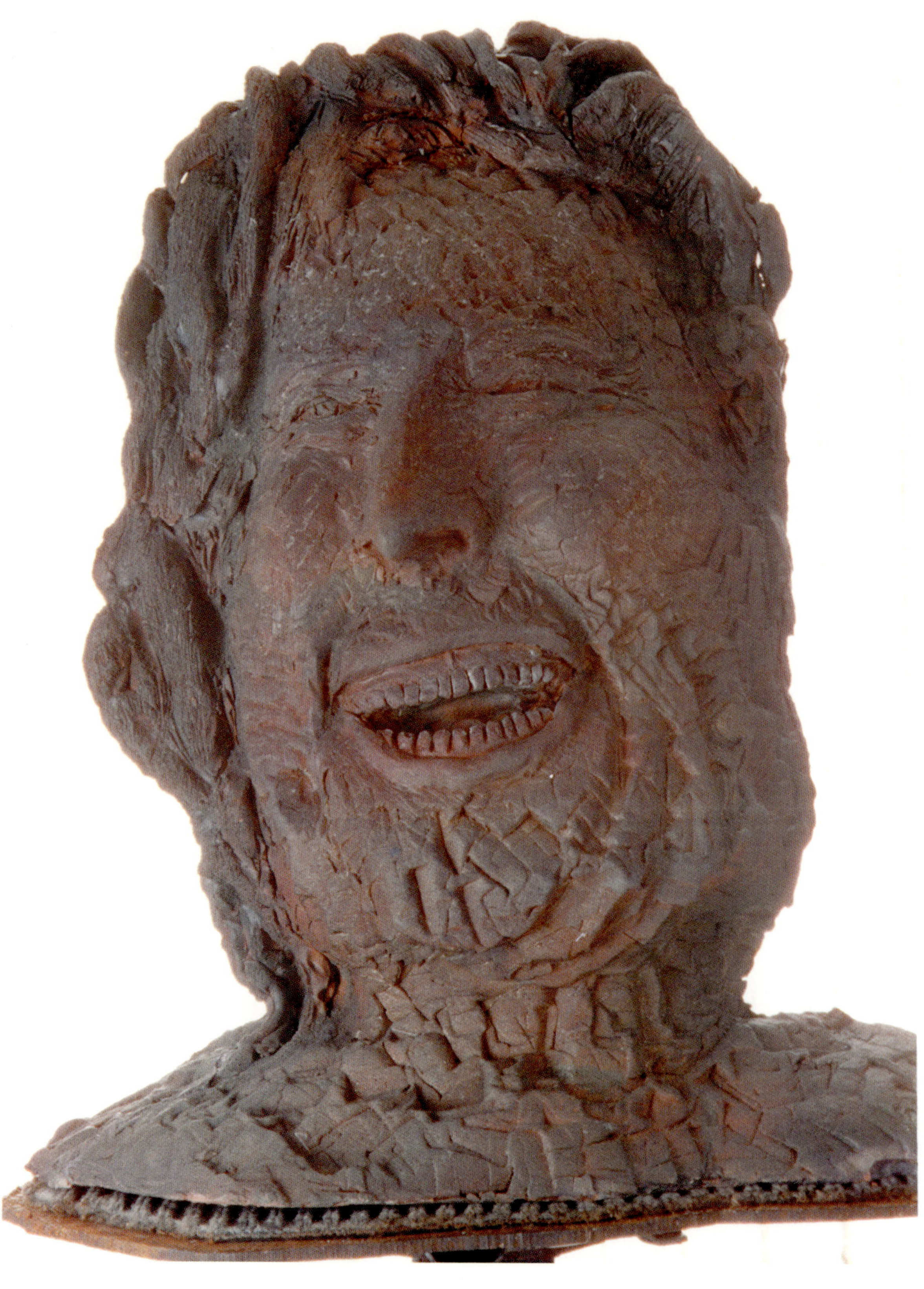

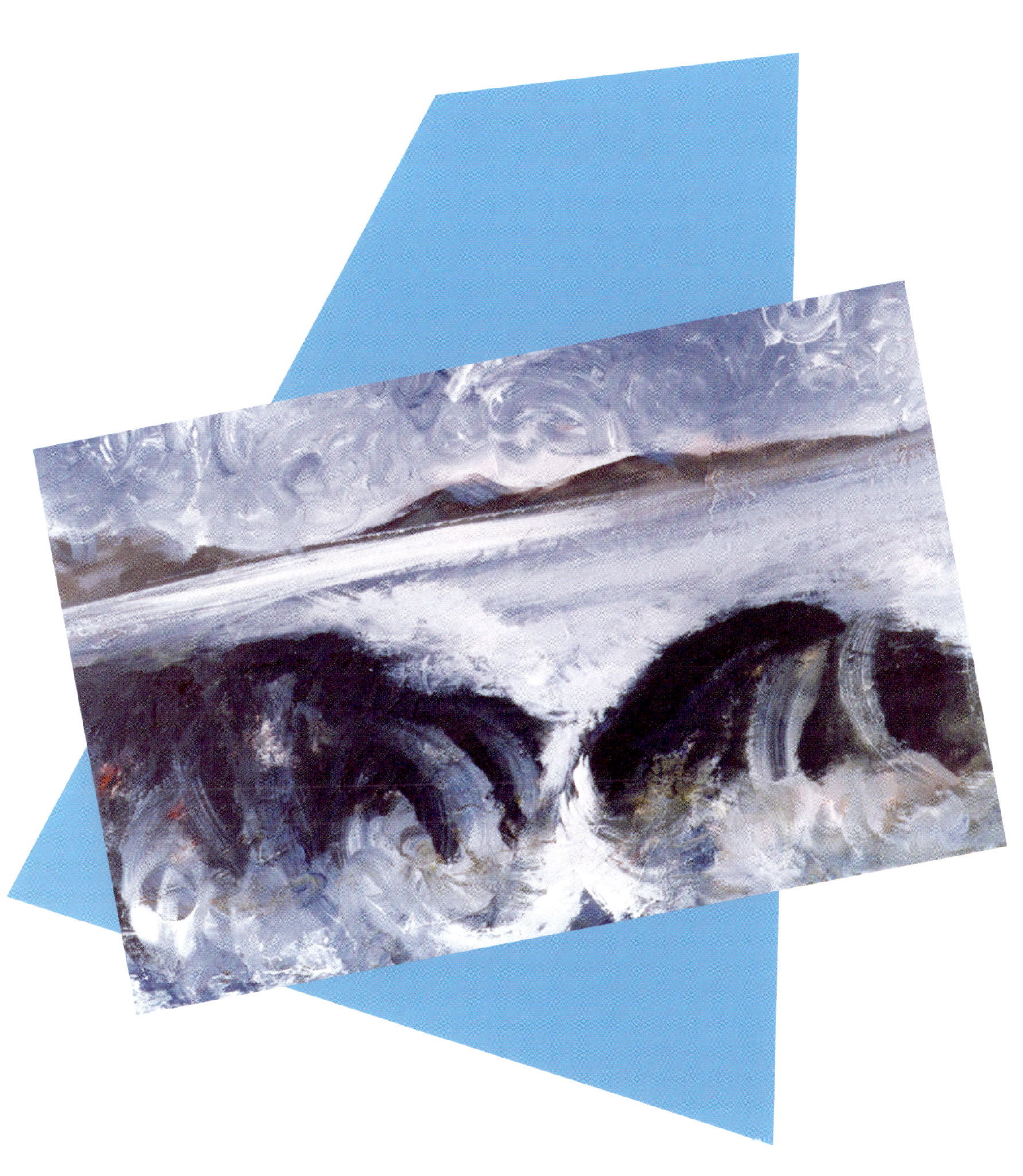

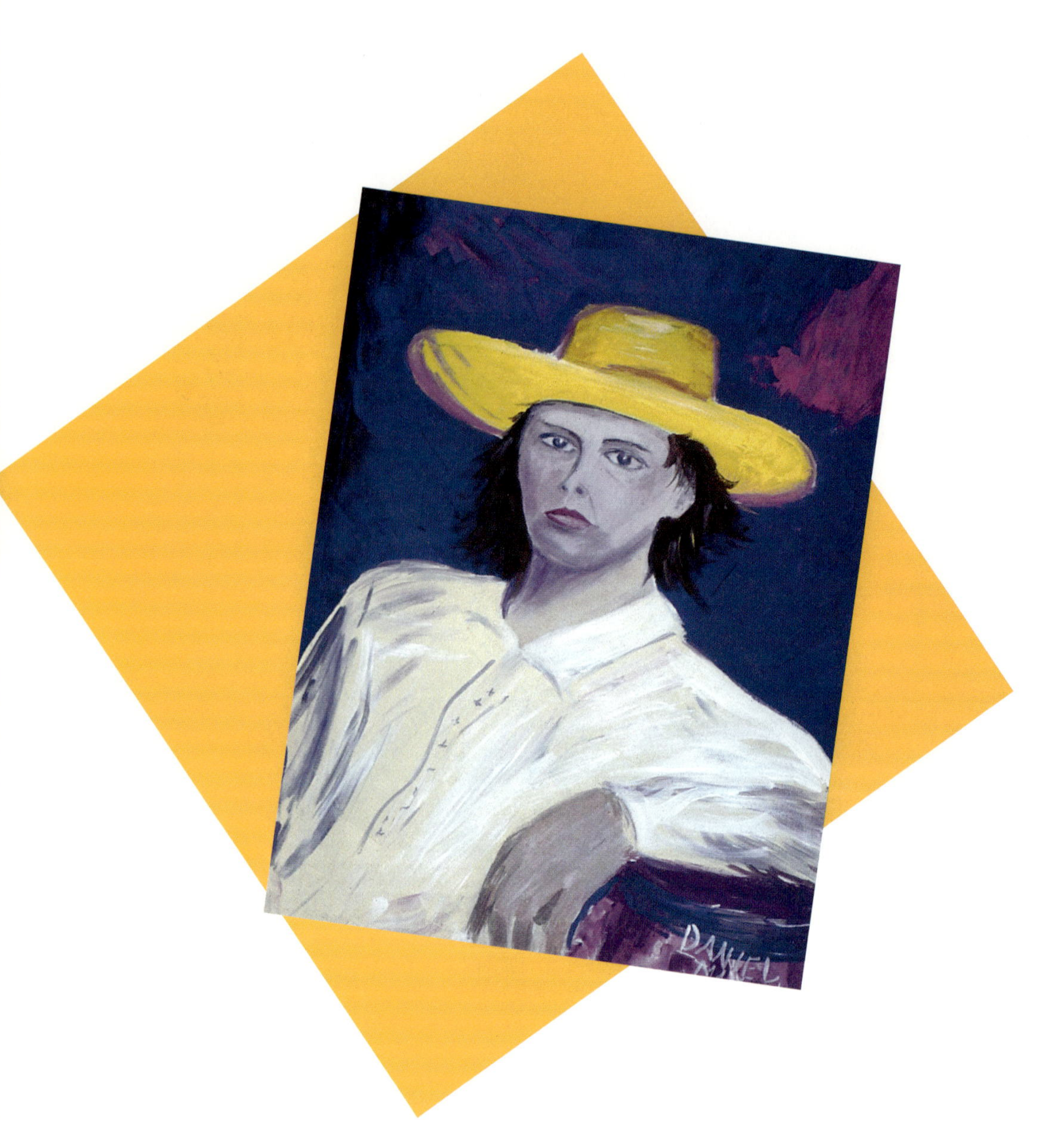

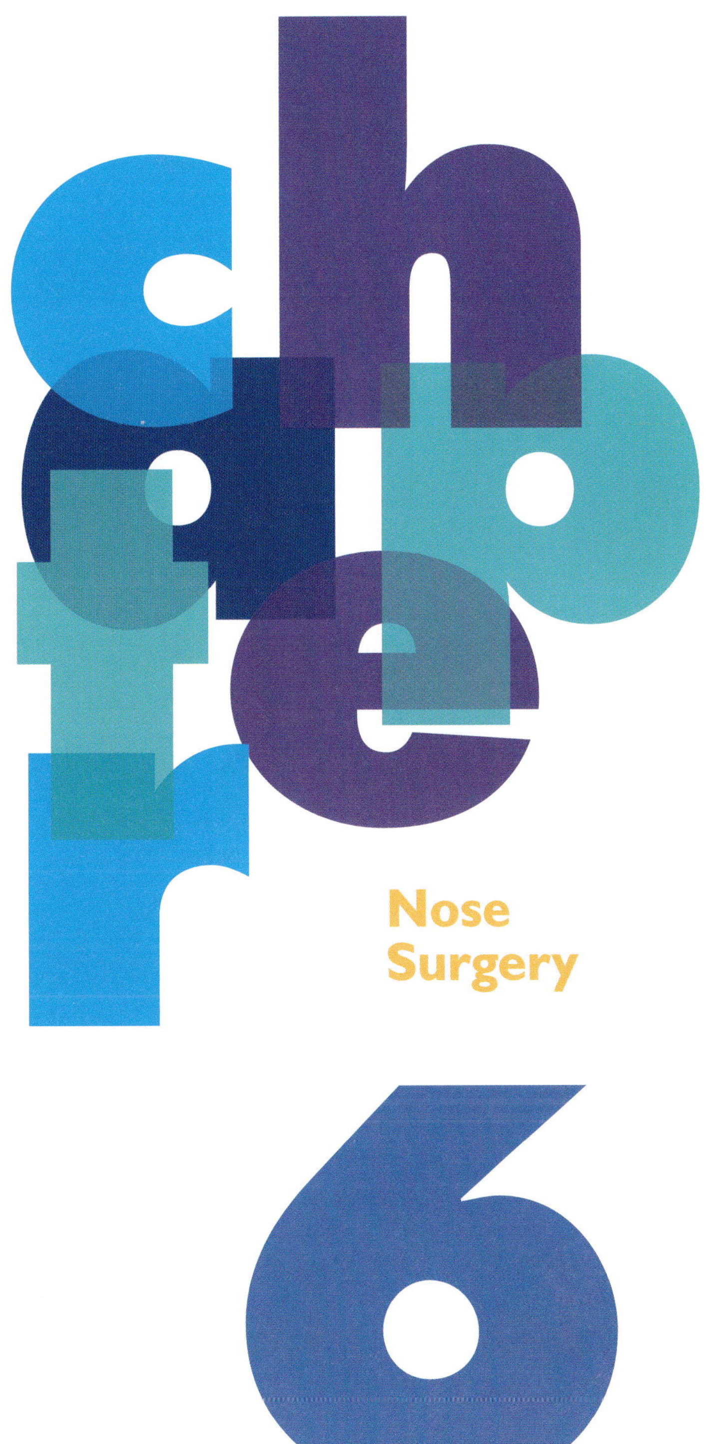

Nose Surgery

Nose Surgery

A rhinoplasty is the surgical procedure used to reshape the nose to improve its appearance, contour and proportion. Nose operations have been performed for over 2,000 years. Some of the earliest recordings appear in the Vedas, the Hindu Holy Book, which describes how surgeons would restore the noses of criminals who had them removed as punishment.

The most prominent of the facial features, the nose can denote our character, as suggested by Leonardo da Vinci, and has been assigned such attributes as nobility and strength. It can also reflect our ethnic heritage and has even been influenced by fashion trends. Noses today more closely fit the individual's face. The style of noses such as the cute, upturned, button nose popular in the 1950s and 1960s has been replaced by graceful and stronger noses that impart confidence.

The reason most people have surgery is to straighten the bridge of the nose, alter the size or shape of the tip, reduce a hump on the bridge or narrow the nostrils. There are also many medical reasons for having nasal surgery, especially for those with breathing difficulties due to blocked nasal passages (deviated septum) or other nasal abnormalities. Nasal reconstruction (more extensive surgery) is performed to correct breathing problems or to restore a nose badly disfigured by injury or disease such as skin cancer.

NOSE SURGERY

Rhinoplasty

Purpose: *To reshape the contour of the nose for a more pleasing shape and proportion to other facial features.*

Includes reducing or increasing the size, repairing deviated septum for improved breathing, removing the bump on the bridge, narrowing the span of the nostrils, and changing the tip and angle of the nose.

Length of procedure: *45 minutes to several hours.*

Anesthesia: *General anesthesia and/or local anesthesia with intravenous sedation.*

Where: *Outpatient surgery or overnight stay*

Recovery: *Swelling and bruising of the nose. Patients wear a nose splint.*

Back to work: *7 – 10 days; Full activities 2 – 3 weeks. Makeup 1 week.*

Risks: *Infection, bruising, swelling, bleeding, reaction to anesthesia.*

Cost: *$5,000 – $8,000*

**(Note: Prices may vary based on physician fees, anesthesia, surgical setting and number of procedures. Data is based on a compilation of sources including Dr. Man.)*

Anatomy of a Nose

The nose is a complex structure of human anatomy — a triangular projection of bone, cartilage, muscle, nerves and skin. Each part varies in texture and thickness. The skin of the upper portion of the nose is thinner and different from the skin of the tip, which is usually thicker.

Improving the appearance and relationship of the nose to the rest of the face, is often performed through incisions made inside the nose. Working through the nostrils, the surgeon separates the outer skin from the underlying bone and cartilage, which is then sculpted to the new shape. The surgeon can remove a hump on the bridge, reshape the tip and reduce the width of the base of the nose by removing small wedges of skin and bringing them closer to the center.

The procedure usually takes between one and two hours, or longer for more extensive reconstruction, and may be done under intravenous sedation or general anesthesia in accredited facilities such as the doctor's office, hospital, or outpatient surgery facility. After surgery a tape, acting much like a splint, is worn for

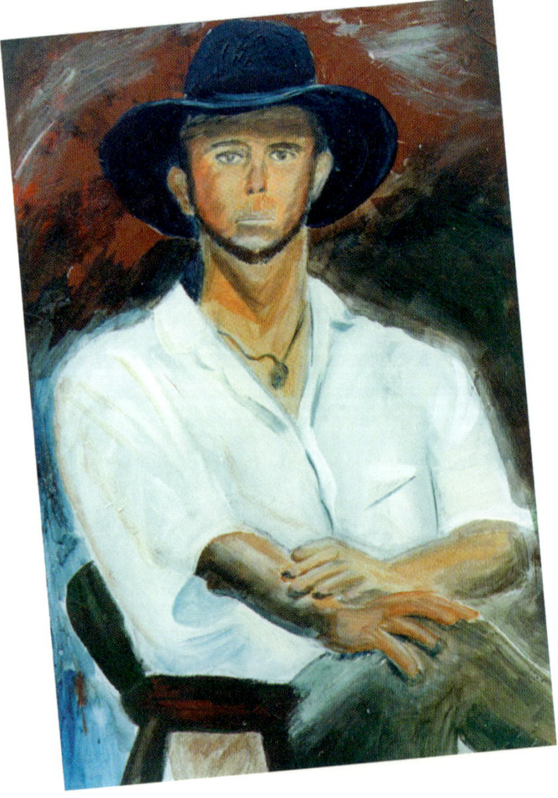

several days. There will be some swelling and bruising, which will disappear after several days. Patients are able to return to work and gradually resume activities in about a week or two.

Before surgery, the surgeon will examine your skin type and thickness, the shape of your nose, its bones and underlying structure, and the shape of your face. During aging, the nose continues to grow, and its skin becomes more fleshy and less elastic. The tip becomes longer and thicker. Patients will be asked what they don't like about their nose and what they expect from surgery. If they've had previous surgery on their nose, this should be brought to the doctor's attention. Breathing problems, allergies to medications and smoking should also be discussed. Smokers will be asked to cease smoking for several weeks prior to surgery.

Age is not usually a consideration, except for children. Rhinoplasties are one of the most common procedures performed on adolescents. It was thought that surgery should be delayed until the age of 16 or 17 or after the growth years. Today, it is generally agreed that teenagers should wait until after their growth spurt which usually occurs around the age of 14 or 15, but surgery can be, in some cases, elected earlier.

Improvement may be dramatic or subtle, depending on the extent of the surgery and the correction required. An obviously disfigured nose will show vast improvement while a minor change, such as removing a slight bump or reducing a tip, may be more subtle. The purpose of having nasal surgery is to have a nose that appears natural and is more in keeping with the other facial features.

For a model, actor, television personality or other person whose work depends on appearance, an acceptable result may require attention to the smallest detail. A nose that is even the tiniest millimeter off — imperceptible to the human eye — may draw unwanted attention to itself. What is unnoticeable to the human eye is magnified by lighting and camera angles. The camera never lies. In this case, this imperceptible flaw can become a serious consideration for a patient whose job requires constant camera scrutiny.

In every case, the decision to have

nose surgery is a highly personal one. For example, one patient who had rhinoplasty was never unhappy with the appearance of his nose, even though he was a magician and performed in front of audiences. He finally chose to have surgery because of his breathing difficulties. He had lived with blocked nasal passages all his life and had only decided to do something about them in adulthood.

Choosing to have a rhinoplasty should be considered carefully, as every surgery carries some risk. Risks include but are not limited to: bruising, swelling, infection, bleeding, reaction to the anesthesia and a less than ideal result. Roughly 5 percent of rhinoplasties require a secondary correction due to aesthetic considerations and unpredictable post-operative healing. Patients should avoid strenuous activities and exercise following their surgery and they should review with their doctor all the risks, expectations and follow-up requirements they can anticipate during their healing process.

NOSE SURGERY

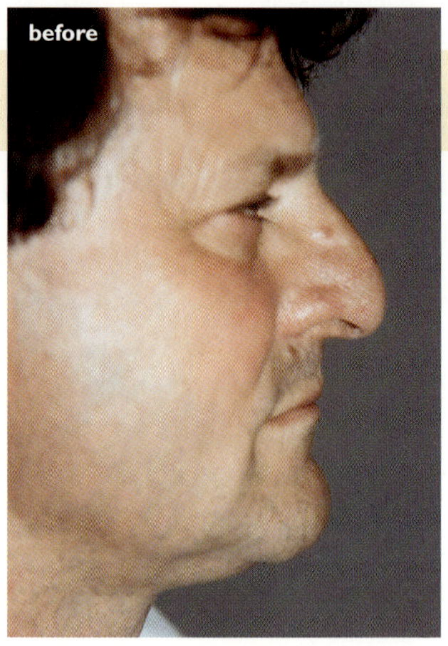

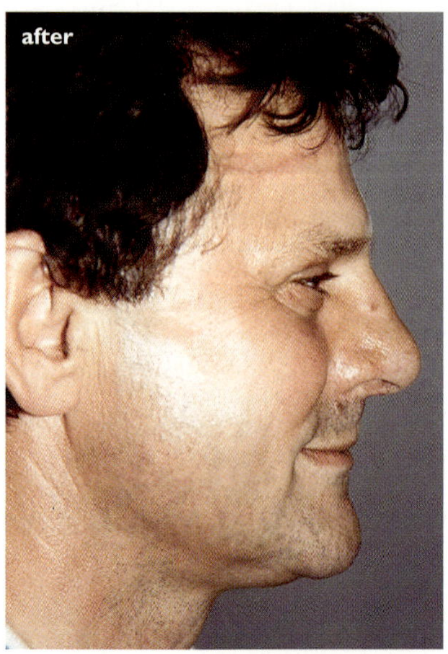

Nose Surgery; Upper & Lower Eyes

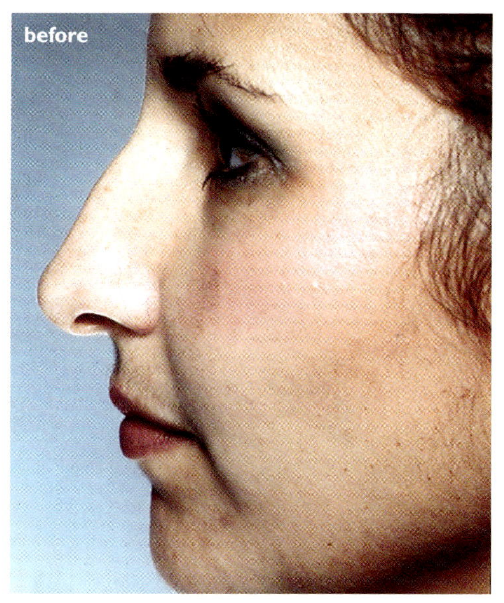

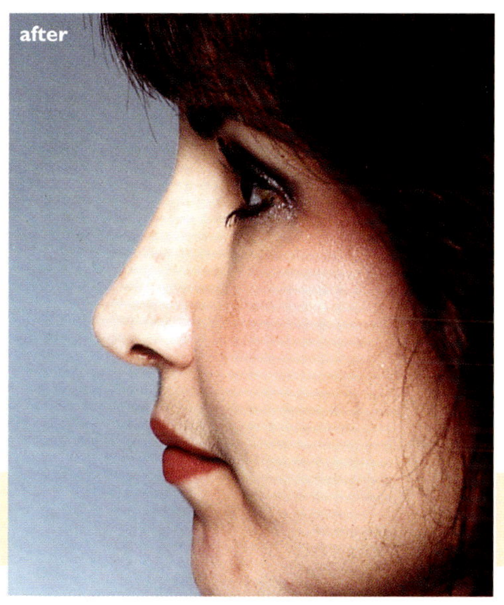

NOSE SURGERY

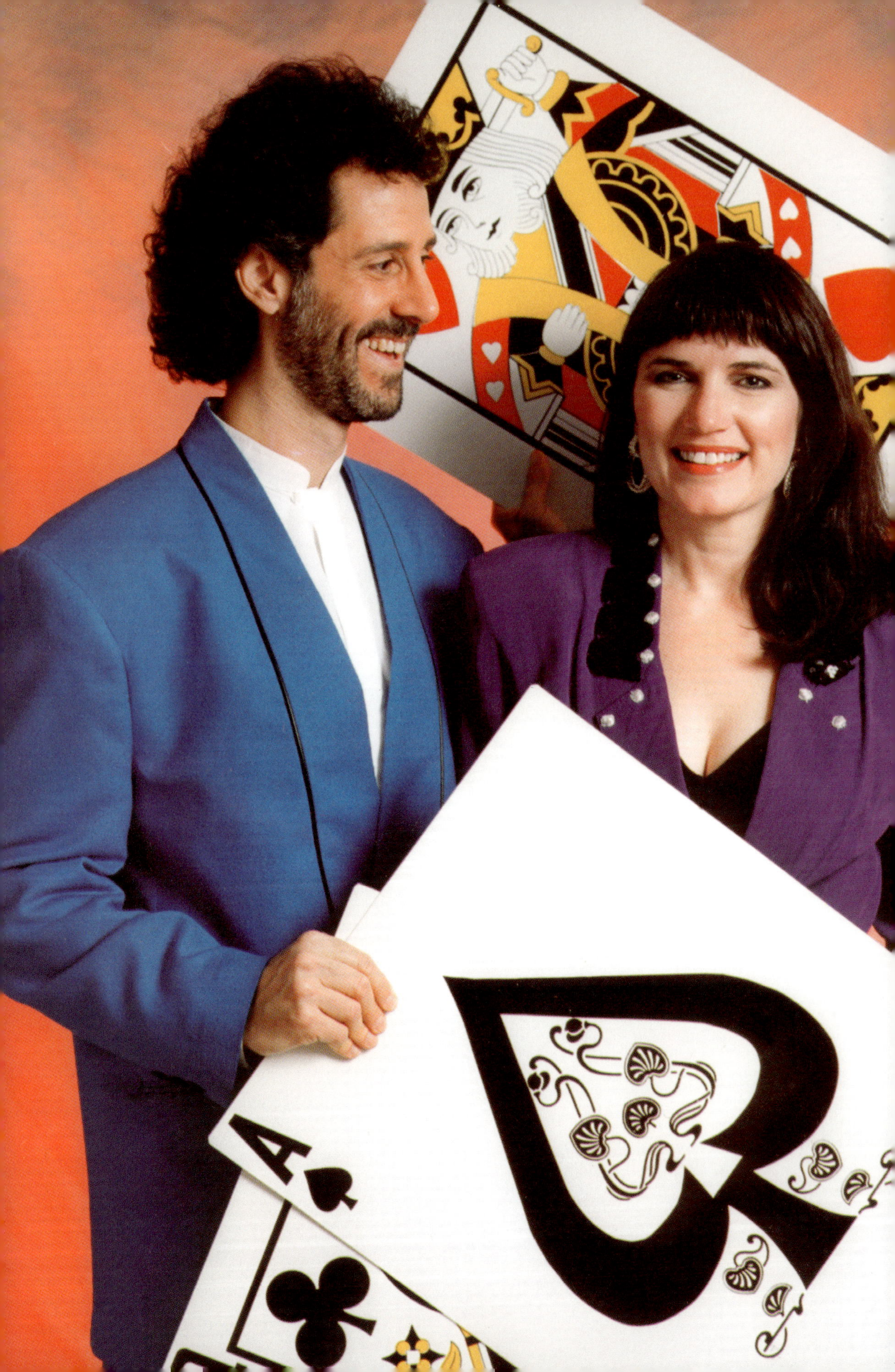

PATIENT PORTRAIT

GARY GOODMAN
NOSE SURGERY
AGE: 36

"I've lived with a deviated septum all my life. Most of the time I couldn't breathe through my nose at all. I had to breathe through my mouth. I'm a full-time magician and illusionist. I make my living performing at children's parties, corporate functions, conventions — sometimes before thousands of people."

"The sound of my voice, the way I project to the audience are all very important. A lot of times when I talked on the phone I sounded like I had a cold. When I talked to clients, people would ask, 'do you have a cold?' I really got tired of being asked that question. I couldn't wait to have this done."

"It was his profile that changed dramatically," explained Jamie, Gary's wife and partner in his magic act. "Gary had major reconstruction and grafting inside his nose. His recovery was what really impressed me. I know, because I had my nose fixed ten years ago. "

"I never had swelling," said Gary. "What I think was really amazing is that I never even had a headache. I never took one Tylenol. I think a lot of people don't have surgery because they think there is a lot of pain and they have to be uncomfortable afterward and lose a lot of time off work. Who wants to go through something painful? To wake up and to not have any pain — not even a headache. That's pretty amazing, especially since I had major work done on my nose."

"It's true, I was expecting some degree of pain, especially from the horror stories everybody told me. Friends told me I was going to be black and blue for weeks and I would have headaches. Years ago, when I was thinking of having this done, I said no because I remembered the stories about the pain, headaches and Jamie's experience. So when my doctor said he didn't do it that way, I thought, great! I don't have to go through what Jamie went through. That was a big plus."

"Afterward I had a very simple little tape splint bandage for about a week. I had to spray inside my nose with saline. I used the two weeks at home to my advantage, practicing new magic routines. Two weeks later, I was back to work. What a difference it has made for me! Being able to breathe easily is great. It's quite a new experience for me after 36 years."

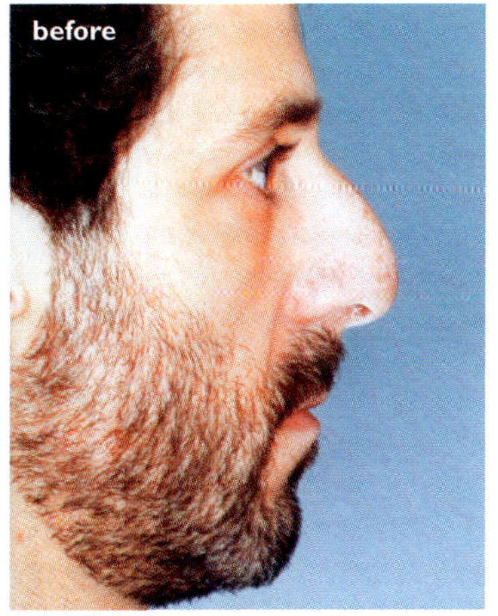

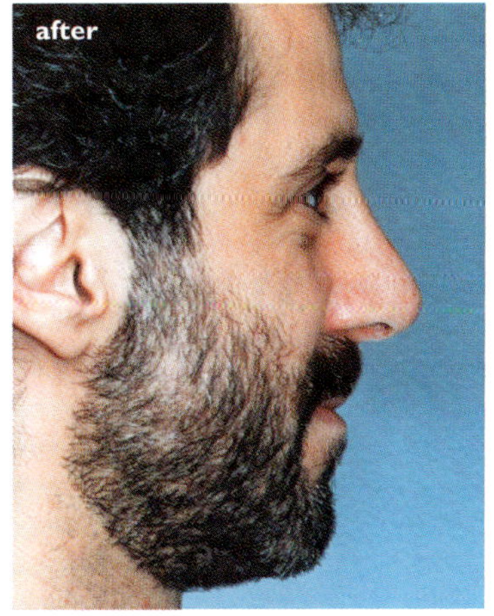

PATIENT PORTRAIT

ALAN WEST
NOSE SURGERY
AGE: 47

Having my nose fixed was something I'd always wanted, ever since I was a 13 and broke my nose playing football with friends. I played an end, and I went out for a deep pass. The ball came and so did the fence. I caught the pass, and the fence caught my nose. The doctor at the time said, though my nose was broken, it would heal and not seriously change my breathing. I really didn't know how it affected my breathing except when I played at sports and found myself having to breathe through my mouth instead of my nose. I never realized that I couldn't breathe through my nose. It was only later that I found out my right nose passage was 90 percent blocked and my left passage was 40 percent blocked. I also had a problem with the size and shape of my nose.

I didn't like my profile. My nose had a big bump at the bridge and was hooked at the end, I think partly from heredity and partly from the football accident. I had periodically mentioned to my wife that I wanted to get the bump on my nose fixed. I looked like I had a beak on my face as opposed to a nose. I was very self-conscious about it, so I made a decision that at some point in my life, I would have my nose fixed. I just needed to get up the nerve to do it. I do not have a high threshold for pain. I was concerned about the stories I had heard years ago about people having their noses fixed, having a black and blue face for weeks and the nose being stuffed with cotton so you couldn't breathe anyway. All those stories I had heard when I was growing up in high school didn't warm me to the idea of getting my nose fixed. But the doctor indicated that the procedure he used worked from the inside out and did not require a rebreaking of the nose. He said he could shave off the bump and restructure the nose from the inside, without leaving me with a packed nose or a black and blue face.

My surgery has increased my self-confidence ten-fold. Now, when I go into a business meeting I don't even think about how my profile looks. I know it looks excellent. In my business, I deal with people on a one-to-one basis and in groups. Your first impression of people is usually the one you keep. If two people apply for the same job, and all things are equal, the better looking person is ultimately going to get that job. It's a subconscious decision-making process. Looks, personality and intellect are all taken into account.

Today, I don't think about my nose. People can't goof on me or call me names and even my youngest daughter, Rebecca, who used to always call me 'The Beak,' can't call me that anymore.

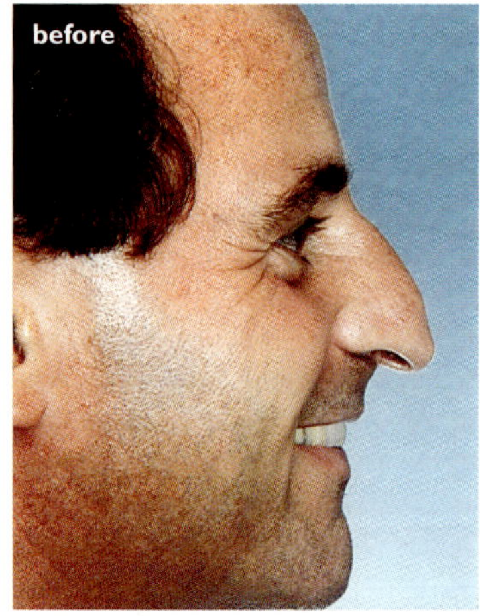

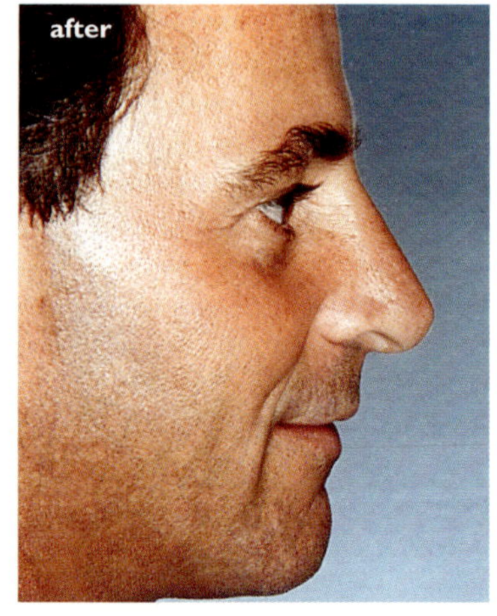

NOSE SURGERY

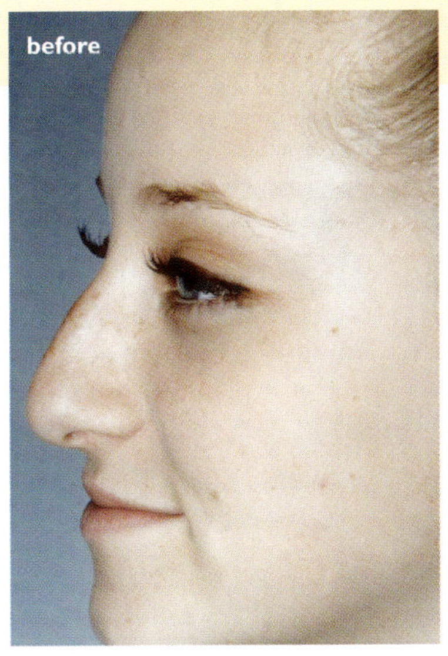

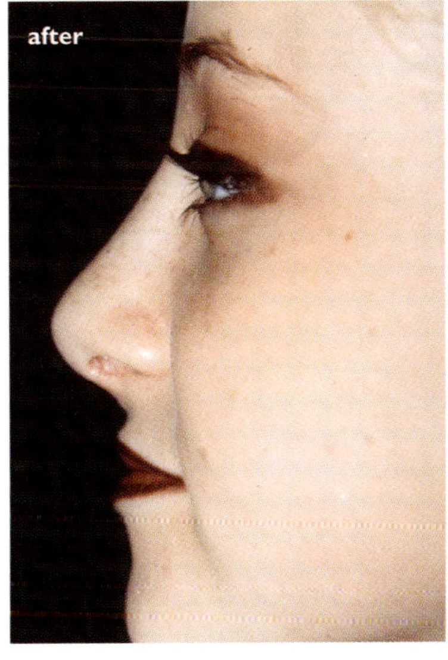

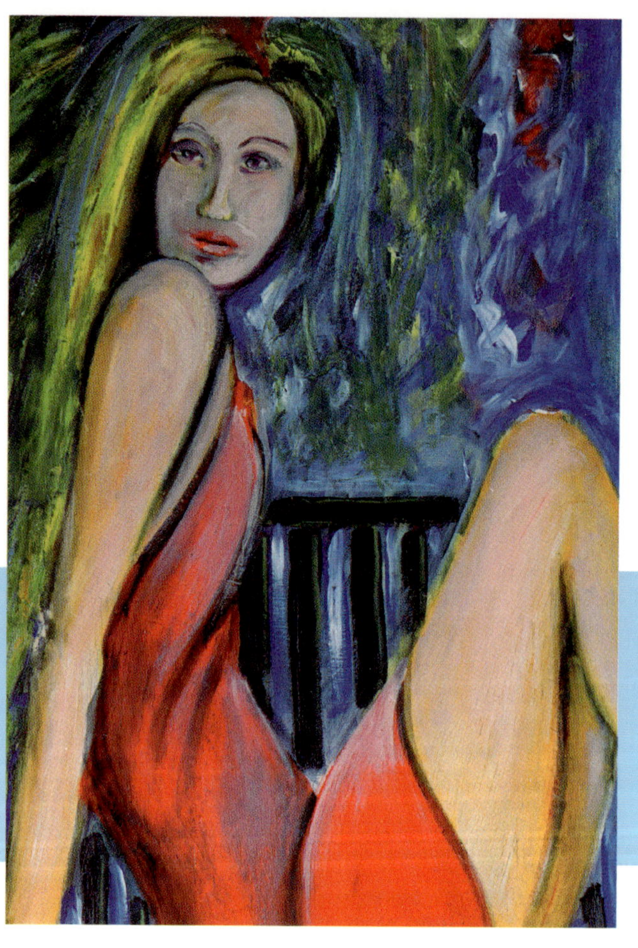

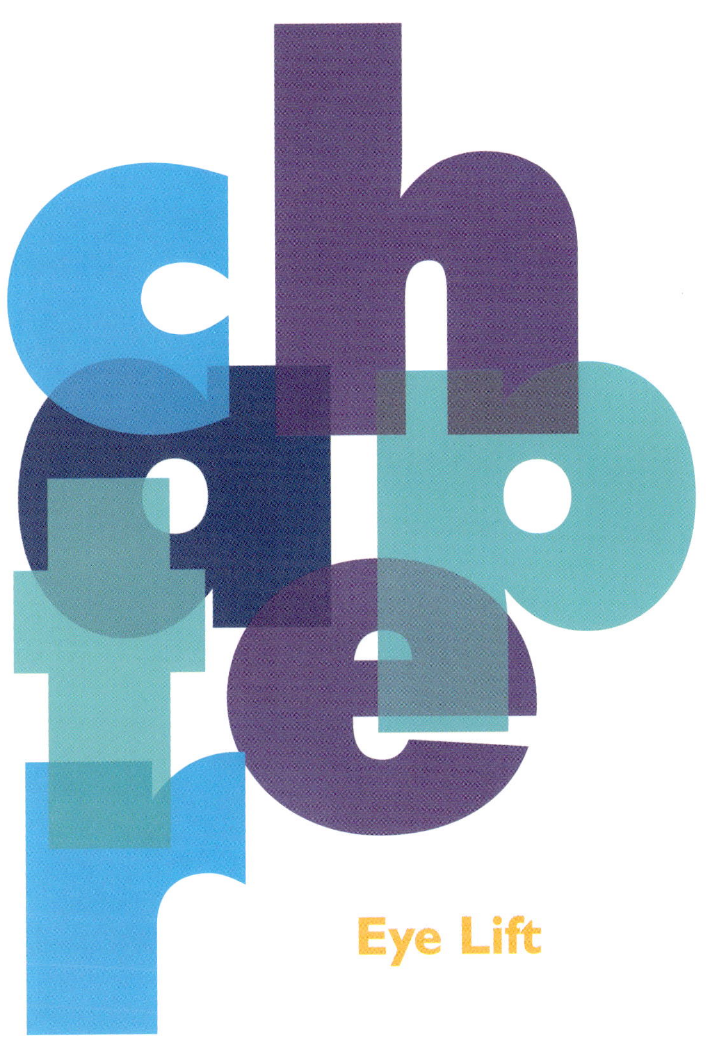

Eye Lift

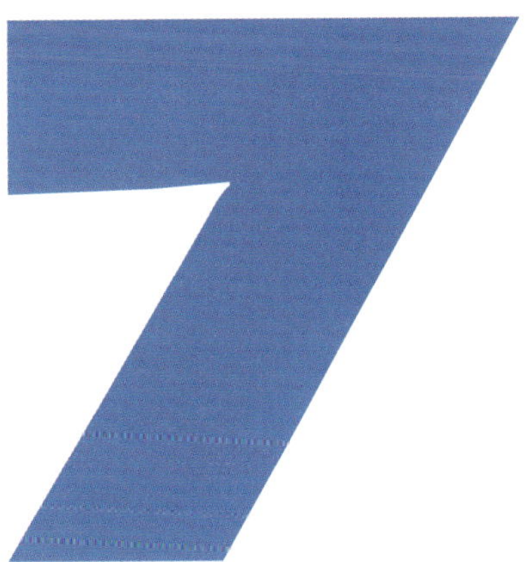

Eye Lift

Eyes speak volumes. Usually they are the first thing we notice about a person. Dark circles, bags under the eyes, and droopy eyelids can give the eyes and face a "tired," puffy look even though you may feel rested and full of energy. There may also be medical reasons that warrant eyelid surgery. Sometimes the upper eyelid skin hangs down over the eye, impairing vision. This is called ptosis of the eyelid. But, whether it is for cosmetic or reconstructive reasons, an eye lift, called blepharoplasty, can return the eyes to a youthful, vibrant, fresher looking appearance.

Surgery of the Eyelids

Eyelid surgery is the second most popular procedure performed by plastic surgeons. It removes excess fat and tissue from the upper and lower eyelids. Today, blepharoplasty is often performed with the use of lasers. The incisions are well hidden in the natural creases of the upper eyelids and inside the lining of the lower lids. Puffy bags under the eyes can be removed at this time. Using the laser, or the peel, the surgeon can resurface areas of the skin such as dark circles and "crepe-paper" skin, which is common under the eyes.

EYE LIFT

Blepharoplasty

Purpose: *To reduce the tired, sad look associated with sagging, droopy eyelids. Also reduces puffy look and bags under the eye by removing excess fat.*

Surgery Length: *1 – 2 hours.*

Anesthesia: *I.V. sedation or local anesthesia*

Where: *Outpatient surgery or overnight stay*

Recovery: *Patients experience swelling, bruising, and tightness of eyelids. There may be some numbness, itching and dryness. Temporary light sensitivity will occur. Back to work: 3 – 5 days; Makeup: 5 – 7 days.*

Risks: *Infection, temporary blurred vision, lid tightness.*

Cost: *$2,700 – $5,200.*

**(Note: Prices may vary based on physician fees, anesthesia, surgical setting and number of procedures. Data is based on a compilation of sources including Dr. Man.)*

Length of Surgery

The procedure is usually performed in the surgeon's office or an outpatient surgery facility under local anesthesia with intravenous (I.V.) sedation. It takes between one to two hours depending on whether both upper and lower eyelids are being done at the same time. Most patients are back to work in several days.

Risks & Complications

Side effects usually consist of bruising or swelling which disappear in a few days to several weeks. There are complications which can occur including infection, blurred vision, dry eye, swelling and scarring, temporary difficulty in closing the eyes while sleeping, lid drooping which can cause the white of the eye to be visible, and, in very rare cases, visual impairment. Sometimes, too, one eye may heal faster than the other.

Hooding/Droopy Eyebrows

Heavy upper eyelids — lid hooding — may be made worse by droopy brows. As skin and muscle tone laxity increases with age, a brow or forehead lift may also be recommended at the same time. Most patients are back to work in several days. Full recovery usually takes between 5 to 7 days. Patients who have a history of dry eye, diabetes, lupus, or Graves' disease are still candidates for this procedure, but may need additional considerations in preparation for surgery. Contact lens wearers are also good candidates for eyelid surgery. Their eyelids can age faster because of the constant pulling down on the lower lids, which makes the skin become loose and lax.

Oriental Eyes

The trend toward Western fashion and products is reflected by the desire for a Western appearance among the Asian cultures. Oriental eyes are characterized by an absence of a crease or fold in the upper eyelid, which gives the eyes a hooded, slit-like appearance. Cosmetic surgery can add creases to the eyes to give a more Western look. As in all people, aging occurs, skin becomes loose and lax, and fat adds to the fullness and hooding effect.

EYE LIFTS

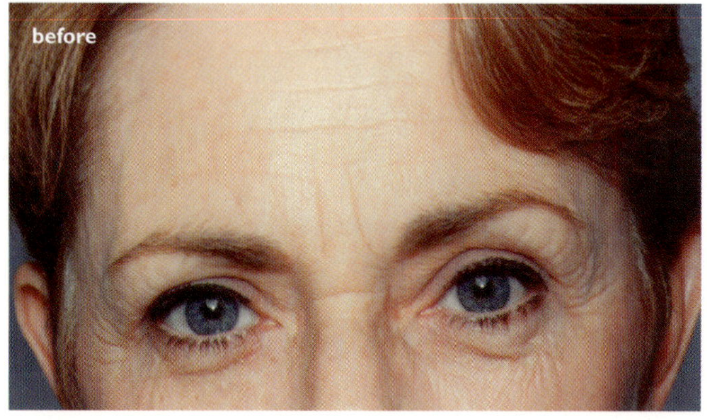

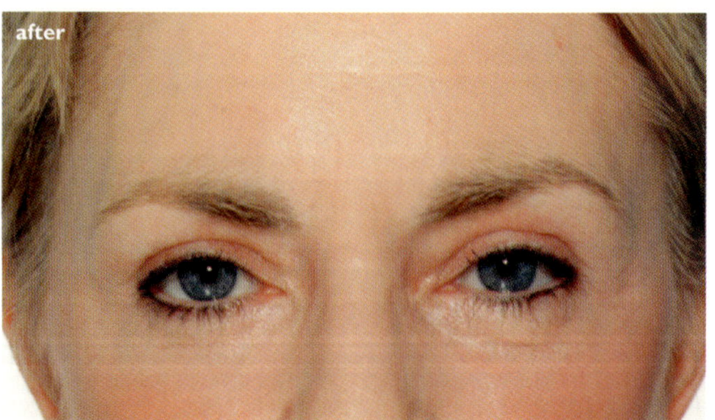

Upper & Lower Eyelids, Cosmetic Laser Surgery. Patient also had face, neck and forehead lift.

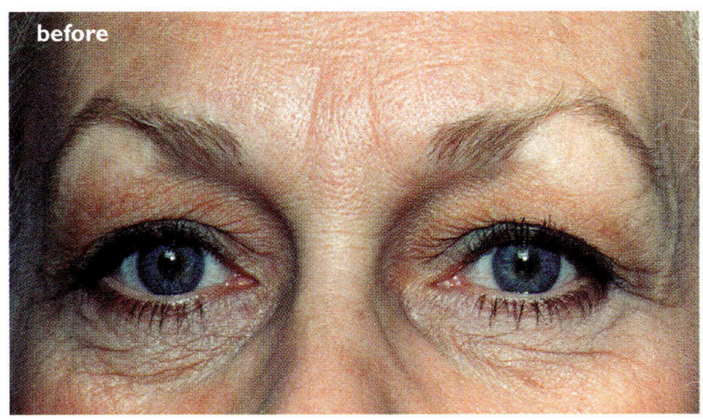

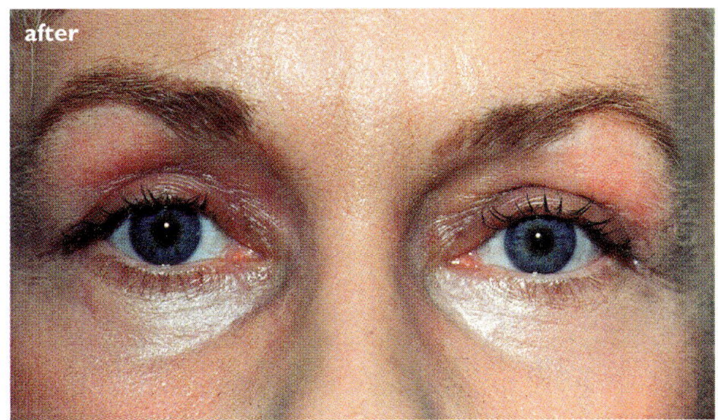

Eye lift and cosmetic laser surgery.

EYE LIFTS

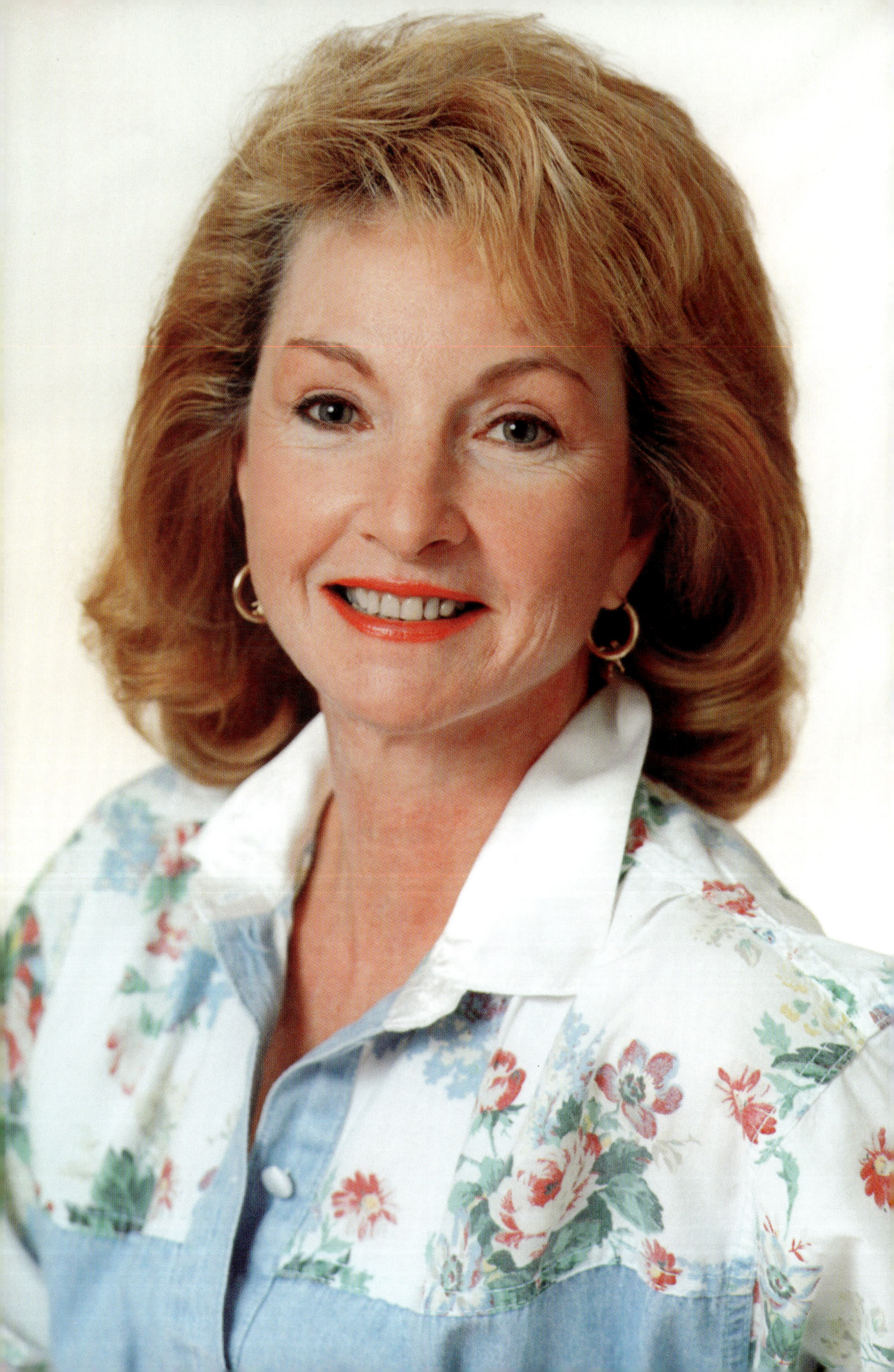

PATIENT PORTRAIT

MARY JANE PACINE
FACE & NECK LIFT, UPPER & LOWER EYE LIFT
AGE: 52

I was married when I was just 16. My husband and I ran a coal strip mine in Pennsylvania, and I had three kids at a very young age. I smoked and I drank and did all those things that are bad for you.

When I was about 48 everything just went. I divorced my husband, moved to Florida, and lost weight. But there I was, with bags under my eyes, jowls, and wrinkles.

I clean other people's houses for a living. I'm not some rich woman who got a facelift because all my friends were getting one. I would be cleaning somebody's big wall of mirror and looking at myself in it and seeing that I was falling apart. I felt that I needed a facelift and needed it badly. I looked terrible and I felt terrible. In the back of my mind, I always knew that when I was 50, I would have a facelift. I wasn't sure how I would pay for it, but I saved up until I could afford it.

I had no qualms about having surgery. But I sure didn't like all of the pre-op stuff I had to go through: the lab work, blood tests for clotting times, the physical, the eye exam, the AIDS test. I didn't like being bandaged or having tubes sticking out of my head the first day after surgery, but ultimately, it didn't matter. Soon all of that was all over. I wanted the facelift so badly that I was willing to put up with all of the discomfort. I knew my looks were going to drag me down if I let them.

I'm not a very patient person. I want everything to be fast, so I don't think I make a good patient. But I was socially acceptable in about three weeks. That really isn't long at all when you think I just had a facelift. I look good. My face doesn't yell out, 'Facelift!' like some others I've seen. The only thing that bothers me now is the little bit of numbness around the lower part of my face, which I'm told will eventually go away. I hope so.

I've changed my life. When I moved to Florida, I stopped drinking and smoking and got a facelift. I'm studying a lot of things, such as yoga, stress management, a Course in Miracles. I'm enriching myself in a lot of ways. For years, fear ran my life. I guess it runs a lot of people's lives, but I had no fear about getting the facelift. I felt ugly. A lot of people think it's vain to have a facelift. But the way I feel now that I've had my surgery, I don't have to think about my looks, and I can get on with my life.

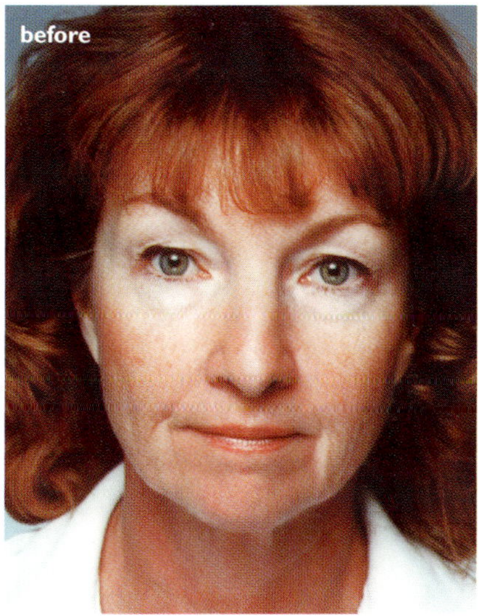

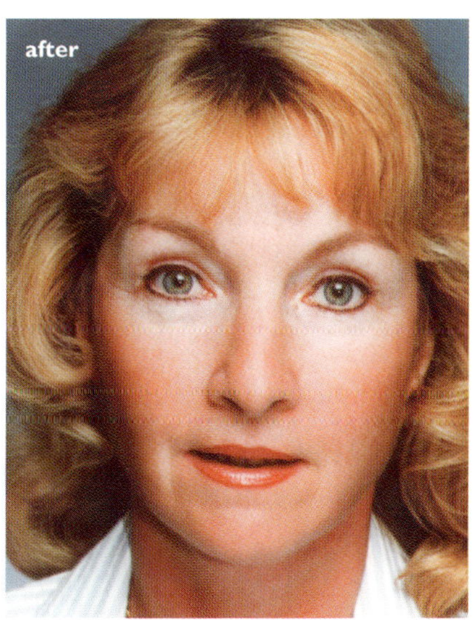

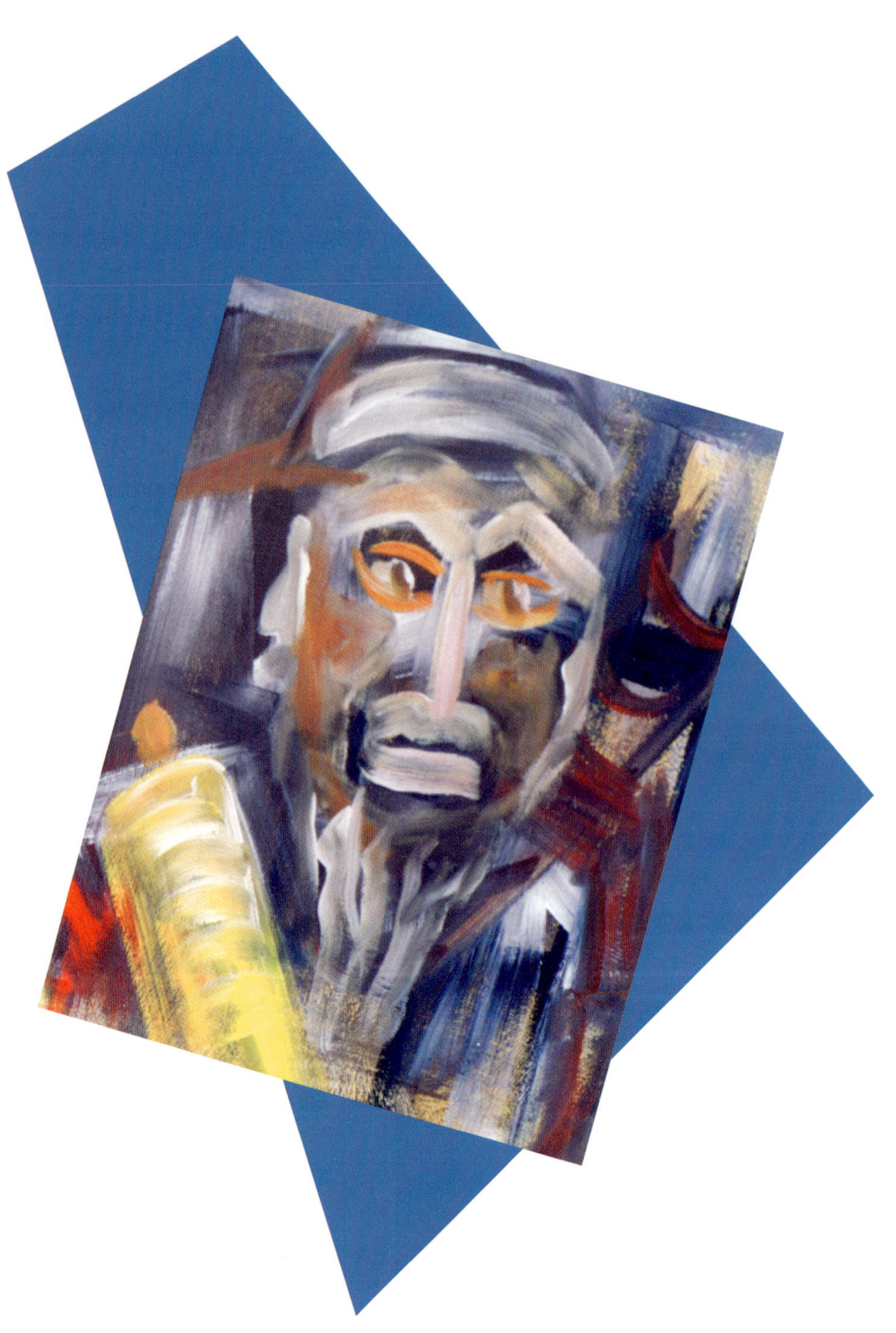

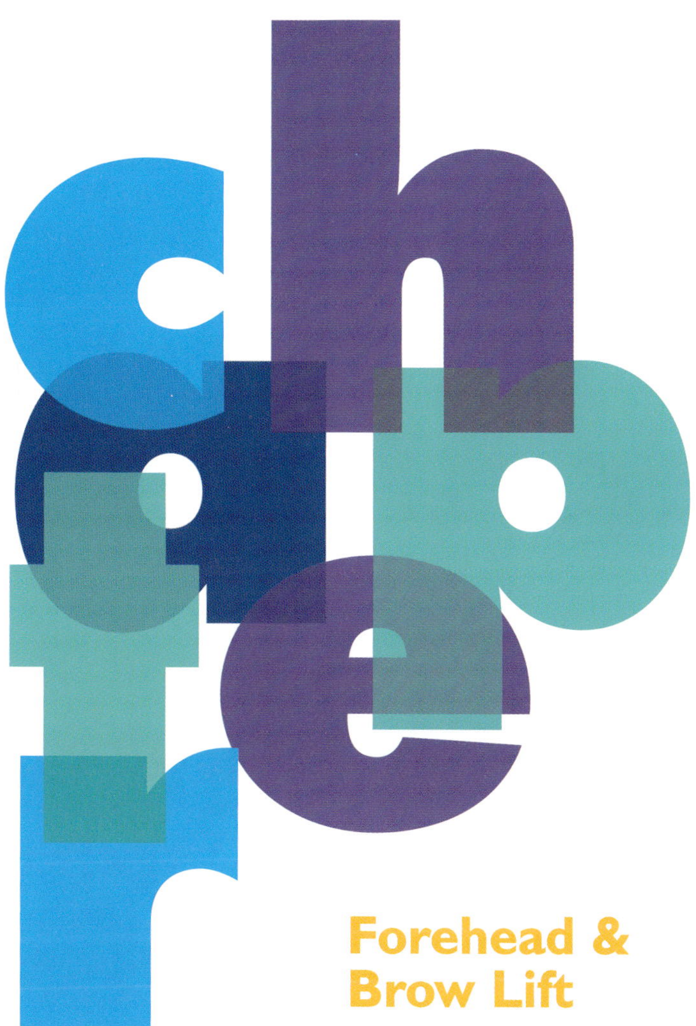

Forehead & Brow Lift

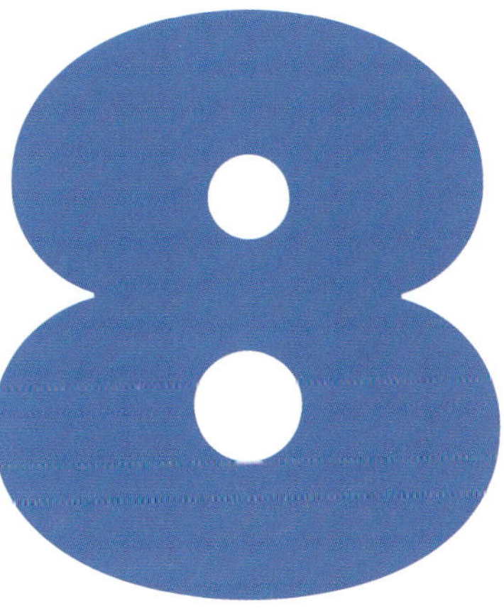

Forehead & Brow Lift

A forehead or brow lift helps reduce creases and frown lines, and correct droopy eyebrows that give a heavy brow look and create hooding over the eyes. The forehead muscles run vertically down the forehead and attach to the eyebrow and eye sockets or orbits. These muscles help maintain the brow position. When the muscles contract, they elevate the eyebrows, creating horizontal lines across the forehead and vertical frown lines between the eyebrows. In a forehead lift, the muscles and skin are tightened in order to smooth the forehead and raise the eyebrows into a more proper position. This procedure is often performed in conjunction with a facelift, eyelid surgery or nose surgery. Frown lines are reduced with collagen injections which fill out the lines or with Botox injections which inhibit the eyebrow muscles from contracting. The results give the face a more alert, rested and youthful appearance.

Forehead & Brow Lift

Procedure: *Forehead & brow lift*

Purpose: *Improves droopy eyebrows, hooding over eyes, forehead creases and frown lines.*

Surgery: *Length is 1 – 2 hours.*

Anesthesia: *General and/or local.*

Where: *Outpatient.*

Recovery: *Temporary swelling, bruising and numbness.*

Risks: *Infection, nerve damage and bleeding.*

Cost: *$2,130 – $4,300.*

**(Note: Prices may vary based on physician fees, anesthesia, surgical setting and number of procedures. Data is based on a compilation of sources including Dr. Man.)*

Endoscopic Forehead & Brow Lift

A forehead lift is performed in the doctor's office or outpatient surgery facility under general and or local anesthesia with I.V. sedation. The traditional approach to a forehead lift is through a coronal incision which runs across the scalp from ear to ear. The procedure requires cutting along the hairline and lifting the forehead skin to reveal the forehead muscles. The eyebrows are brought into a higher position and the excess scalp skin is removed and the flap is sutured to its place.

New advances using the endoscope have simplified this procedure. The endoscope has been used since the early 1970s in many types of surgical procedures including bladder and hernia repair and knee and joint surgery, among others. As in other surgeries, the endoscope gives the plastic surgeon an inside and close-up view of the surgery site without the need to make major incisions. The endoscope is inserted through tiny 1/4- to 1/2-inch incisions. The surgeon is able to view the forehead muscles under video magnification and insert special surgical instruments to release the muscles and fix the brow in a better position. The patient benefits by having fewer incisions, which means fewer chances of scarring.

This is important for those who have thinning hair, high foreheads or receding hairlines. Using the endoscope there is also less bleeding, less pain and quicker recovery.

Length of Surgery

The forehead lift takes from one to two hours, and is usually performed in an outpatient facility, under general anesthesia or I.V. sedation. Patients may experience numbness, bruising and swelling. Complications can include trauma to local nerves, infection, localized hair loss. Patients are usually back to work in several days, in the case of endoscopic surgery, and a week to ten days for traditional forehead surgery.

Frown Lines

Frown lines may also be reduced by injecting collagen or fat into the lines and creases to fill them out. These injections may be repeated several times, since a portion of the collagen and fat is absorbed by the body. Botox injections offer another means to reduce frown lines by inhibiting the eyebrow muscles from contracting. Botox is injected to the muscles which causes them to relax, smoothing out the vertical lines. The results last up to six months, sometimes less, at which time the procedure can be repeated.

FOREHEAD & BROW LIFT

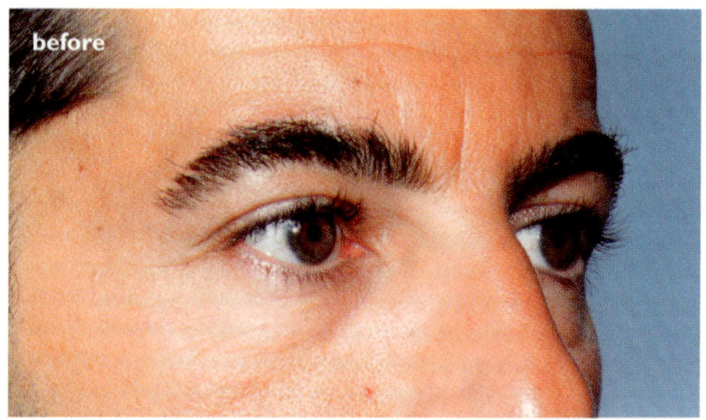

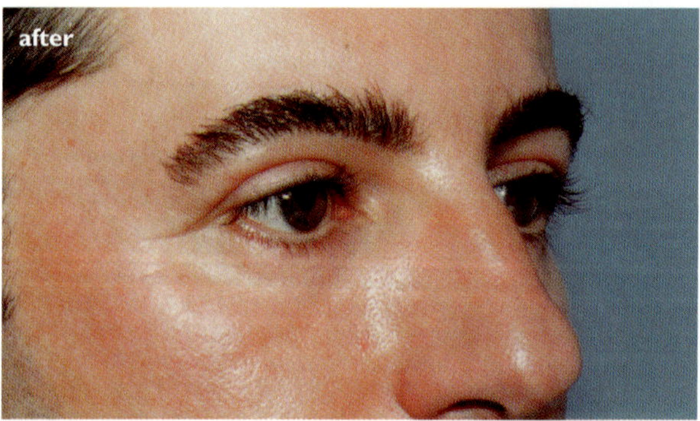

Forehead Lift, Upper and Lower Eyes, Liposculpture, Full Face Laser, Botox

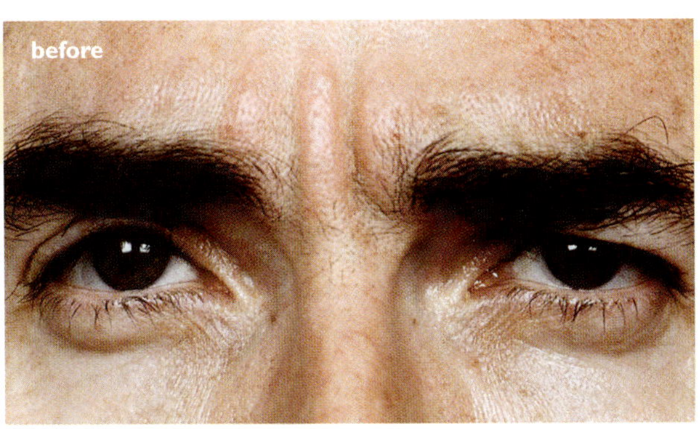

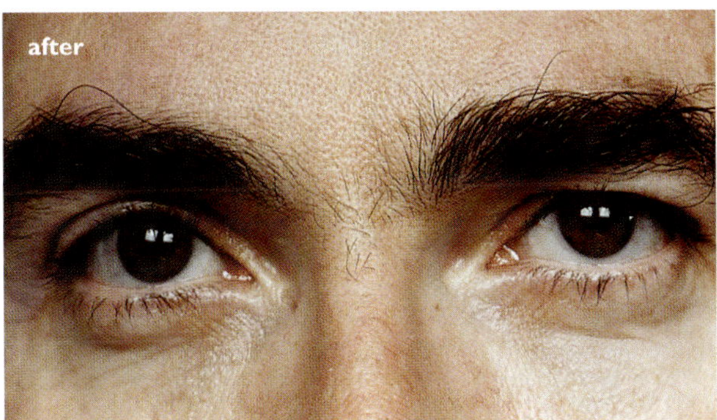

Botox Injection

FOREHEAD & BROW LIFT

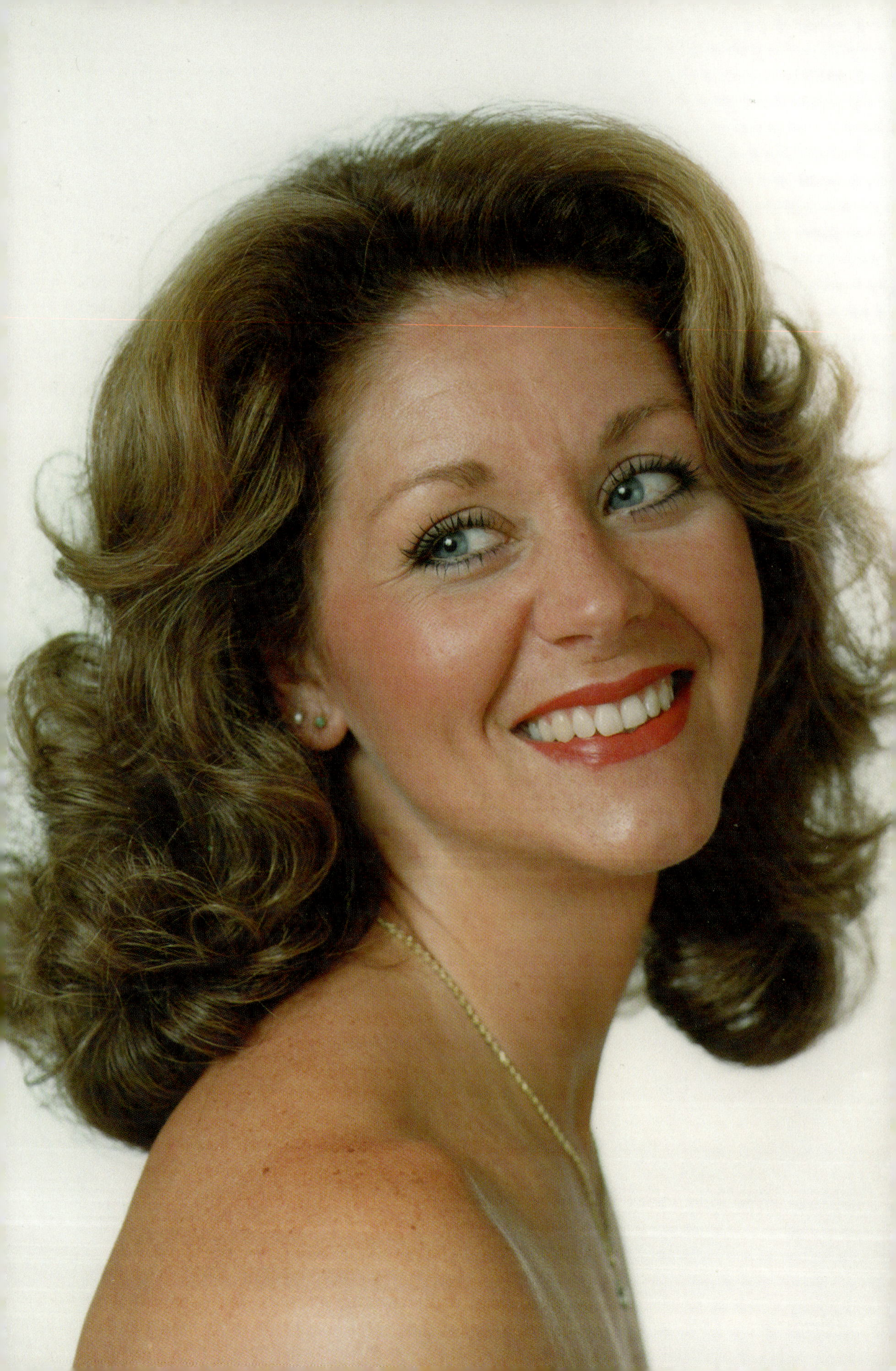

PATIENT PORTRAIT

DIANE ZAPACK
FOREHEAD LIFT
AGE: 39

Since I work with young people in the performing field, I feel it is important to look good. It is hard to see by the pictures, but I had deep frown lines and creases on my forehead. Now, they are gone. I tried collagen, but it didn't last. Surgery was the best way for me to go. A lot of people thought I was too young for plastic surgery, but you have to do what you think is right for you. I look and feel a lot younger — and that's important to me.

I'm an aerial artist. At the age of 16, I auditioned for Ringling Brothers & Barnum and Bailey Circus. After graduation from high school, I packed my bags and was off to the Big Top. I spent the next 12 years travelling across the United States and other countries. Six of those years were with Ringling Brothers, and the remaining time included performances in my own flying trapeze and trampoline act and two years as part-owner of a circus in South America.

I needed a break from all the hustle and bustle of showbiz, so I came back to the States and studied to be a firefighter and paramedic. I worked at that job for about seven years. During that time, I was offered an opportunity to teach aerial work in my spare time. I really enjoy teaching and plan to continue my love of aerial artistry by helping young people.

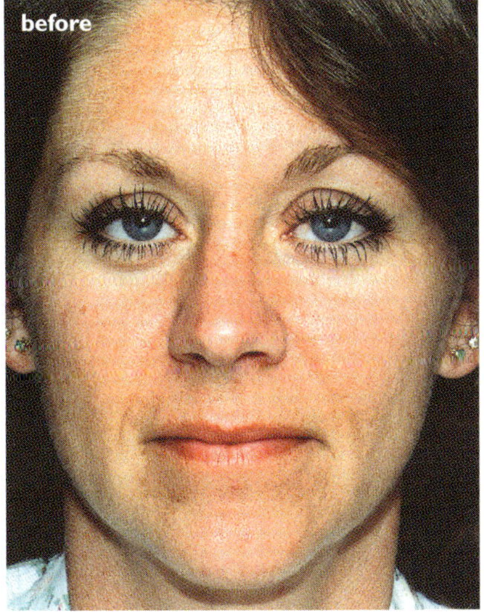
before

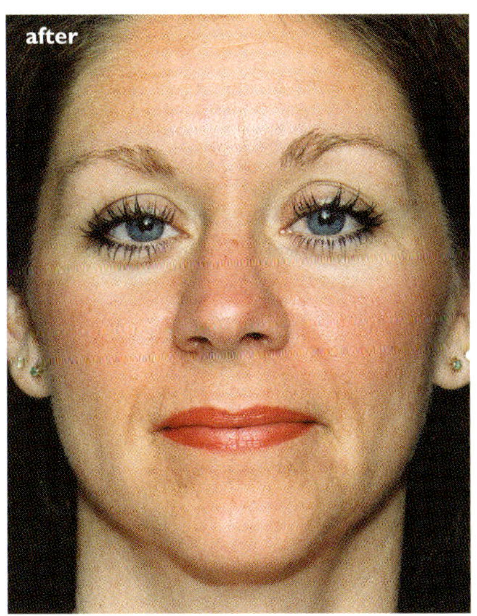
after

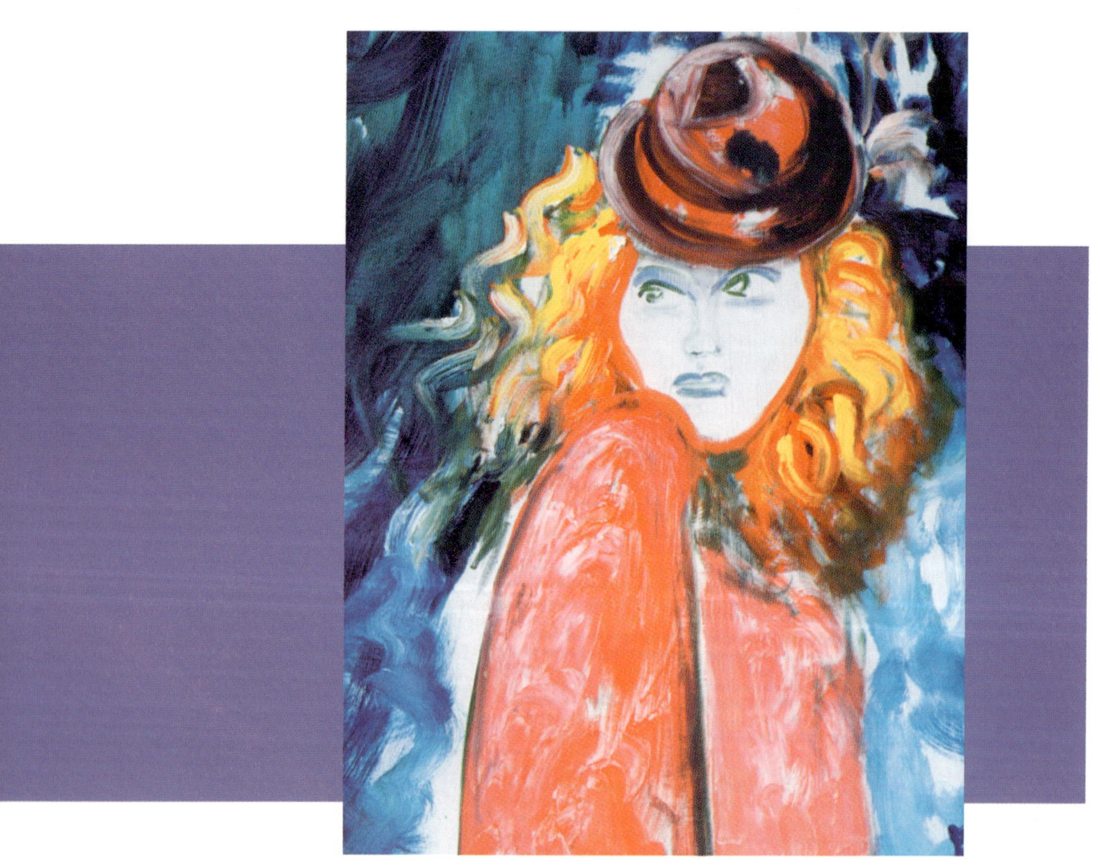

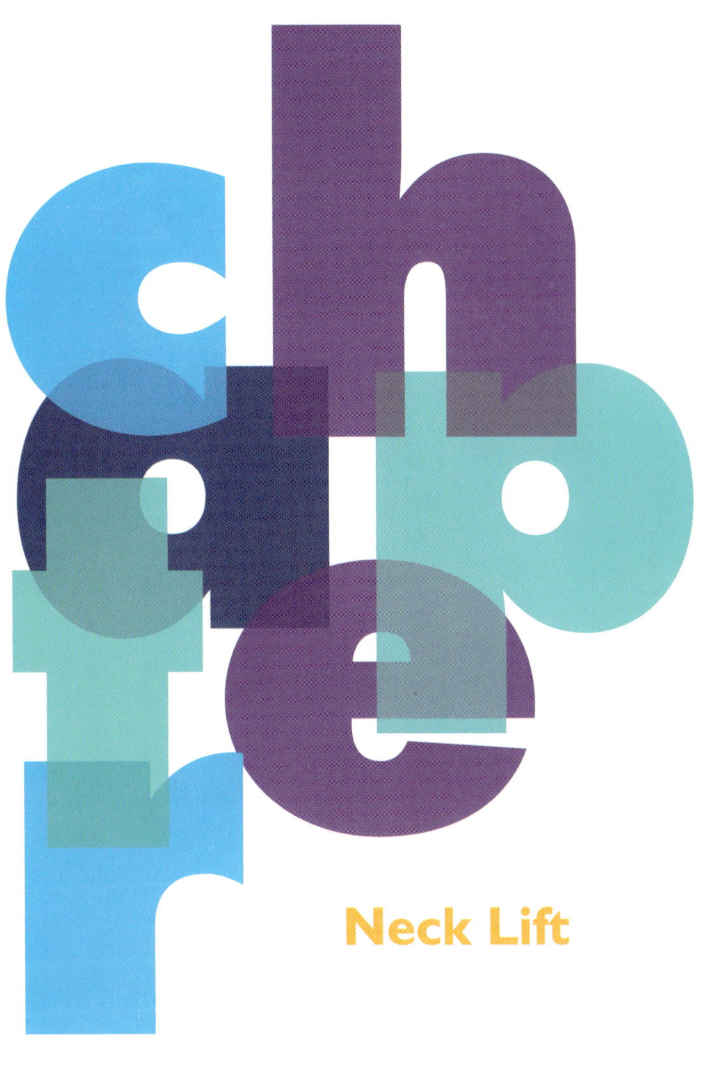

Neck Lift

Neck Lift

Today, a much greater emphasis is placed upon the neck in facial rejuvenation. No matter how beautiful and youthful the facial features are, if they are not poised on a youthful neck, much is lost. The combination of a young-looking face and a droopy neck, like aging hands, are tip-offs as to a person's true age. A neck lift may be included in a facelift or may be performed separately. A youthful neck has a well-defined jaw, depression under the chin, visible thyroid cartilage and muscle border, and a 90-degree neckline angle.

As we grow older gravity and aging cause the skin of the neck and lower face, particularly under the chin, to sag. Jowls result from loose muscles and fat deposits along the jaw line and the neck. Fat, which is naturally deposited under the chin in the upper part of the neck, loses its support and causes a short, wide neck. In many cases, "turkey gobbler" deformity develops. This condition is caused by weak muscles and bands which further weaken the shape and structure of the neck.

Neck Lift

Purpose: *To remove excess skin and fat under the neck by tightening muscles and redraping skin. Improves neck, jaw line, cord-like structures in the front of the neck, and corrects double chin.*

Surgery length: *2 – 3 hours.*

Anesthesia: *General and/or local with I.V. sedation*

Where: *Outpatient.*

Recovery: *Numbness, swelling, bruising.*

Risks: *Infection, loss of sensation, scarring.*

Cost: *$4,000 – $5,500.*

**(Note: Prices may vary based on physician fees, anesthesia, surgical setting and number of procedures. Data is based on a compilation of sources including Dr. Man.)*

Surgical Correction

In the neck lift, fat can be removed through various methods which tighten the muscles and redrape the skin. Submental lipectomy is a method which combines cervical defatting and muscle tightening. In this procedure, an incision is made just beneath the chin which allows for excess fat and skin to be removed, muscles to be tightened, and for excess skin to be trimmed.

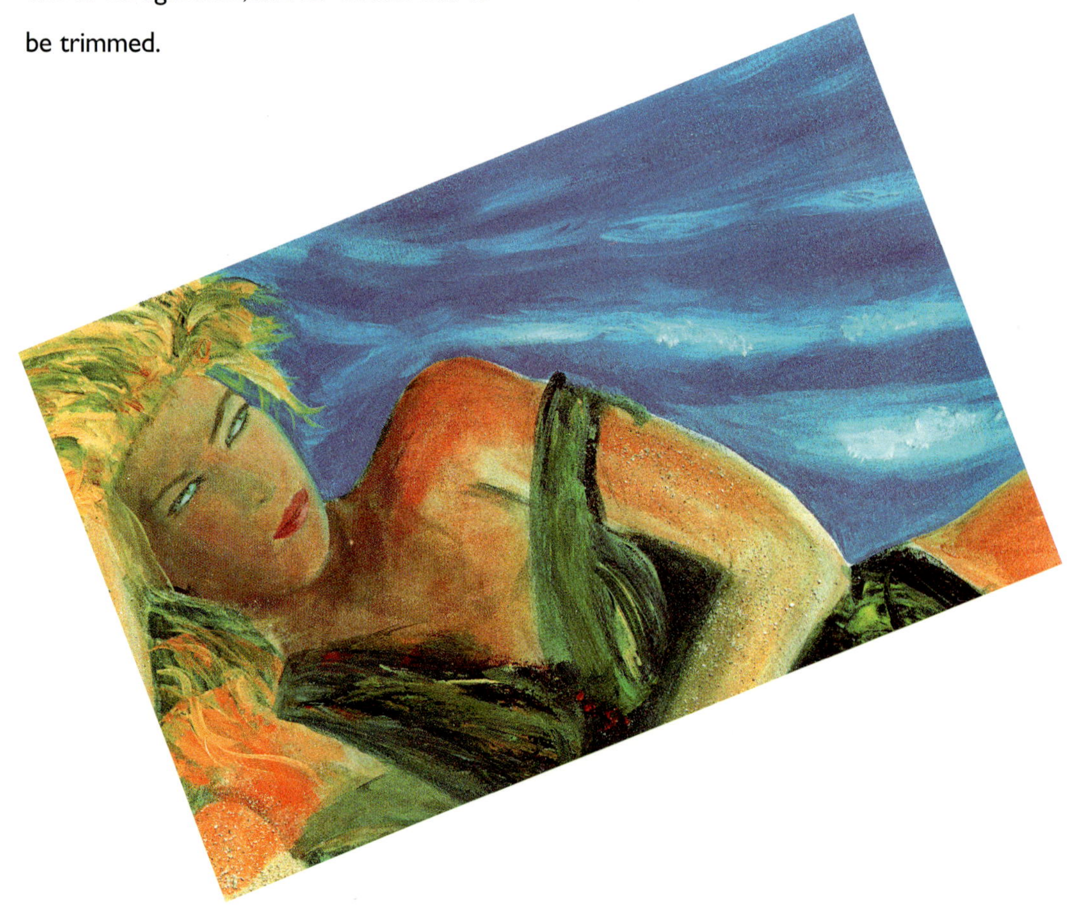

Endoscopic Technique

Endoscopic techniques may also be used to tighten muscles and remove excess fat. In this case, two or three small incisions are usually made in the neck and behind the ear. These incisions assist the surgeon by providing access to the muscles and fatty areas which are tightened and removed. Complications may include bruising, swelling, numbness, loss of sensation, infection, poor healing, bleeding and nerve damage. As in any surgery, patients should discuss all the risks beforehand. Though a neck lift is not a substitute for a facelift, it has its appeal to those patients who want to defer a larger procedure. Sometimes neck lifts can also be done with liposculpture and laser resurfacing.

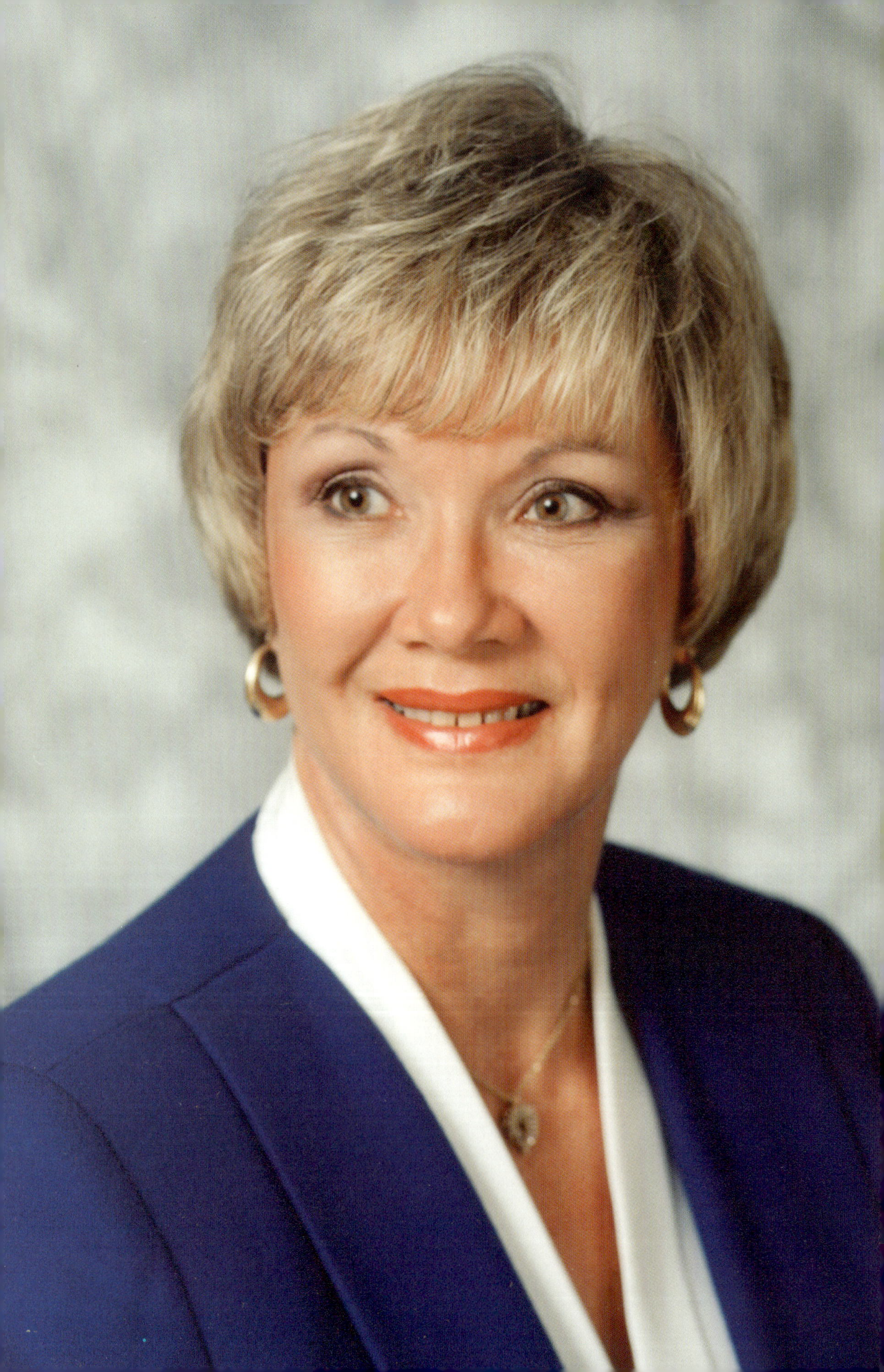

PATIENT PORTRAIT

JEAN RICHMAN
FACE, NECK, FOREHEAD LIFT; UPPER AND LOWER EYES; LIPOSCULPTURE
AGE: 44

I was curious so I went to the plastic surgeon. I was thinking I would get my eyes done. But, the doctor said I needed more. I was shocked when he said I needed a facelift. But, he was right. After the consultation I kept looking at my eyelids. Just doing my eyes was not going to help. I had jowls and lines around my lips. When he told me what he could do, I couldn't wait to have surgery. I wanted to have it the next day.

I never realized I had jowls or lines. I always thought you had a facelift in your fifties. Now I realize you can do something without waiting till the lines and sagging gets worse. After my surgery, even my doctor couldn't believe how really good I looked. I changed my hair style before one of my follow-up appointments. The office staff had not seen me in a couple of weeks and they didn't recognize me. The results were incredible even though I was still a little swollen two weeks after surgery.

That was what really amazed me — the recovery time. I was wearing makeup and going out two weeks later. I was looking at my wedding pictures. I think I look younger and better today than I did then. My husband is amazed. I look so natural. people think I look different but they don't really know why.

My eye lift was a big concern to me because of my contacts. Before my eyes were done, my contacts used to bother me. Now they don't. They are more comfortable. Before my surgery I said to my eye doctor, "Is this going to affect my contacts?" My eyes have always been dry. My doctor had a hard time fitting me to contacts. I thought that because of my eye surgery that my lids were going to be tighter. But, I was surprised. The surgery is so natural I can wear my contacts all day even better and more comfortably than before.

I am an executive with a top management company. How you look is important to your career. In the sales seminars they always say dress for success. If you have only one suit, make sure it's the best. I believe your face is your best suit. So you want it to look as good as you can. My husband and I work together. Now, I've got him thinking about his looks. I even have him hooked on facials.

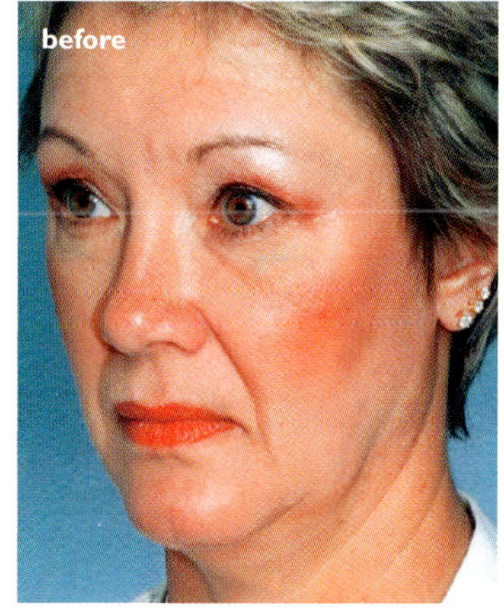

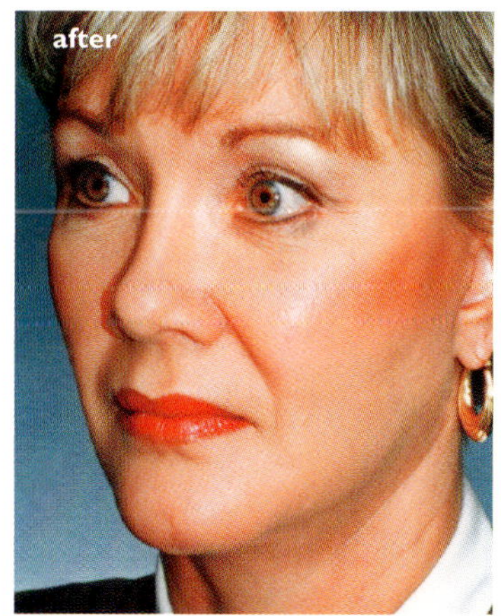

NECK LIFT

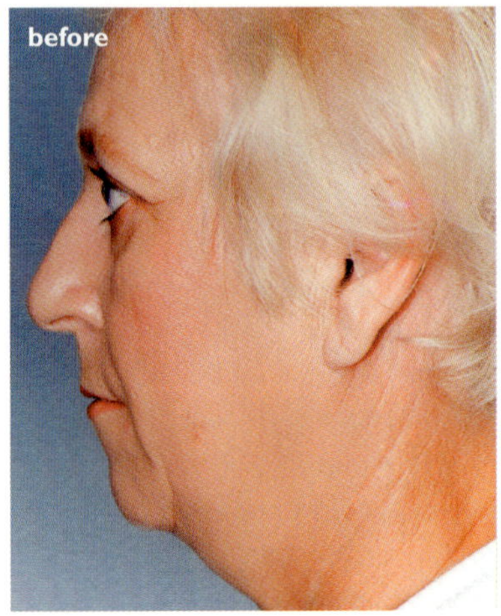

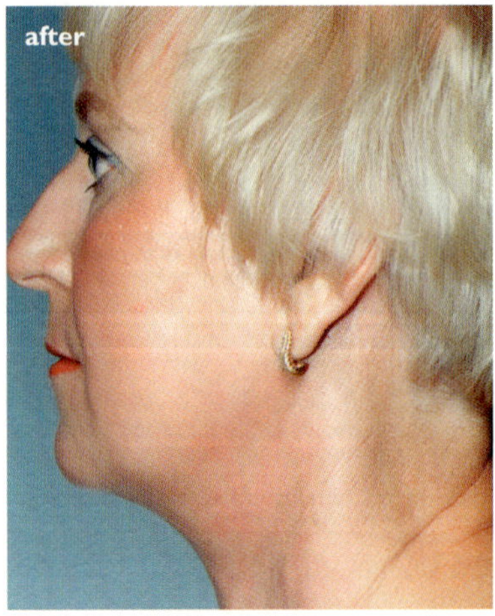

Neck Lift and Cosmetic Laser Surgery.

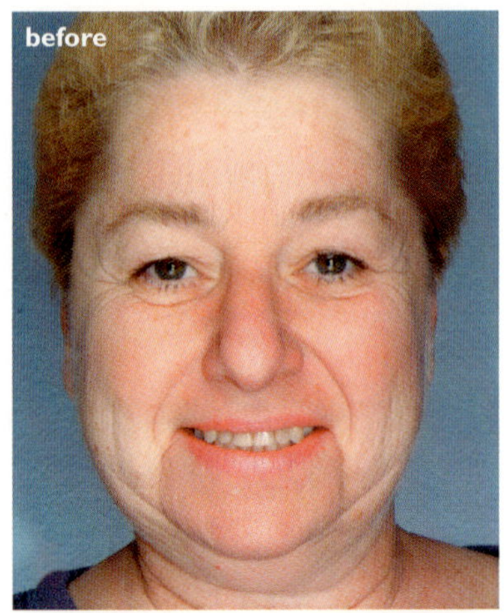

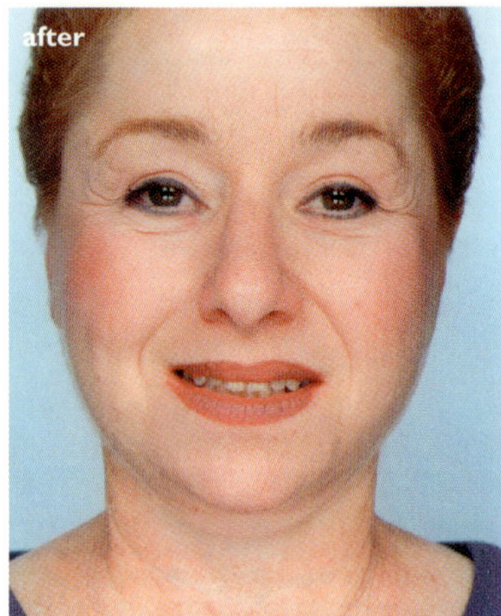

Patient before and after Face, Neck, Forehead & Eye Lift; and Laser around eyes.

PATIENT PORTRAIT

SUSIE KIRKLAND

FACE & NECK LIFT, UPPER & LOWER EYE LIFT, CHIN IMPLANT

I'll never tell my age again. I'm just a kid in a grownup's body. I work hard and I play hard, and I'm having a wonderful time. Before I had my surgery I didn't have any confidence, but that sure has changed! Saturday night I went to two different parties. I'm busy — going out, having fun, dating and working in real estate. I do lots of things I wouldn't have dared do before my surgery. I go out a lot now. I get all dressed up. I put beads in my hair, different things like that. Before my surgery I would never have done anything to call attention to my face. Now I want to call attention to my face. I'm single and looking, and I'm having a lot of fun while I'm waiting for Mr. Right to come along. I don't want an old man; I want a young one. I like to look and when I look, they look back because I am lookin' good! My mother is just amazed at the change in me and in my personality. I feel so good about myself now. My surgery has made the whole world my playground.

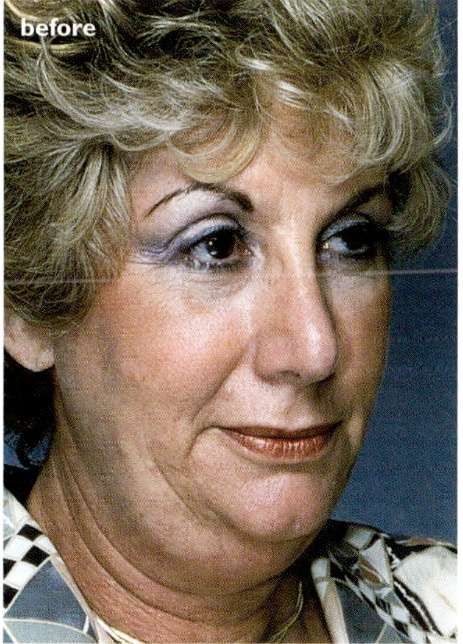

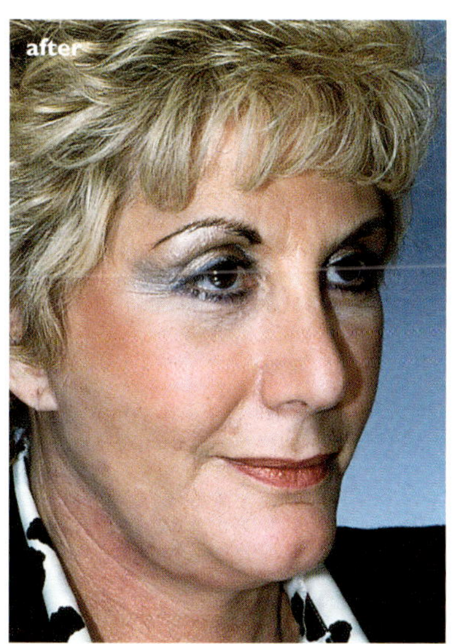

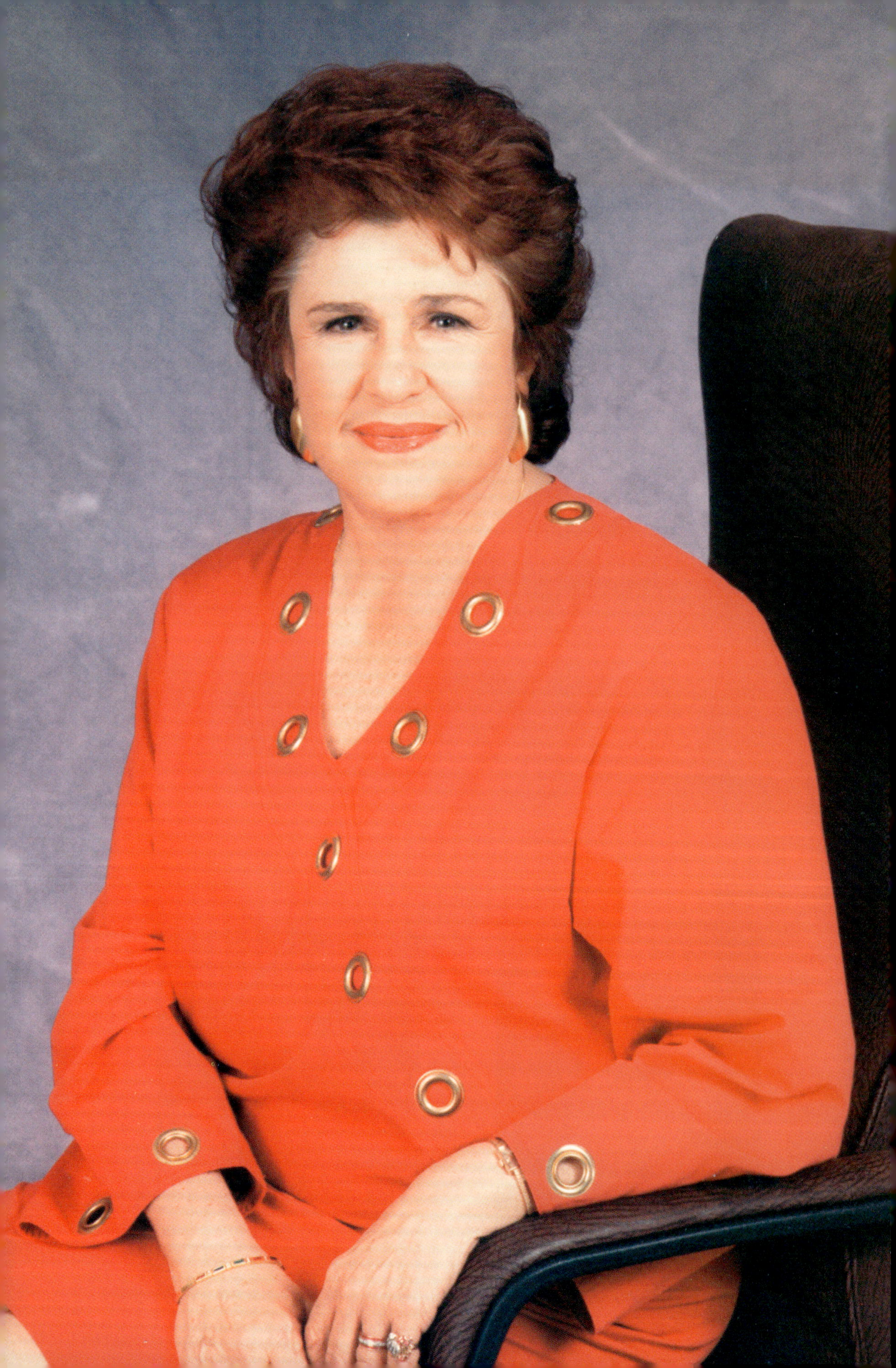

PATIENT PORTRAIT

SELMA CAPPON
FACE & NECK LIFT, FOREHEAD LIFT, UPPER EYE LIFT, SKIN REJUVENATION PEEL
AGE: 68

I think I am very lucky. I have a lot of natural gifts. I have good bone structure, good teeth – I think I was a workable object. My husband and I are healthy, energetic people. My husband loves the way I look and he loves showing off his"young" wife. When I see how my husband looks at me after 47 years of marriage, it assures me that my decision to have the facelift followed by the Skin Rejuvenation Peel was absolutely correct.

Friends have said,"I didn't know you were so vain." To this I have responded,"I'm not vain and I'm not arrogant. I just want to improve myself, to do what pleases me." This was something I wanted. I don't see anything negative in being the best I can be.

Some people don't care how they look. I want to appear the very best possible. I really disliked my neck and my double chin, which runs in my family.

I didn't do it for anyone else. I did it for me. I was very influenced by Joan Rivers, who was very willing to share her plastic surgery with her public. She really influenced me to make the decision to do something about my appearance. I'm thankful that there are doctors who can help people in this way.

When I had my peel I was happy to stay at the surgical center. It was like being in a cocoon. There were six of us there at the same time.We all had chemical peels. We were told to keep our faces still and not laugh. Well, I have to tell you, we had so much fun, we were laughing all the time. When you stay at a recovery center where the doctor has personally hired all the people there and has control of how things are done, the progress of your recovery is under constant observation and more likely quicker than if you immediately opted to stay in a large hospital or went home. I went into that cocoon like a caterpillar and came out feeling like a butterfly.

I'm in my senior years now and boy, it hurts to say that! I feel very fortunate at this time in my life to have the ability physically, emotionally, and financially to do something which I wanted and from my point of view needed. I have absolutely no regrets.

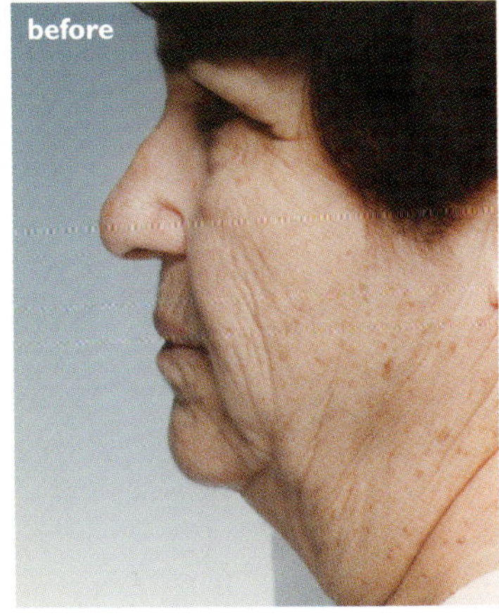
before

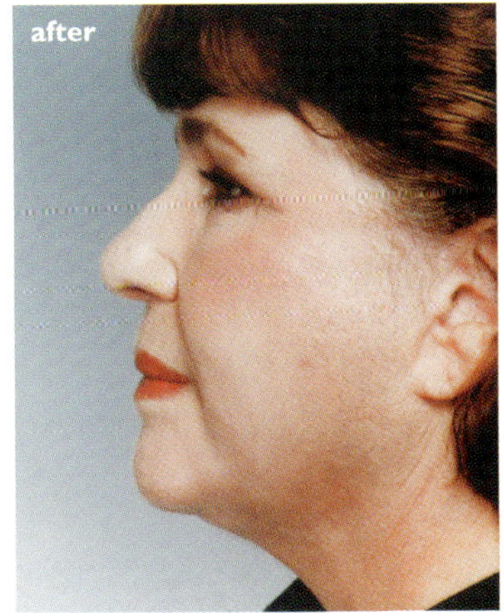
after

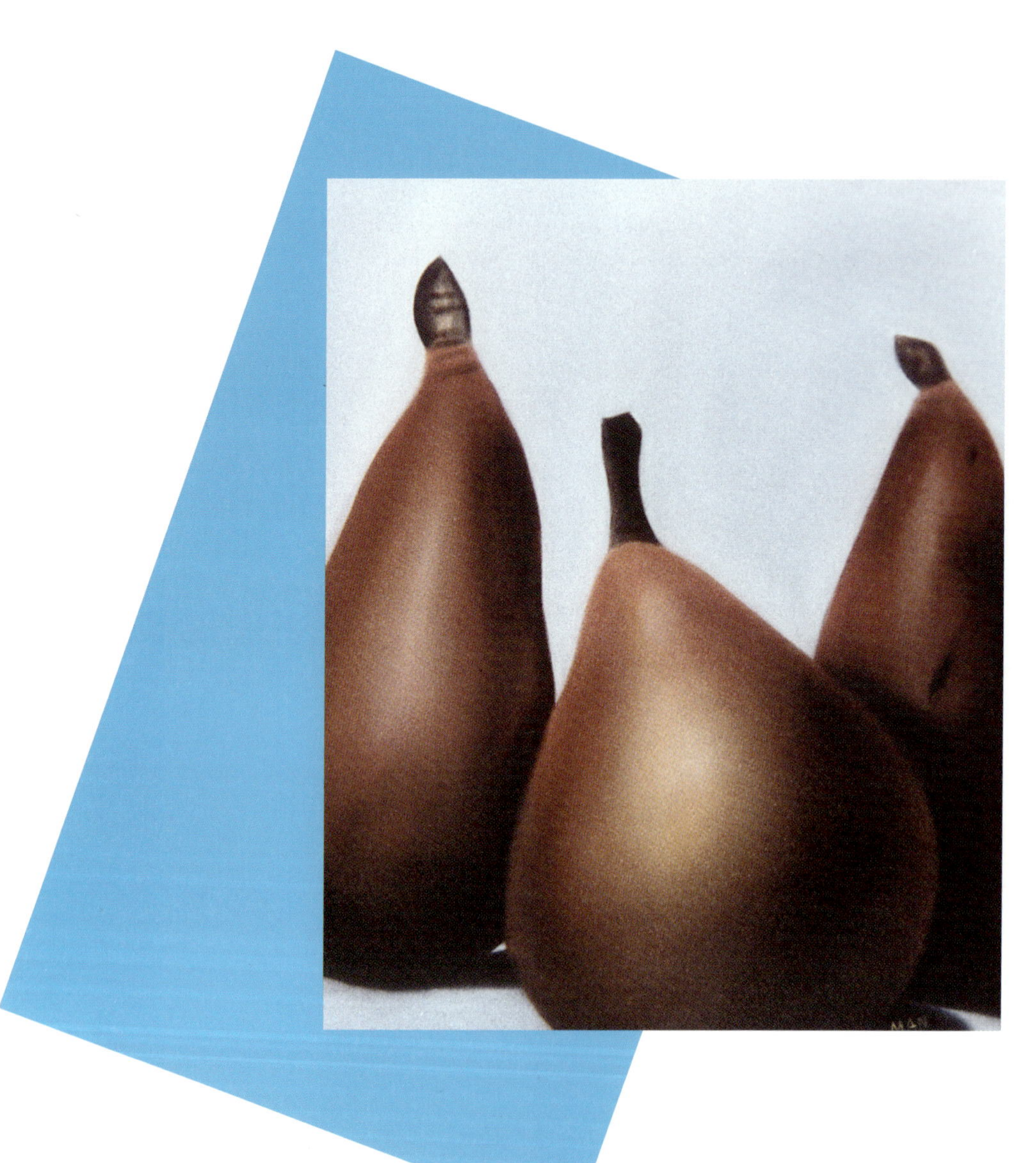

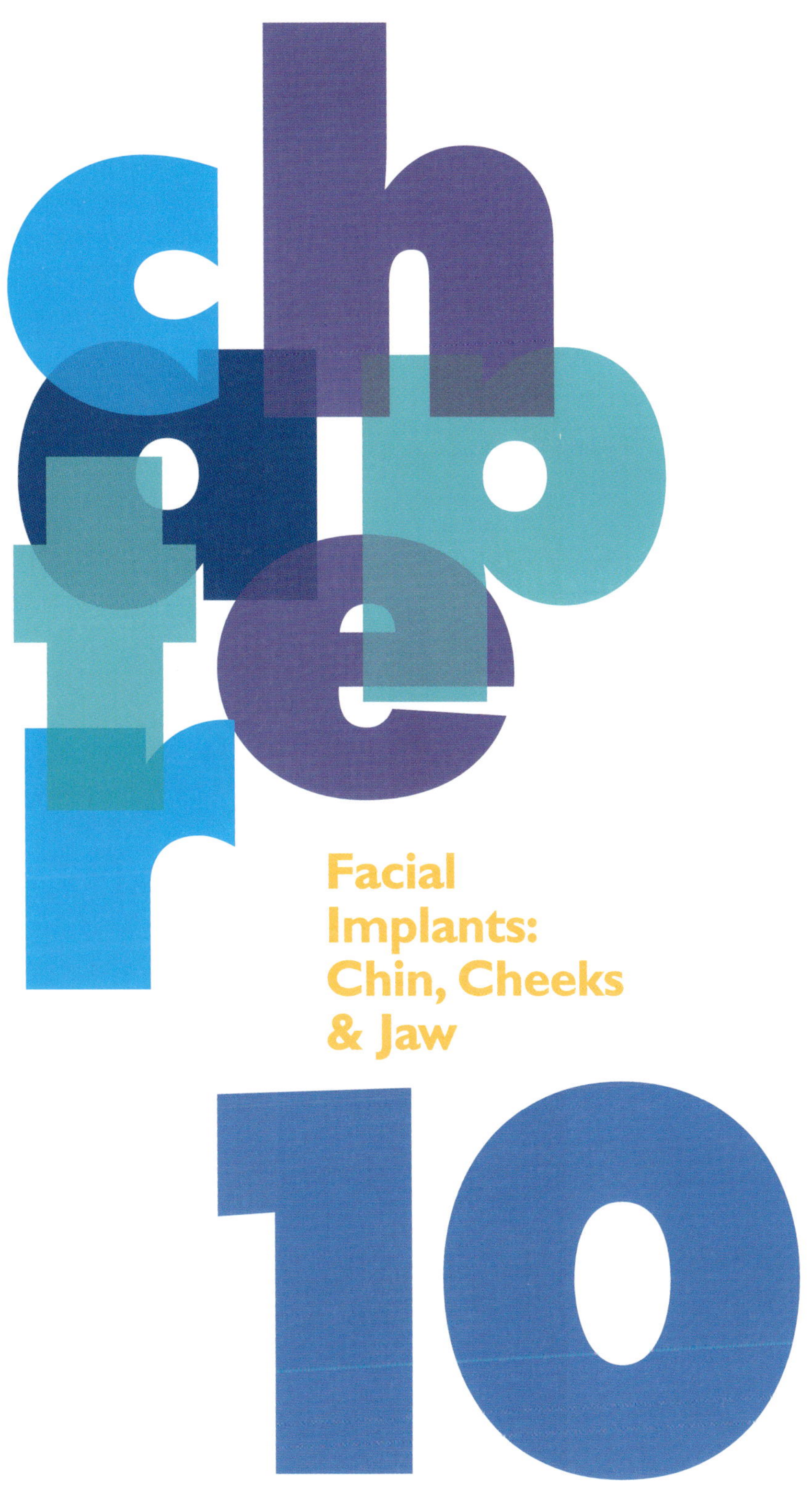

chapter 10

Facial Implants: Chin, Cheeks & Jaw

Facial Implants

Chin, Cheeks & Jaw

Beauty may be in the eye of the beholder, but there are certain facial features most people include in their definition. For example, when we describe the perfect model, our description will usually include high or prominent cheekbones. We often attribute health to rosy, round cheeks, as in a baby or young child.

The cheeks provide balance and help to fill out the middle portion of the face. In our youth, our cheeks are fuller. But as we age, the fat pads, which fill out the cheeks and give them their plumpness, change position, fall, flatten and disappear.

There are several ways to add definition and fill out the cheeks. The easiest way to build up the cheeks is at the time of the facelift. Your surgeon may recommend cheek implants, or liposculpture, fat injections using fat harvested from your own body.

Cheek Implants

Cheek implants are comprised of silicone and shaped to fit over the bony prominence of the cheeks. Implants are

Facial Implants

Purpose: *To change the shape, contour and balance of the face using special implants designed for specific areas including cheeks, chin and jawline.*

Surgery length: *30 minutes to 2 hours.*

Anesthesia: *General or local anesthesia with I. V. sedation.*

Where: *Outpatient surgery.*

Recovery: *Patients have termporary discomfort with swelling, bruising, stiffness, and numbness. In the case of jaw surgery, patients will be unable to fully open the mouth for several days.*

Risks: *Infection, hardening of scar tissue around the implant and shifting of the implant.*

Costs: *$2,000 – $8,000.*

(Note: Prices may vary based on physician fees, anesthesia, sessions required and surgical setting. Data is a based on a compilation of sources including Dr. Man.)

most often inserted through incisions inside the mouth. The surgeon makes a small incision inside the mouth and creates a pocket over the cheekbone where the implant will be placed. The entry site is then closed with dissolving sutures.

Post Operative

After surgery, the cheeks will feel stiff and numb for a few days. Chewing may be uncomfortable, but this will subside in a couple of weeks. Because of the risk of infection, antibiotics are prescribed after the surgery. Surgery lasts roughly one hour and is performed under local anesthesia with intravenous sedation, usually in the doctor's office. It may also be performed in an outpatient surgery setting or in the hospital. In some cases, it may be performed under general anesthesia.

Liposculpture

Liposculpture, or fat injections, are excellent ways to restore youth of the face. Using fat harvested from the patient's body, the surgeon injects various areas to give them a plump look. The procedure may need to be repeated in order to build up volume, and to compensate for the fat that is absorbed by the body. Liposculpture is very useful in correcting aging and loss of volume in areas of brows, tear trough, cheeks, nasalabial folds and lips, pre-jowl areas and underneath the jaw.

Chin Augmenation

The chin helps define the profile. Chin implants are often done in conjunction with a facelift or nose surgery. The chin implant makes the chin more prominent and gives balance to the face. A chin implant is inserted most commonly through a small incision underneath the chin or inside the mouth. As in cheek surgery, the procedure is usually done on an outpatient basis in the surgeon's office. It takes about one hour to complete the surgery.

After surgery the chin may feel numb or aching for one to two weeks. If the implant was inserted through the lower lip, the mouth will also feel stiff. Swelling may last for one to two weeks. Soft foods should be considered during this time. Stitches inside the mouth will dissolve or be removed by the surgeon after the first week. If you have stitches under the chin, they, too, are usually removed in about a week, or less. Complications include infection, and asymmetry caused by shifting of the implant.

In some severe cases, chin augmentation surgery may be required to alter the shape, as in cases when the chin recedes or is not evenly proportioned. The chin may be lengthened or shortened through several techniques that require the jawbone to be cut and reset.

Jaw Implants

A "Kirk Douglas" style jaw, with its wide, square shape, has been associated with a manly look, but it has also been associated with strength and strong character. The jaw gives our face its definition and provides balance for the face and neck. For women, too, a strong jaw has been associated with beauty as depicted in pictures of models with their wide, square jaws.

Jaw implants are one way to increase the angle and width of the jaw. These types of implants are not as common as chin implants and are mostly done on young people. As in chin and cheek implants, this procedure carries a rare risk of infection and misplacement.

The procedure is most often performed under local anesthesia with I.V. sedation in the doctor's office. Bruising, swelling and numbness will last for several weeks and the jaw will feel stiff, which can make opening and closing of the mouth temporarily uncomfortable. Soft foods and a liquid diet are recommended at this time. Patients usually go back to work after a week, though some are not comfortable going out until the swelling and bruising have subsided. Detailed instructions regarding brushing the teeth and resuming normal activites should be discussed by your doctor.

PATIENT PORTRAIT

RANDI RHODES
NOSE, FOREHEAD, EYELIDS, CHIN IMPLANT & LIPOSUCTION, NECK LIFT AND EAR PINNING
AGE: 37

I'm a comedian. My name is Randi Rhodes and I'm South Florida's "Goddess Of The Radio." My job is to talk to people every day and crack jokes. But the story I'm about to share isn't funny. I have hidden behind my hair for a total of 37 years so people could not see my face! I can still hear my mother yelling at me, "Randi, get your hair out of your face!" — even 20 years after I moved out of my parents' home! Hiding was second nature to me. Okay, it was first nature. In fact, I chose a career in radio and became a radio personality because it is a non-visual medium and I could crack my jokes while hiding behind the microphone. Self-deprecation became a big part of my act.

In my job I talk to people all day long. They knew my voice but they rarely saw my face except in glossy billboards and when I was required to make personal appearances. Yuk! I hated personal appearances. Personal appearances were very painful for me because invariably someone would say to me, "Oh, you're Randi Rhodes", like they couldn't believe it was me. One day a lady commented, "Well, hon, you don't look that bad, you shouldn't put yourself down so much." The pain of hearing those kinds of comments over and over again was devastating. Men were often the cruelest even though they didn't mean to be. They would say something like, "Hey, I like me a big gum-chewing girl with big hair and a set on her … too bad about that 'radio face', eh honey?" I became very bitter.

I also had another problem. I secretly wanted a career in television and the movies. Yeah, me the one who always hid. So I decided to have plastic surgery.

I went to see Dr. Man. He gave me a hand mirror and asked me to look at myself. Then he asked me to describe what I wanted to change and why. He drew my nose and explained the changes he would make. Then he looked at my chin and neck and asked me to follow along in the mirror. He explained how the face is divided into three parts which should be in proportion and harmony. He spent a long time explaining things to me and then he brought in this book which he held in his hands like a proud father or artist sharing his portfolio. He showed me the before and after photos explaining the various procedures he had done. They all looked amazing and with his help I finally began to see the person that I felt was inside me waiting to be brought out. I became very excited and wanted to see this new person staring back at me in the mirror.

Sometimes I wonder where I found the courage. Before my surgery I would ask myself, "Why are you doing this?" I knew three days after my surgery I would look in the mirror and scream, "Why did you do this to yourself." But I also knew three weeks after I would be asking "Why did you wait so long in the first place?"

I will never regret the decision to have plastic surgery and am comforted by the thought that I will never have to hide behind my hair or my microphone. I look forward to public appearances and who knows … maybe one day the movies?

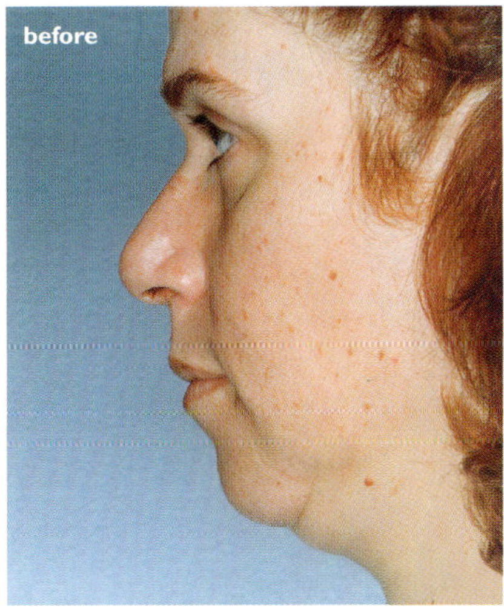

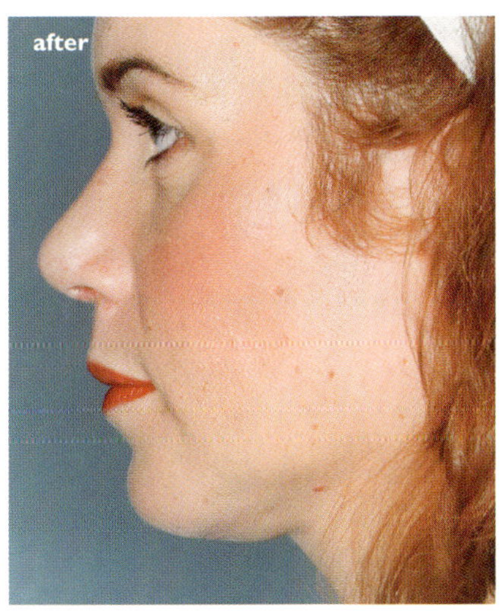

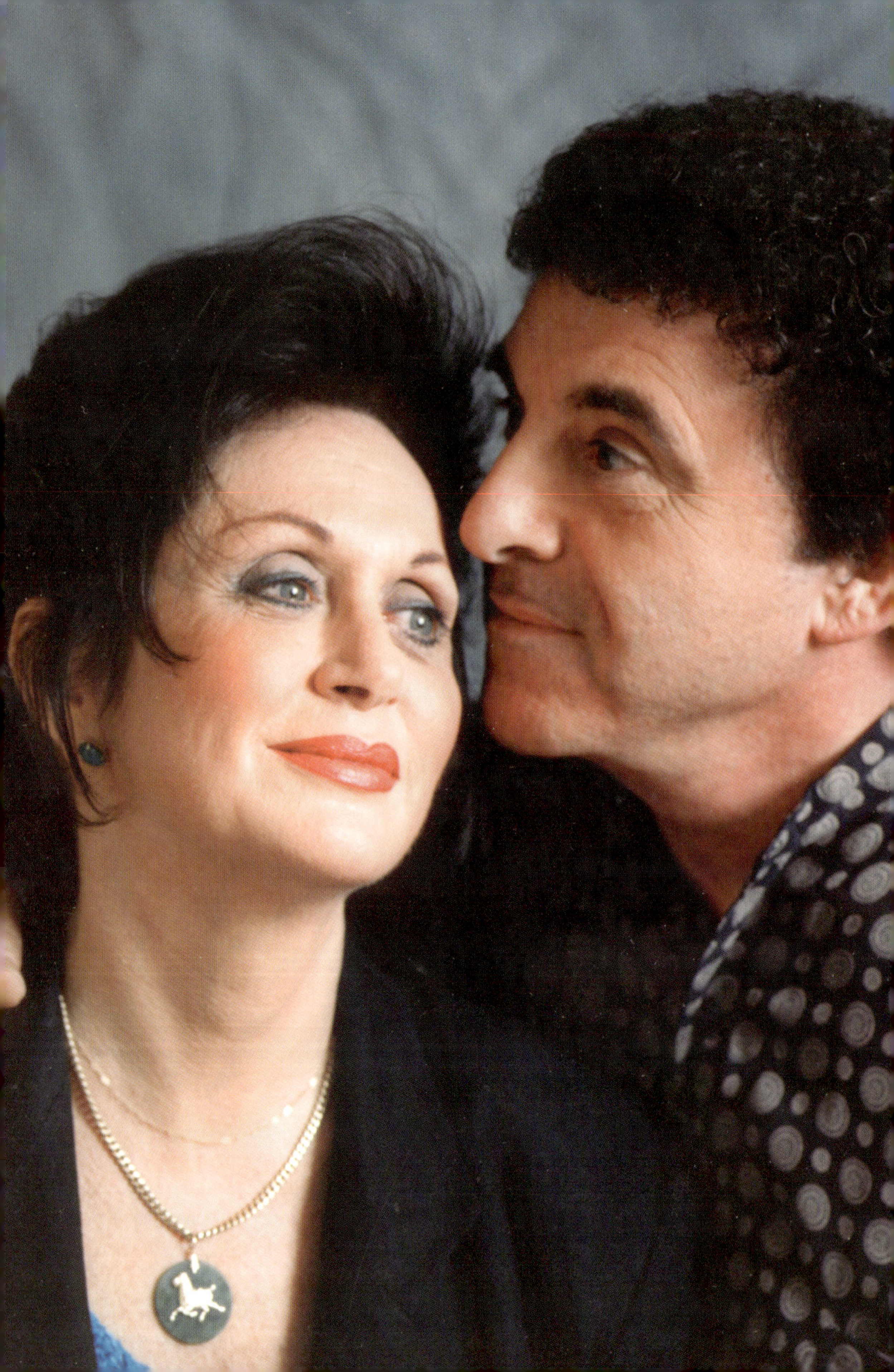

PATIENT PORTRAIT

ELIZABETH MERCURIO, SKIN REJUVENATION PEEL, CHEEK AUGMENTATION, ROBERT MERCURIO, FACELIFT & NECKLIFT

"I feel as if I got the benefits of a facelift without actually having one," said Elizabeth Mercurio, even though it was her husband Robert who actually had facelift surgery. "Not only did I lose the lines on my face, my skin feels and looks tighter. When you look at my photos you can see that my nose is higher. The distance between my nose and my upper lip is shorter. It's absolutely astonishing. It's like magic. I'd like to have my whole body peeled. If the doctor would just fill a tub with those chemicals, I'd jump right in."

Robert said, "The bottom of my face was swinging back and forth when I walked. Those folds were just slappin' from side to side, I could feel them. Everyone told me how tired I looked. I absolutely hated it. Every time someone would say to me, 'Say, Robert, you feeling OK? You sure look tired,' I wanted to punch them. Now I don't hear that anymore. If I had known how easy it was I would have done it years ago. There was absolutely no pain."

Robert continued: "I had a whole facelift and I wasn't black and blue at all. The doctor gave me some kind of lotion that I put on my face for a week before my surgery to minimize the swelling and the discoloration. Not only that, I didn't have any pain, not even a headache. I've only got small scars and my sideburns are just slightly closer to the front of my ears, I like that." Elizabeth smiled, "Right after the surgery, you look so good that I forgot just how bad you looked before. Then – I look at the 'before' photos and I can't believe you waited so long. I'm a very tidy person," continued Elizabeth. "I like everything neat. I wouldn't wear unpressed clothes, so why should I wear a wrinkled face? I wanted to have cheek implants to bring my cheekbones up but the doctor convinced me to have fat injections instead. The doctor said it was better to use the body's own material."

"The fat injections last a long time and there is no foreign body reaction with the fat. What convinced me though, is that he said the fat injections would give me a more natural look then the cheek implants. Now I know he was right. And just take a look at Robert, now he looks like he looked twenty years ago," she said.

"That's right. I see pictures in our old albums and I think, 'Yeah, that's how I should look.' Friends don't know about my facelift. They can't quite put their finger on what is different. They say, 'You've lost some weight, Robert.' I just agree with them. I say, 'Right I lost a few pounds," he said. "You did," laughed Elizabeth. "You lost at least two pounds from your neck."

"Or they ask, 'Been on vacation, Robert?' And I say, 'That's right. I did, had a great time.' "I hated how I was looking. I would look in the mirror and all that I could look at was this 'stuff' hanging there. No matter how much weight I lost I always looked fat and jowly." Robert shook his head, "I see so many men looking like old hound dogs, with all this flesh flapping over their shirt collars. Men shouldn't be shy about getting something done. It's as important in business for men as it is for women to look good. People should look as young as they feel. It builds confidence, it certainly built mine. You need that edge against younger competitors."

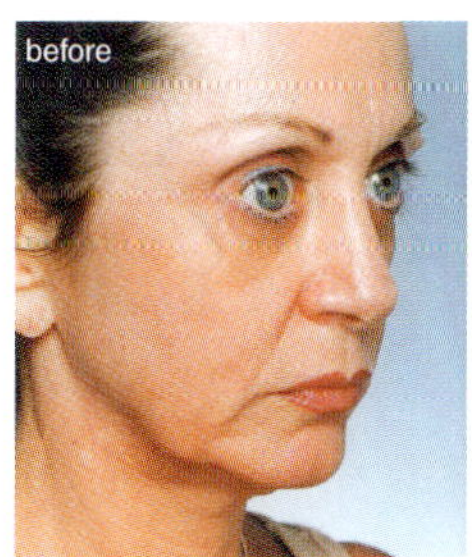
before

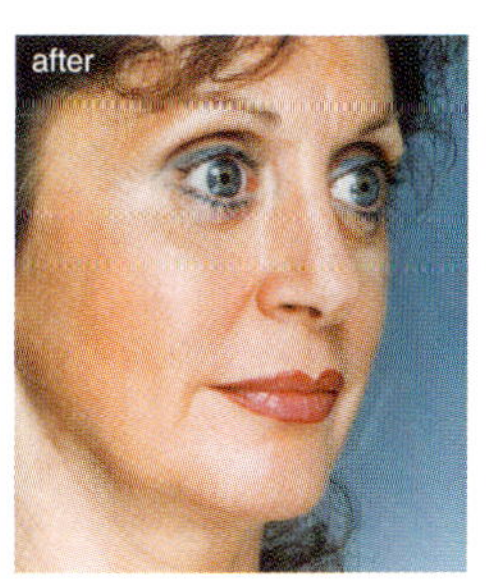
after

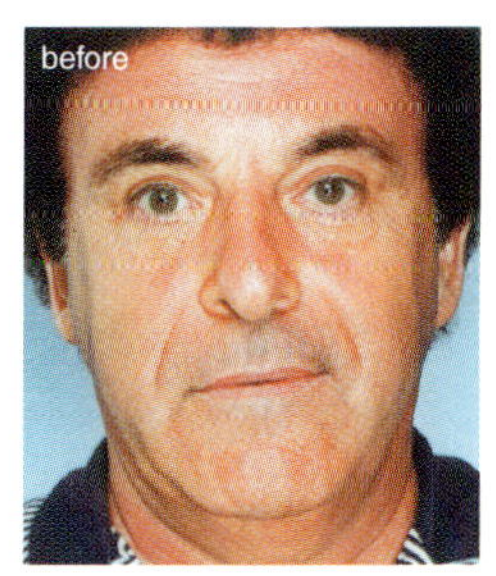
before

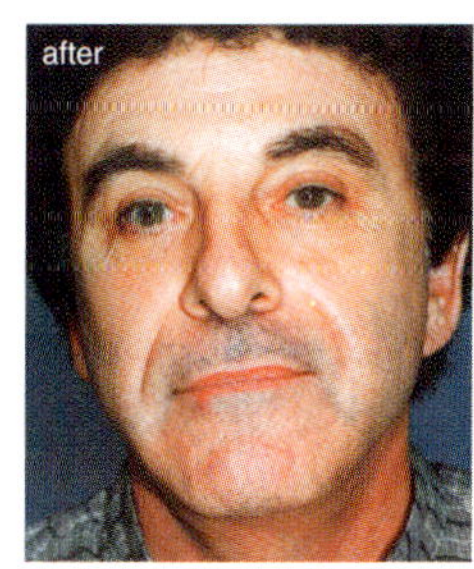
after

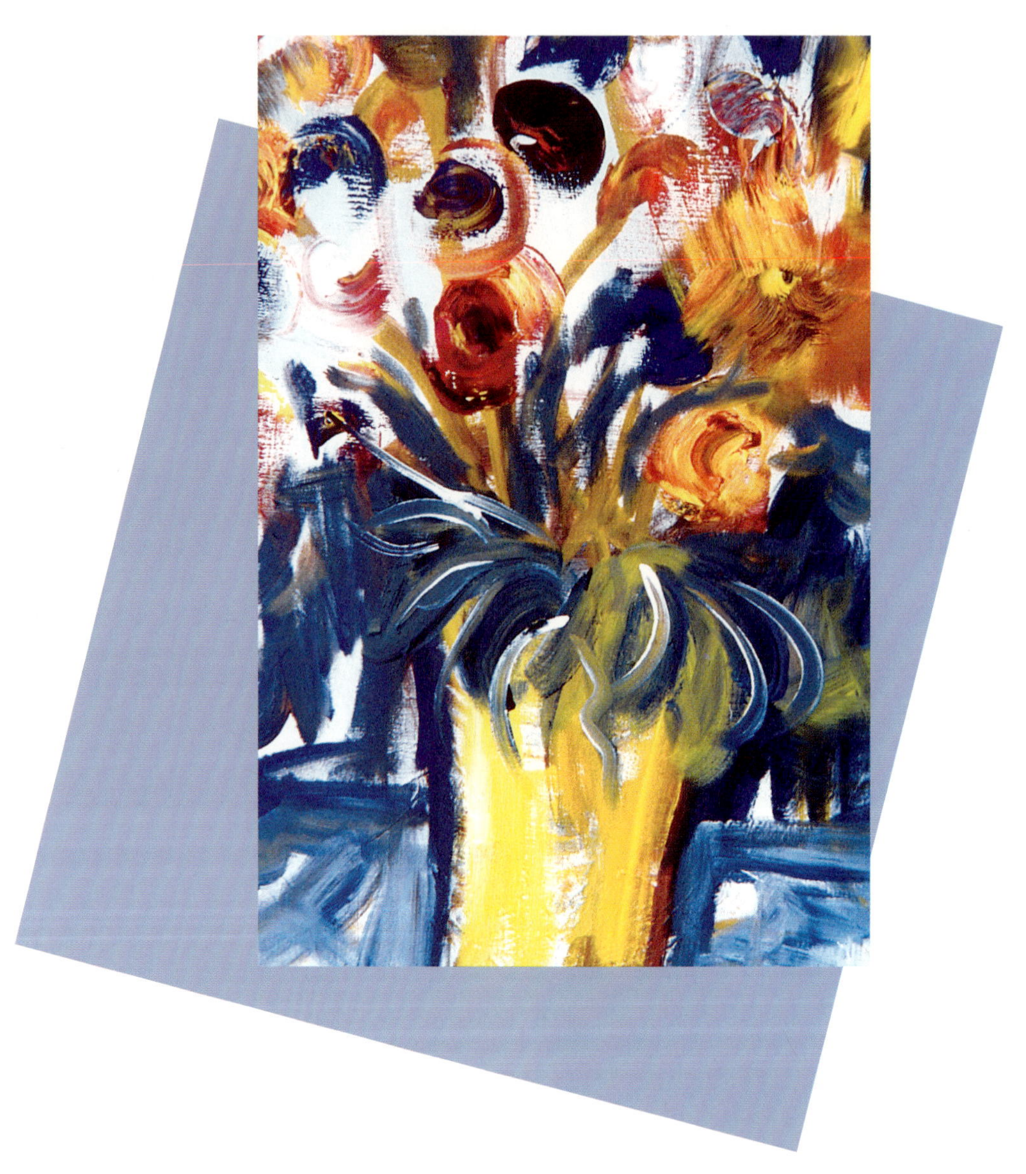

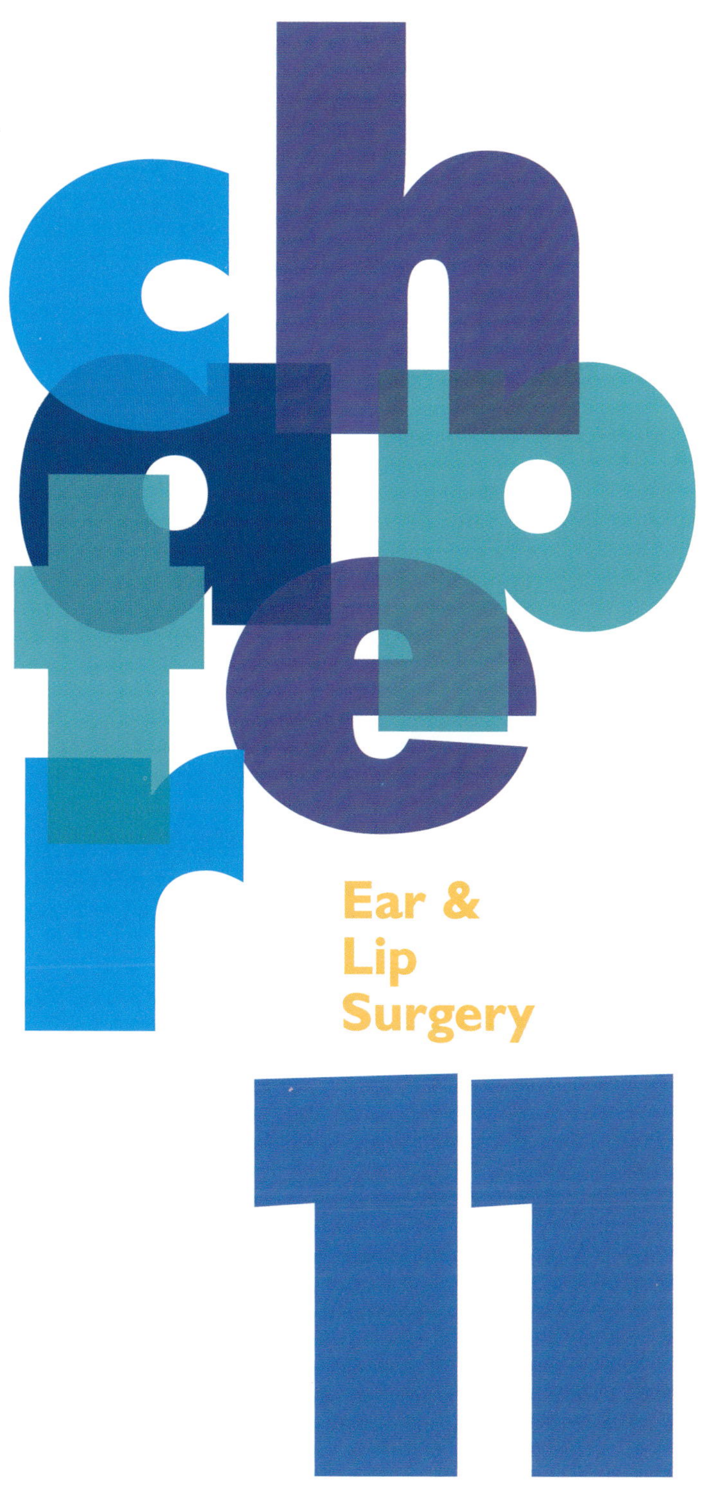

Chapter 11

Ear & Lip Surgery

Ear & Lip Surgery

Otoplasty is a procedure performed to correct disproportionately large, protruding ears. Unfortunately, children and adults can be adversely affected by big ears. In Western cultures, very large ears may even be considered a deformity. In the Orient and the Far East, large, protruding ears can be considered an omen of good luck.

In the case of a child, otoplasty may be undertaken in the very early years, usually after age four, so that the child may avoid emotional stress often encountered in school. The ear is comprised of skin and cartilage. At about the age of five, most of the ear growth has neared completion, and the child and the parents may consider surgery.

Otoplasty is usually done under general anesthesia or I.V. sedation in a hospital outpatient surgery facility or in the physician's office-based surgery center. The procedure can take several hours and usually requires the surgeon to remove skin and cartilage from the back of the ear. Sutures are placed behind the ear and over the repaired cartilage. Scars are usually well concealed.

At the end of the procedure, a bulky dressing is applied for several days. Patients are usually up and about in a day or two following surgery. Patients are usually back to school in a week, while

Ear Surgery

Otoplasty

Purpose: *To reduce the size of large prominent ears and set them closer to the head.*

Surgery length: *2–3 hours.*

Anesthesia: *General and/or local anesthesia with I.V. sedation.*

Where: *Outpatient surgery, or overnight stay.*

Recovery: *Swelling, bruising, and numbness. Back to school, work in 5–10 days. Full activities, 1–2 months.*

Risks: *Bleeding infection, scarring and uneven or mismatched ears.*

Cost: *$3,000 – $4,500*

**(Note: Prices may vary based on physician fees, anesthesia, surgical setting and number of procedures. Data is based on a compilation of sources including Dr. Man.)*

adults can return to work sooner. A special dressing is worn for several days after surgery. Stitches are usually removed after five to seven days. During this time, the ears will appear swollen and red. Numbness is also common and may persist for several weeks. Complications may include bleeding and infection. Fortunately, these are rare.

Lip Surgery

When we are young, our lips are full and have a youthful pout. As we grow older, the upper lip begins to lose its fullness. The distance from the tip of the nose to the upper lip becomes greater and begins to lengthen as the lip drops downward. The vermilion border, often called the "cupid's bow," flattens and becomes thin. When viewed from the profile or side, the lips begin to shift in a vertical, downward line.

A lip lift may be recommended by itself or at the time of the facelift, since aging lips will appear incongruent when other facial features have been made more youthful.

Lip Surgery & Plumping

Purpose: *To increase the volume and contour of the lips.*

Surgery: *Lip lift and plumping with fat, collagen injections, alloderm graft.*

Anesthesia: *Local or I.V. sedation.*

Recovery: *Swelling, bruising.*

Risks: *Allergic reaction, infection.*

Cost: $2000 – $4,500

**(Note: Prices may vary based on physician fees, anesthesia, surgical setting and number of procedures. Data is based on a compilation of sources including Dr. Man.)*

Lip Lift

Shortening of the upper lip is accomplished by removing an area of skin between the nose and upper lip. The incision is made along the base of the nose and scars are usually minimal and hidden. Sutures are removed after several days. As in all surgery, complications such as swelling, bruising, infection and scarring can occur but are very rare. Risks should be discussed in more detail with your surgeon before you decide on surgery.

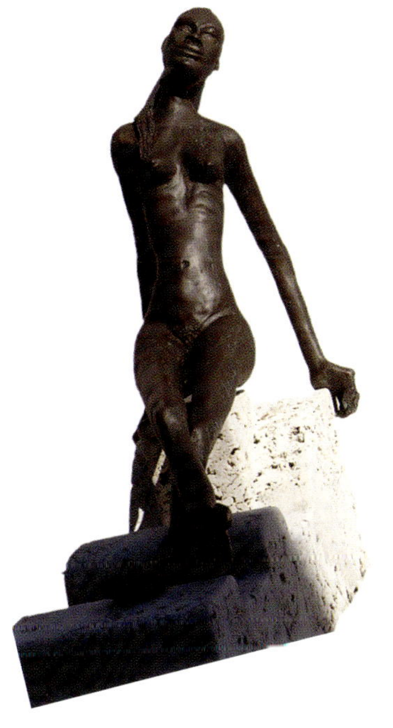

Collagen/Fat Injections

Another popular means of increasing the fullness and natural pout of the lips is using collagen, fat injections or Alloderm grafts. Collagen and fat injections are discussed in more detail in Chapter 12.

LIPS

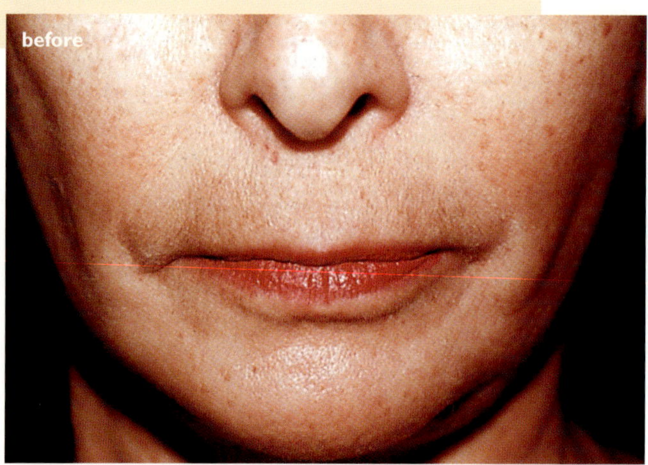

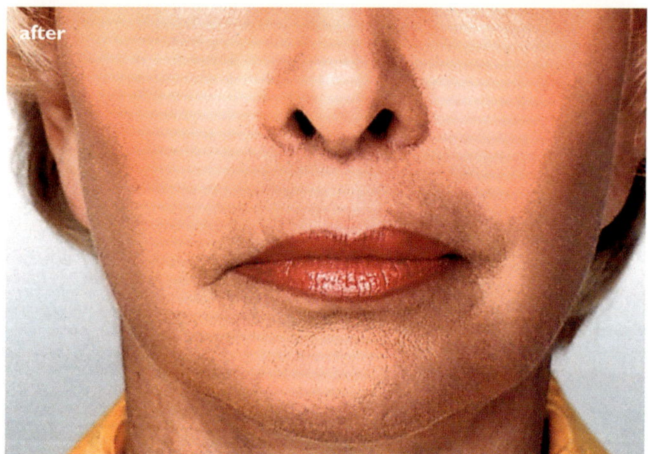

Lip Lift; Liposculpture, Full Face Laser

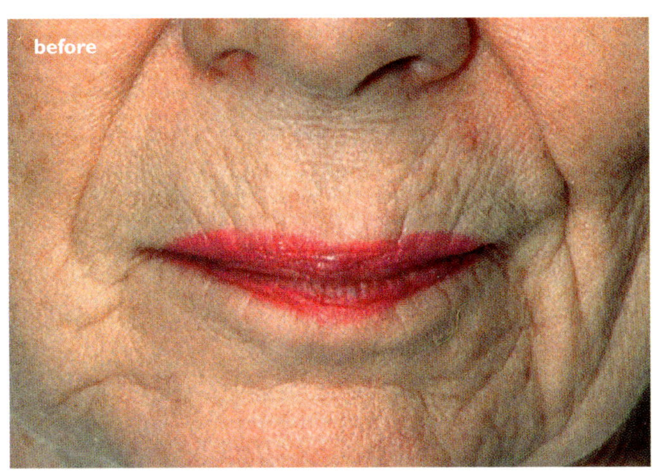

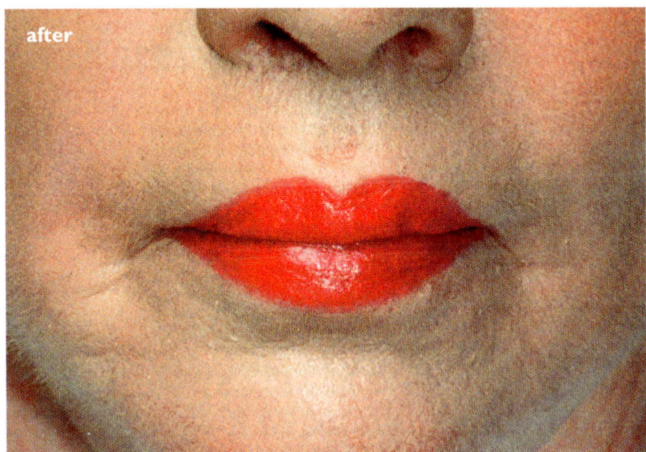

Liposculpture to Lips and Face; Face, Neck and Forehead Lift; Upper and Lower Eyes; Full Face Laser

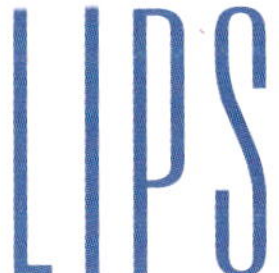

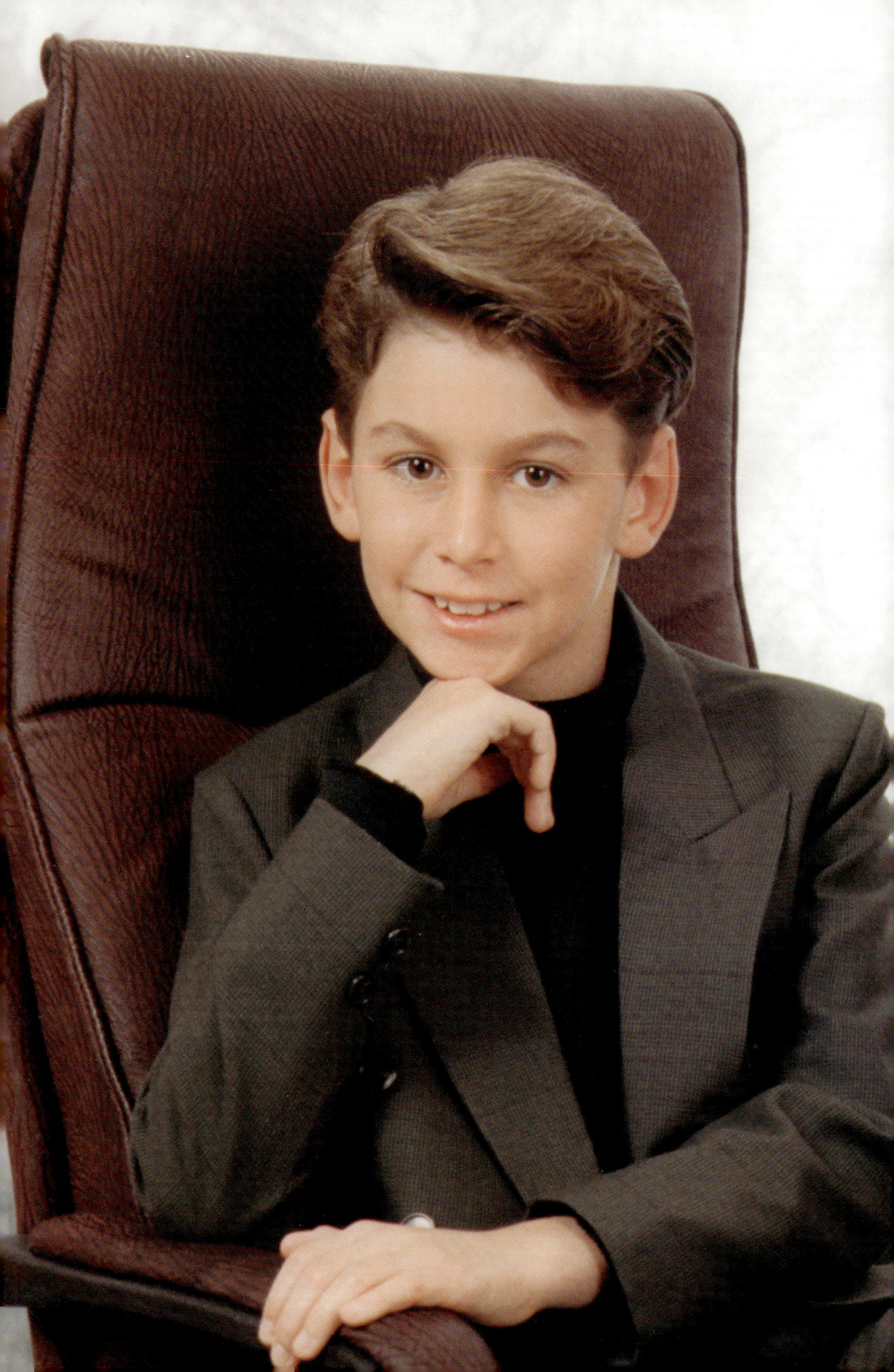

PATIENT PORTRAIT

ANDREW DURGEE
EAR SURGERY
AGE: 11

"Dumbo! Dumbo!" That's what the school kids called him.

"Everybody made fun of me," said Andrew Durgee. According to his mother, Andrew's ears were his most prominent feature. "The teasing got so bad he was having trouble getting along at his preschool," said Mrs. Durgee. "He became very aggressive and started getting poor grades. We realized this might scar him emotionally, so we took him to a psychologist. There, he drew a picture of himself with these huge ears. It became very evident he had a poor self-image. So we decided it was important to go ahead and do something while he was young, so he wouldn't have to suffer. The doctor agreed and said he should have surgery before he started regular school. So that was how we spent his summer before entering elementary school."

Andrew said, "I wasn't really scared until I got to the operating room, where they put a big mask in front of my face. That was the last thing I remembered until I woke up and saw a big dinosaur my Aunt Kim had left for me. I don't remember any pain. The only bad thing was the itching. I had my head all wrapped up to keep my ears flat so they could heal. I was bored from having to stay inside two weeks. My mother decided one day that I could bring a friend along and we would all go to the movies.

"That was when I started itching. Right in the movie theater. I didn't know I was doing it, but I had pulled on the bandages and my ears started bleeding. My mom called the doctor right away, and we had to go and have the bandages taken off a little early. After the bandages came off, my ears were real flat. The doctor asked me, 'So, what do you think?' I said I didn't like the color, but I liked that they didn't stick out anymore."

"Andrew's ears were still black and blue, but they healed beautifully from that point on," said a proud Mrs. Durgee. "Today, Andrew is a different young man. He has taken up modeling like his sister, Alexis, and he even acted in a movie called Heli-Kids. It's an educational video for children about helicopters."

"Making a movie was a lot of fun. But, I think I would like to be a veterinarian when I grow up," said Andrew, smiling. "Then I could help take care of sick animals. I have a cat named Maggie and two hermit crabs. Maybe I'll get other animals too."

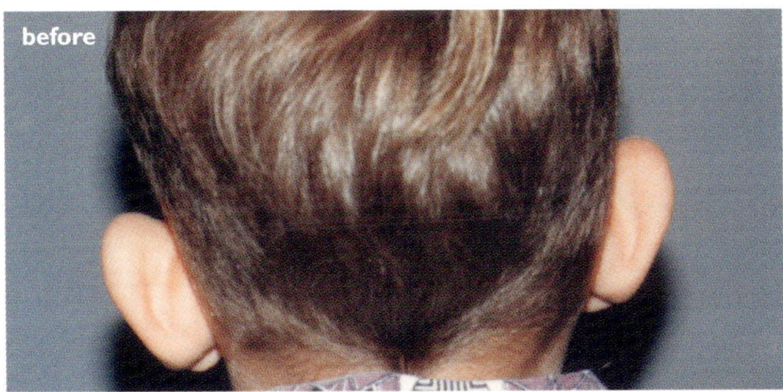
before

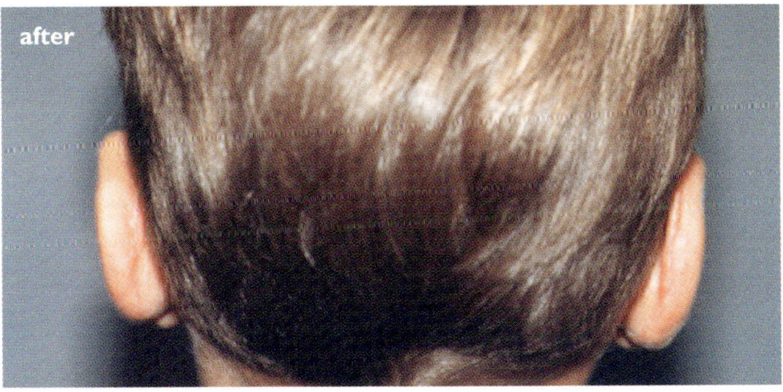
after

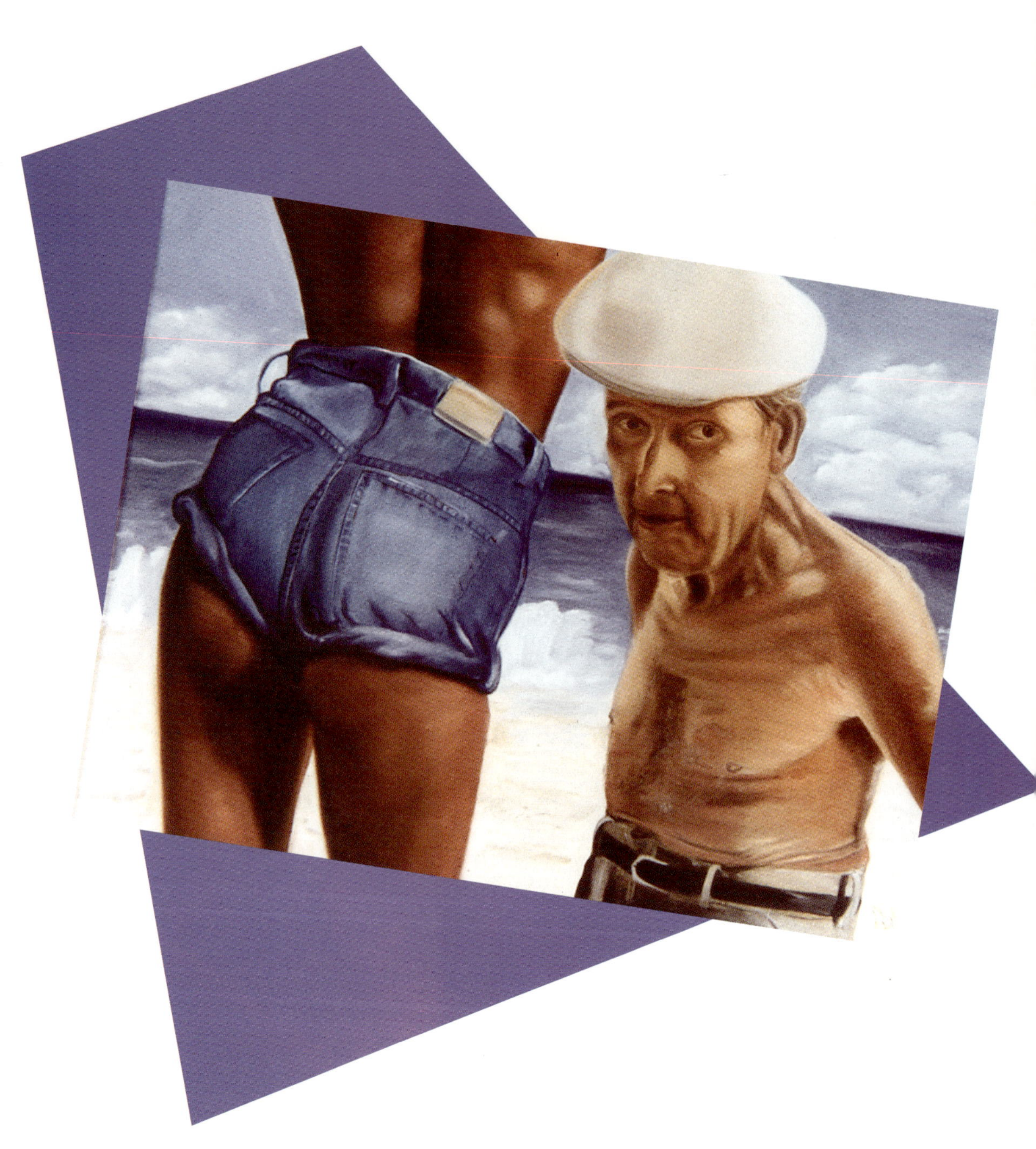

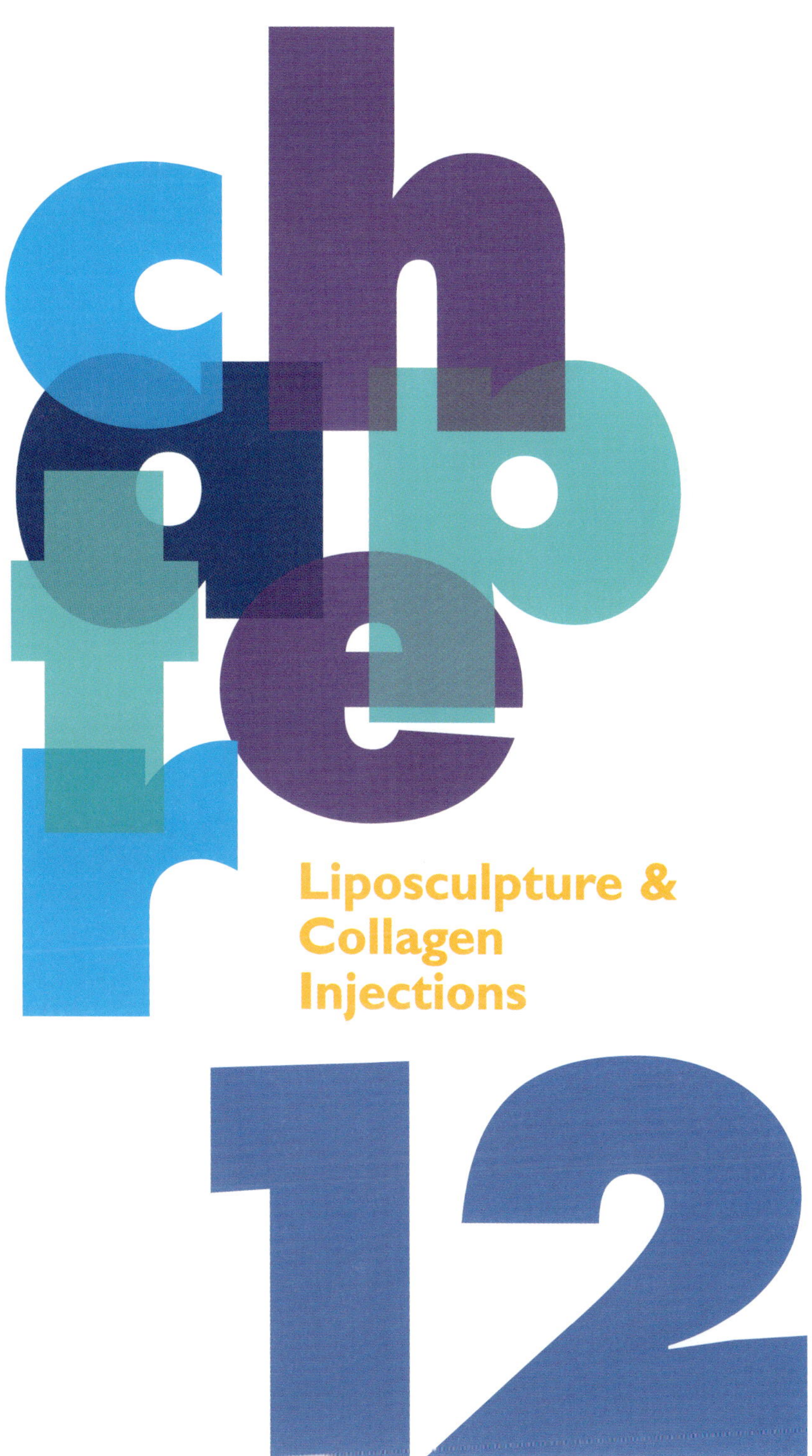

Liposculpture & Collagen Injections

Liposculpture & Collagen Injections

Collagen is a natural protein found in certain tissues of the human body including the skin, muscles, tendons and bone. Collagen provides a network of connective fibers that give our skin its support and elasticity. As we grow older, this connective tissue is weakened and the skin becomes less resilient and elastic. A lifetime of smiling, frowning, smoking or worrying becomes evident as our face forms grooves and lines in the skin. Sun exposure cause further deepening of these lines and wrinkles.

Collagen Injections

Collagen replacement restores the collagen that is lost due to sun damage and aging in the skin and helps plump up and reduce lines. The procedure uses refined animal collagen found in cows, which is very similar to human collagen. Collagen is injected directly into the skin to help smooth out facial lines, including smile lines, frown lines, lip lines, crow's feet around the eyes, smoker's lines, and facial scars.

Prior to treatment, the doctor will ask for a medical history and perform a skin

Liposculpture & Collagen Injections

Purpose: *To plump up lines and sunken areas, add fullness to the areas such as nasolabial folds, lips and scars. Several treatments may be required.*

Procedure: *Length 15 minutes to 1 hour.*

Anesthesia: *Local or none.*

Where: *Outpatient.*

Recovery: *Temporary stinging or burning sensation.*

Risks: *Infection and allergic reaction. Both fat and collagen injections can cause irregularitites in the skin's contour.*

Costs: *$500 – $4,500.*

(Note: Prices may vary based on physician fees, anesthesia, sessions required, and surgical setting. Data is based on a compilation of sources including Dr. Man.)

test to see if there are any allergies or reactions to the collagen. Complete correction may require several treatments, depending on the skin type, area being treated, and the patient's age.

The treatment takes minutes in the doctor's office. Several injections are needed, since the collagen material is eventually absorbed by the body.

Liposculpture

Aging of facial features is evident in the decreased volume and projection of the brows, cheeks and smile lines, as well as the lips. Filler materials such as Alloderm®, Gortex®, SoftForm®, are used to fill up depressed areas in the skin such as wrinkles and scars and can also be used in lip augmentation Replacement of the lost volume with one's own fat is a sound solution with reasonable longevity. Liposculpture is an excellent option for those seeking to increase volume or to minimize facial lines, wrinkles and scars. Fat is taken from one area of the body where it is less desirable and injected into areas such as the cheeks and lips to make them plumper and to fill out wrinkles and fine lines such as lip lines, frown lines and crow's feet.

Fat is more advantageous for injection than collagen since it comes from the patient's own body and usually lasts longer. This procedure begins by gently suctioning and collecting fat. In men, it is usually harvested from the abdomen. In women, it is taken from the abdomen, hips, buttocks, thighs or knee area. If significant amounts of fat are needed, the donor site may look somewhat flattened, a desirable result when it is taken from the abdomen and buttocks. In the case of the hip, thigh or knees, both sides should be considered donor sites in order to maintain symmetry. Approximatly 60 percent of the fat may be absorbed after the first treatment, over three to six months. However, the 40 percent improvement is very significant and long-lasting. The procedure is performed under I.V. sedation and with local anesthesia.

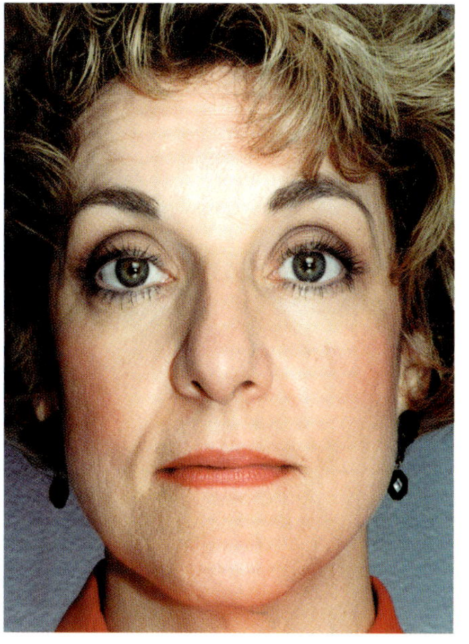

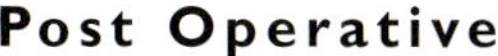

Post Operative

After the procedure, some lumpiness where the fat has been injected may be noticed. The area being injected will be swollen and tender, and there may also be some bruising and temporary discomfort. Sometimes an antibiotic prescription will be recommended. Most of the initial swelling will subside in one to four weeks. The bruising should be gone in a week or two. Persistent redness should be brought to your doctor's attention.

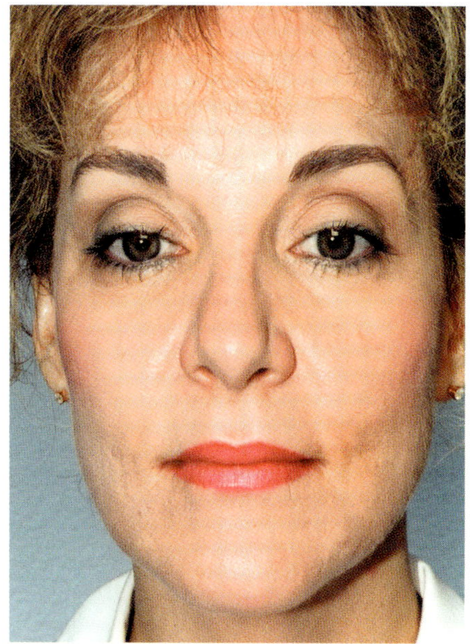

Fat injections to face; tca peel

Patients can usually resume normal activities in a few days. In some cases, patients will be asked to wear compression garments, which look much like a girdle. These are usually worn for several days to several weeks, in order to reduce swelling.

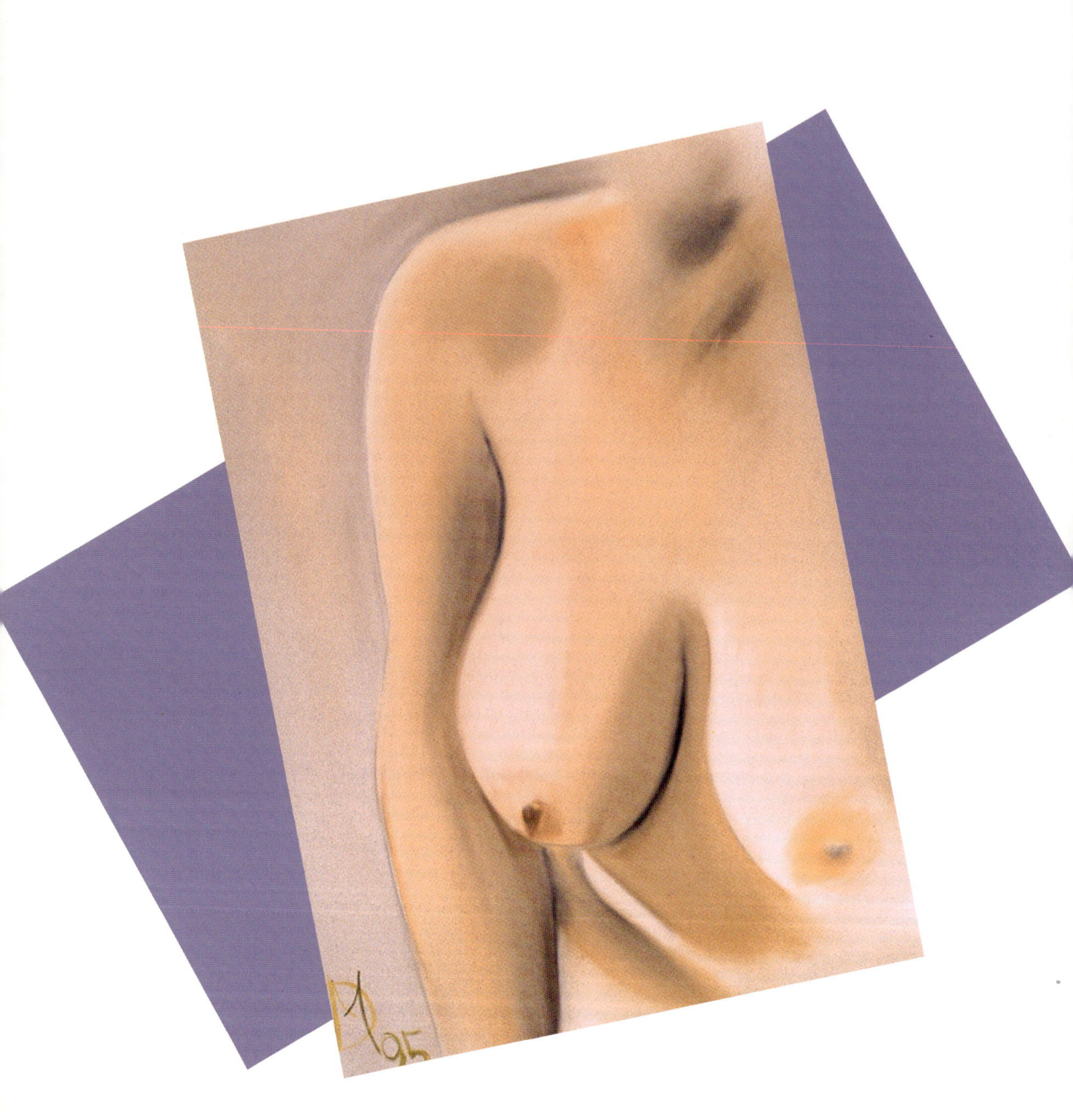

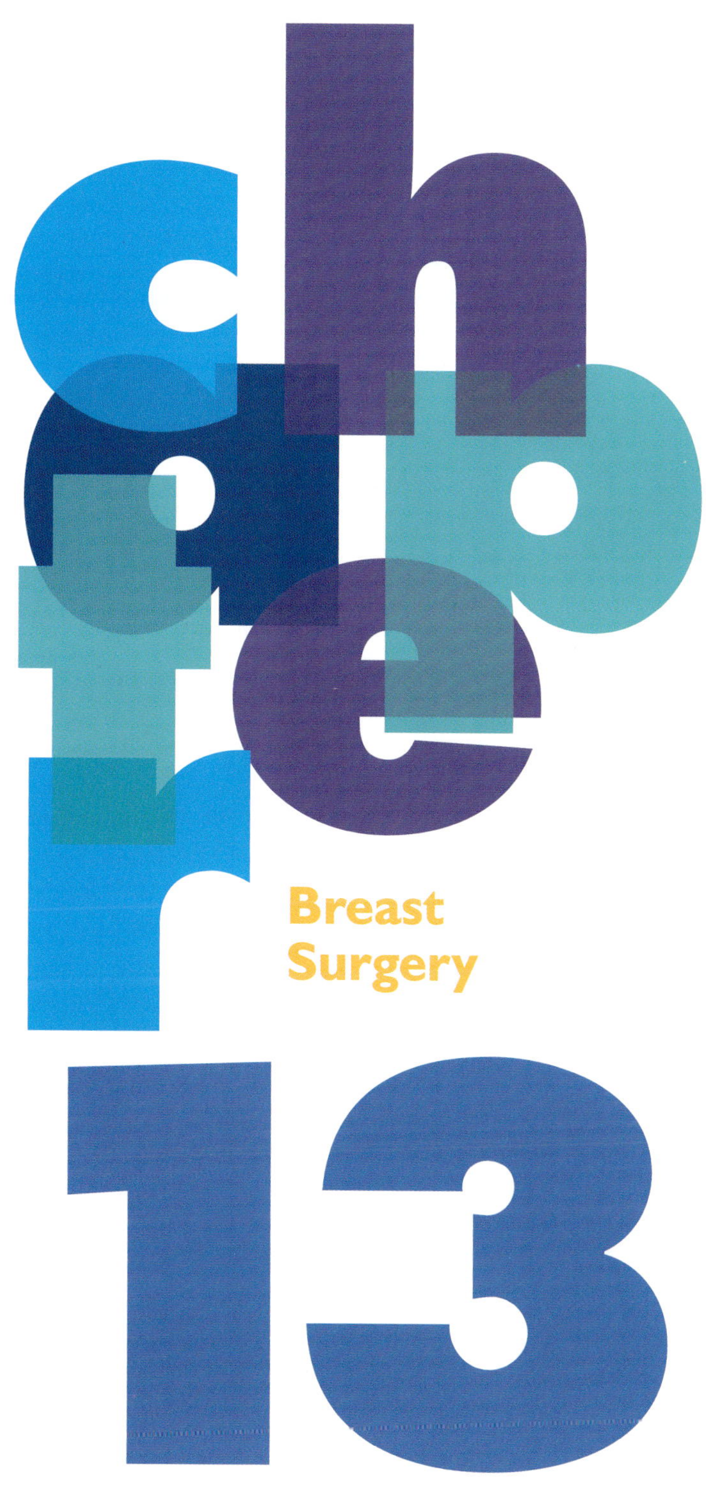

Chapter 13

Breast Surgery

Breast Surgery

Breast sizes and shapes vary greatly among women, and there is no one perfect size or shape. Emotionally and psychologically, a woman's sense of self-esteem and of being a woman is often associated with her breasts. There are many types of breast surgeries. Breast augmentation, increasing the size of the breast, is the most common. Other breast surgeries include: breast reduction or decreasing the size of the breast; breast lift to correct sagging breasts; breast reconstruction after mastectomy; and surgery to correct congenital birth deformities including non-symmetrical breasts.

Breast Augmentation (Implants)

Some of the reasons why a woman may decide to have breast augmentation are to increase the size of small or underdeveloped breasts, to reshape and enlarge breasts that have lost their shape and fullness after child-bearing or aging, or to create symmetry between breasts of differing sizes or shapes. The surgeon accomplishes this with the placement of a breast implant. If the breasts have sagging of the gland and skin, this can also be corrected at the same time with another procedure called a mastopexy, or breast lift.

Breast Enlargement

Augmentation Mammaplasty

Purpose: *To increase the size and shape of the breast using artificial implants.*

Surgery length: *1 – 2 hours.*

Anesthesia: *General*

Where: *Outpatient surgery or overnight stay.*

Recovery: *Temporary soreness, swelling, breast sensitivity and loss of nipple sensation.*

Back to work: *1 – 2 weeks*

Full activities: *2 weeks to a month.*

Risks: *Bleeding, infection, hardening of the implant, rupture, asymmetrical breasts and scarring.*

Cost: *$4,000 – $8,000*

**(Note: Prices may vary based on physician fees, anesthesia, surgical setting and number of procedures. Data is based on a compilation of sources including Dr. Man.)*

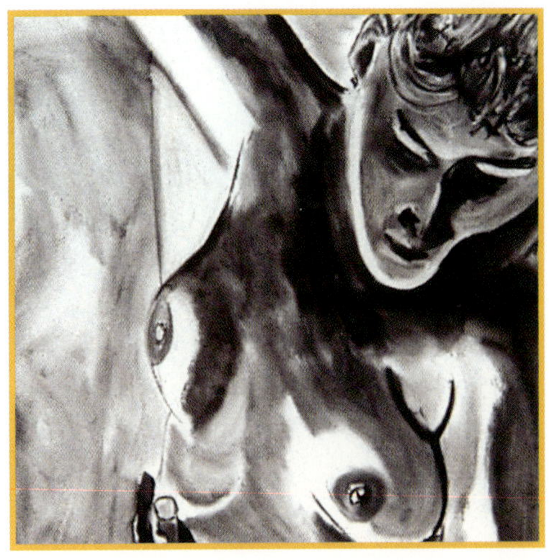

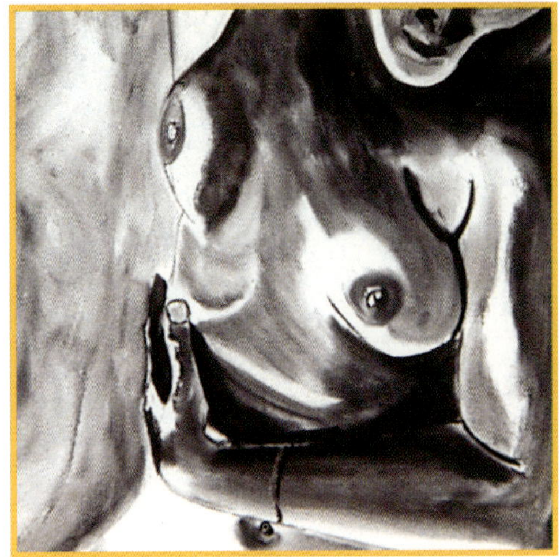

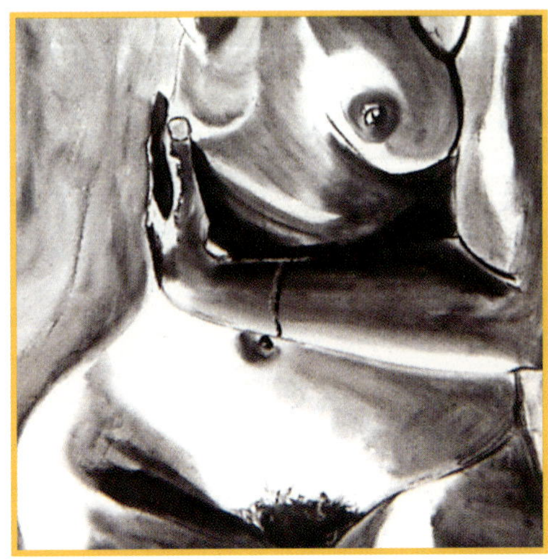

Breast Implants

Breast implants come in many sizes and shapes and consist of two types: a silicone pouch with an inner filling of silicone gel; or a silicone pouch filled with a saline solution (salt water).

Silicone is a bio-compatible material that has dozens of medical uses besides breast implants. It is used in artificial joint replacements, in cardiac pacemakers, in syringes and medicines, and in hundreds of non-medical substances with which we come in contact every day, including food, plastic products, clothing and even the furniture we sit on. Silicone gel-filled breast implants are currently available only to women who are undergoing breast reconstruction after a mastectomy (breast removal), or to patients who are having revisionary surgery to remove implants that have hardened or ruptured.

The Surgery

During breast augmentation surgery, the saline-filled implant is inserted through an incision either under the breast, in the crease where it meets the chest wall (called the inframammary incision); around the nipple and areola, called the periareolar incision; or through the armpit, referred to as the axillary incision. In each case, the incision scar is well hidden in the skin fold or bra line. The implant is surgically placed in a pocket located inside the breast either behind the breast tissue or behind the breast muscle. The procedure takes approximately one to two hours and is performed under general anesthesia in an outpatient surgery facility such as the doctor's office, sometimes with an overnight stay.

After surgery the breast may be tender and painful to the touch, and nipple sensation may be reduced, but should return after a period of several weeks to several months. There will also be some swelling and bruising, which will disappear. Some complaints include hardening of the implant, called capsular contracture, and deflation of the implant due to rupture and leakage of the saltwater (rare).

Capsular contracture, or hardening of the implant, is a condition that results when scar tissue forms around the implants making it feel painful and hard to the touch. In order to reduce the chance of hardening of the implant, patients are instructed in massage and exercise techniques.

Breast Reduction

For many women, large oversized breasts can be physically uncomfortable, causing back and shoulder pain, breathing problems, and restriction in motion. Large breasts can also be a source of embarrassment, especially for young women who experience excessive breast development during puberty.

Breast reduction is a procedure that reduces disproportionate, oversized breasts. Surgery involves removing skin, fat and glandular tissue, and relocating the nipple and areola to a more appropriate position. The areola can also be reduced at the same time.

Breast Reduction

Reduction Mammaplasty

Purpose: *To reduce oversized, large and sagging breasts.*

Surgery: *Length 2 – 4 hours*

Anesthesia: *General and/or local sedation.*

Where: *Outpatient surgery.*

Recovery: *Swelling, bruising and numbness. Permanent scarring.*

Back to work: *2 weeks. Full activities 3 – 4 weeks.*

Risks: *Bleeding, infection, loss of sensation, and asymmetrical breasts or uneven position of nipples.*

Cost: $7,000 - $9,000

**(Note: Prices may vary based on physician fees, anesthesia, surgical setting and number of procedures. Data is based on a compilation of sources including Dr. Man.)*

Breast Lift

After pregnancy and nursing, and often as a result of aging, a woman's breasts may begin to droop and sag. A breast lift will reposition the breasts into a more pleasing position and provide for a more pleasing contour. During the procedure, the surgeon will make several incisions outlining the area of skin that will be removed above and below the nipple. The nipple will be moved to a new, higher position, while the excess skin above and below the nipple is removed and the breast reshaped. The procedure takes roughly two to four hours, and is performed in an outpatient surgery facility.

Breast Lift

Mastopexy

Purpose: *To reshape and reposition the breasts.*

Surgery length: *2 to 4 hours.*

Anesthesia: *General and/or local with I.V. sedation.*

Where: *Outpatient or overnight stay.*

Recovery: *Temporary swelling, numbness and bruising.*

Back to work: *1 – 2 weeks.*

Full activities 3 – 4 weeks.

Risks: *Bleeding, scarring, tissue loss, infection, uneven nipple position, loss of sensation in breasts and nipples.*

Cost: *$7,000 – $9,000*

(Note: Prices may vary based on physician fees, anesthesia, sessions required and surgical setting. Data is based on a compilation of sources including Dr. Man.)

Breast Reconstruction

Purpose: *To restore a natural looking breast after mastectomy with the use of implants or through flap reconstruction such as the tram flap which does not use implants.*

Surgery Length: *2 – 5 hours.*

Anesthesia: *General.*

Where: *Hospital, inpatient.*

Recovery: *Discomfort and swelling.*

Back to work: *4 – 6 weeks.*

Full activities: *Several months.*

Risks: *Scarring, infection, capsular contracture in the case of implants. Loss of flap & abdominal weakness*

Cost: *$10,000 – $ 20,000*

(Note: Prices may vary based on physician fees, anesthesia, sessions required and surgical setting. Data is based on a compilation of sources including Dr. Man.)

Breast Reconstruction

Breast reconstruction can be an important part of recovery for women after a mastectomy. Years ago, when a woman had a mastectomy, she was given few options. Either she was told she had to live with the disfigurement, be fitted with a prosthesis or have a breast implant.

The most common reconstruction technique utilizes breast implants. This reconstructive procedure involves several stages, the first stage requires the insertion of a tissue expander, which is gradually filled with saline in order to stretch the skin. This prepares the breast for the final stage, insertion of the permanent implant.

Many women today want breast reconstruction, but some don't want implants, preferring natural reconstruction. The solution is natural breast reconstruction using flaps of muscle and skin taken from the back, abdomen or buttocks.

The tram flap (Transverse Abdominal Island Flap) has become very popular. It is really two procedures in one: a tummy tuck and breast reconstruction. This procedure uses a woman's own body tissue to form a new breast without implants. The procedure involves taking tissue and muscle from the abdomen and transferring it under the chest wall to the mastectomy site, where it is shaped and sutured into place. A nipple and areola are added at a later time, completing the new breast. After the new breast is shaped and sutured, the abdominal skin is then stretched and tightened in the same procedure that is used in most tummy tuck operations

It was developed by several plastic surgeons who were challenged to find a method of breast reconstruction that reached such goals as:

1) creating an aesthetically pleasing contour and natural-feeling breast
2) creating a visually pleasing breast that looks natural
3) finding an acceptable donor site
4) creating symmetry with the other breast

Not all women are candidates for the tram flap procedure. The best way to find this out is to consult with a plastic surgeon who has extensive experience performing these procedures and talk to patients who have undergone them.

The new breast will not replace the missing breast in all aspects. It may look like a natural breast, but sensation will vary and some scarring will remain.

BREAST ENLARGEMENT

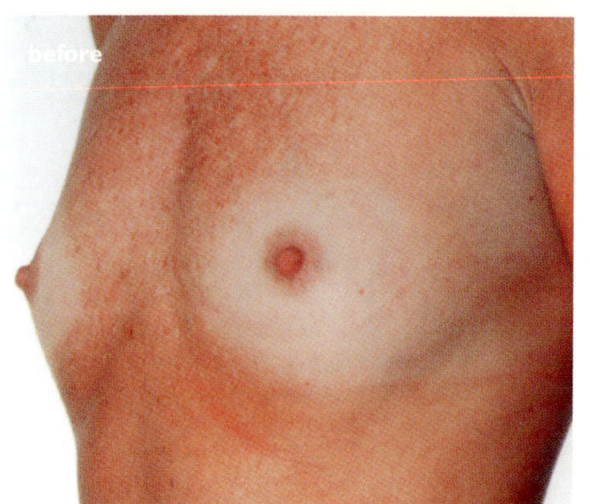

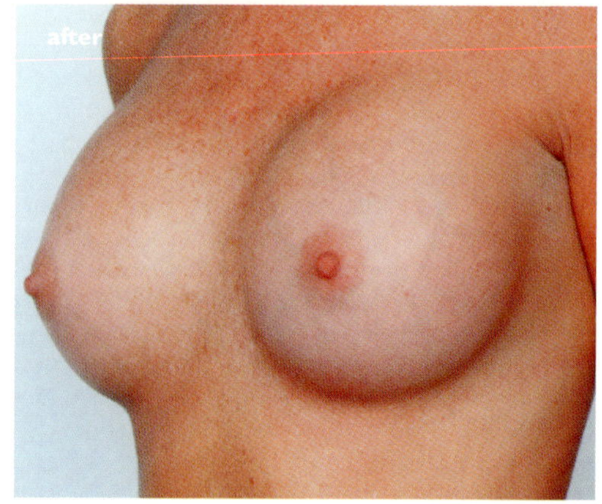

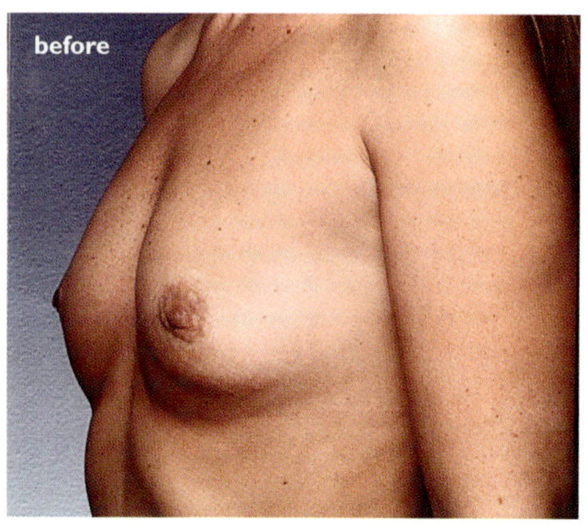

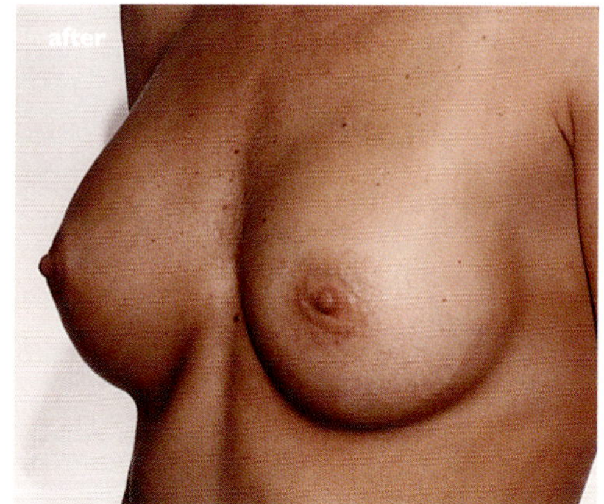

BREAST ENLARGEMENT

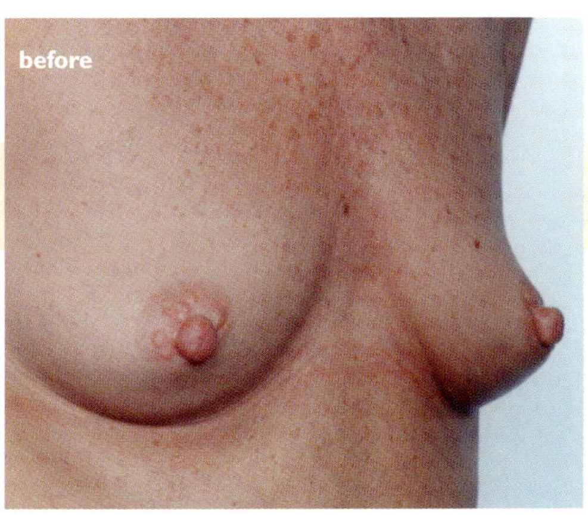

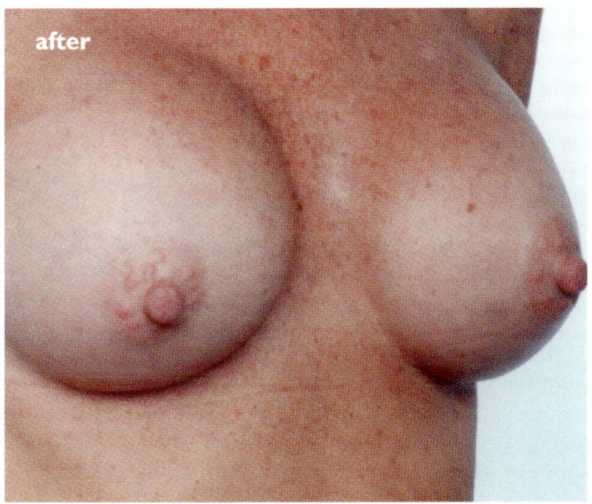

BREAST REDUCTION

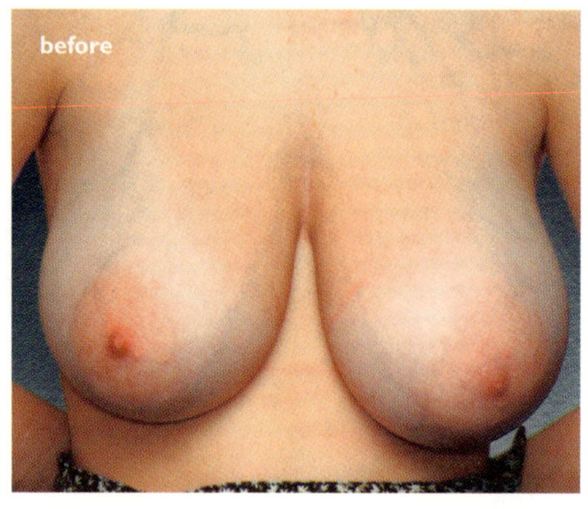

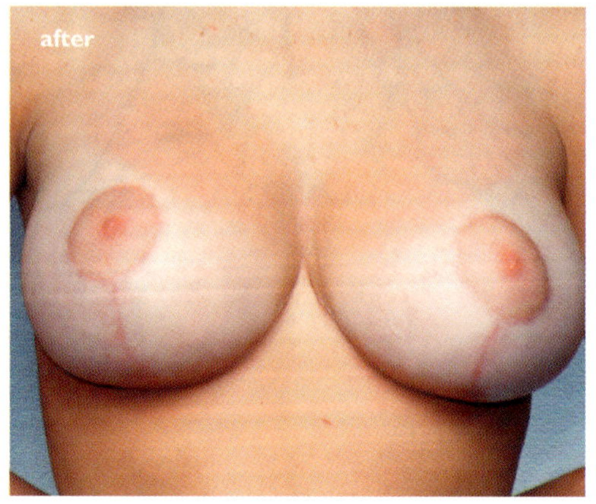

BREAST RECONSTRUCTION (TRAM FLAP)

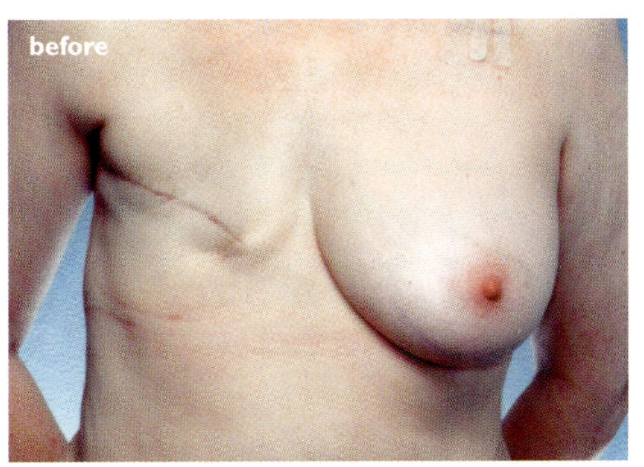

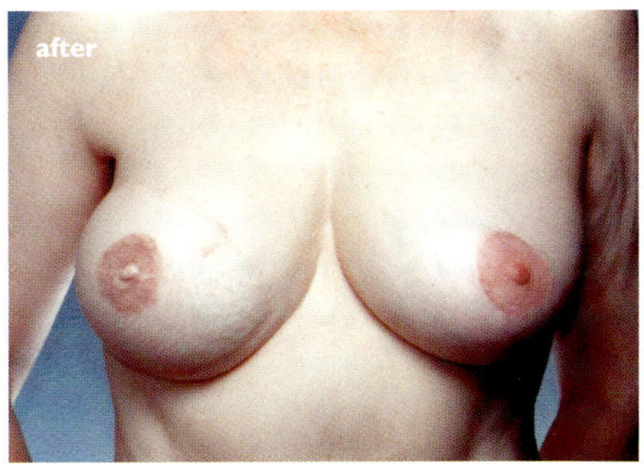

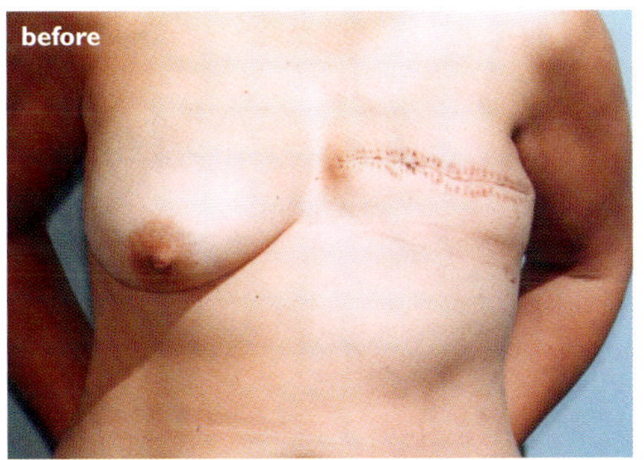

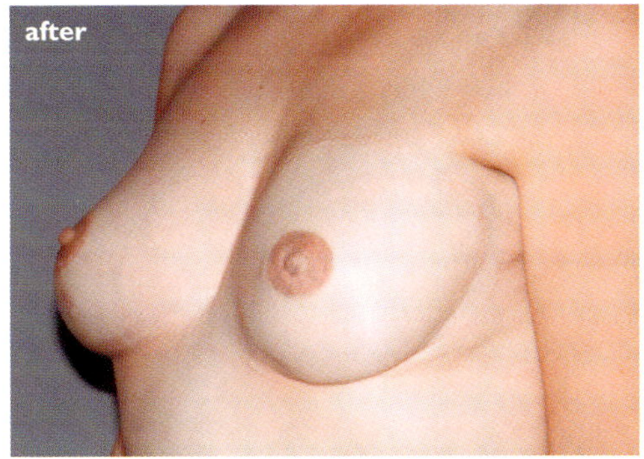

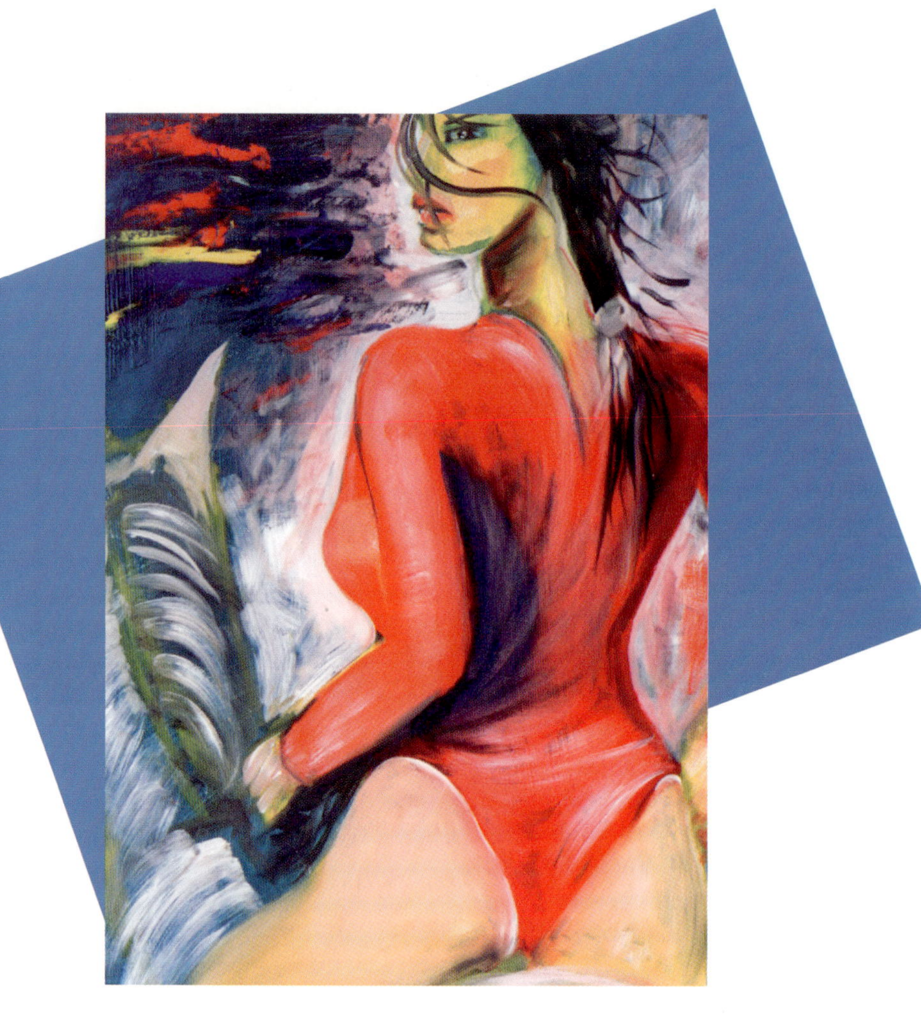

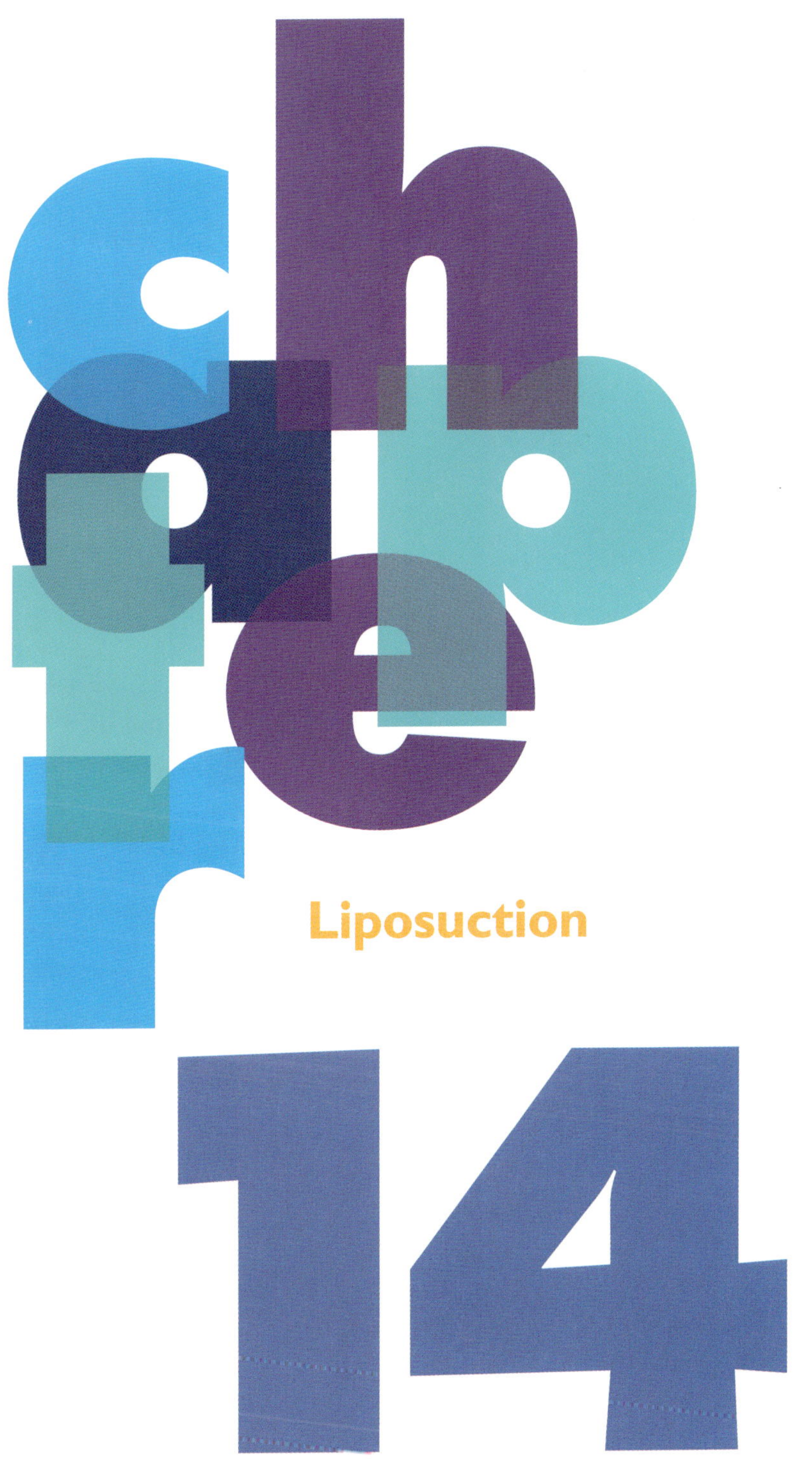

Chapter 14
Liposuction

LIPOSUCTION

The ability to mold flesh into a more pleasing form is truly the essence of plastic surgery. A sculptor works with stone and clay. A plastic surgeon molds human flesh. As we grow older, our fat to muscle ratio increases as our metabolism slows down. Most people experience a thickening of the mid-portion of the body. Physicians also recognize that, for some people, no matter how much they exercise or diet, certain areas of fat remain. Fat deposits, such as "saddle-bag" thighs, are a good example, in which fat is localized to specific areas that make the body appear out of proportion.

Though not a replacement for sound eating habits, diet and regular exercise, liposuction is a process that can remove unwanted fat from the body. Prior to the introduction of liposuction, surgeons could cut out fat, but it resulted in ghastly scars. It wasn't until the early 1970s that a procedure was developed to remove fat without scarring by literally vacuuming it away. Introduced by a French plastic surgeon, liposuction, also called fat suctioning, or suction-assisted lipectomy, helped usher in a new era for plastic surgery. Finally, there was a means to surgically alter the body shape with minimal scarring.

Modern plastic surgery has benefited tremendously from the introduction of lipo-

LIPOSUCTION

Ultrasound Suction Lipectomy

Purpose: *To remove stubborn, hard-to-lose fat.*

Surgery Length: *1 – 2 hours, depending on how many areas.*

Anesthesia: *General, spinal or local sedation.*

Where: *Outpatient or overnight stay.*

Recovery: *Bruising, swelling, tenderness.*

Risks: *Infection, lumpy skin.*

Costs: *$2,600 – $3,600 or more depending on how many areas are being treated.*

**(Note: Prices may vary based on physician fees, anesthesia, surgical setting and number of procedures. Data is based on a compilation of sources including Dr. Man.)*

suctioning. It is now used almost routinely in a wide range of procedures from neck and face lifts to breast reduction. Fat suctioning can remove unwanted fat deposits from other areas as well, including the back, hips, buttocks, neck, arms, abdomen, knees or ankles. Men typically collect extra fat in areas around the waist called "tires" or "love handles," and in the chest and the neck.

Women have a tendency to store fat on the hips, buttocks, thighs and abdomen. Liposuction contours and helps reshape the body. For example, the leg, which is thick at the top, can be made to look longer by suctioning under the buttocks. Body builders have also benefited from this technique.

Liposuction has evolved over the years and is dramatically improved from the early days. Using a syringe and needle (Tumescent technique), the surgeon makes a tiny, one-quarter inch incision in the area of fat that is being removed. The area is then filled with large amounts of saline to decrease the bleeding and gently suctioned with a narrow cannula and a syringe until the desired shape is achieved.

Ultrasound Suction Lipectomy

The most recent developments in liposuction use ultrasound to emulsify the fat prior to being suctioned out. Ultrasound (soundwaves) break up the fat turning it into a liquid or emulsified form so that it can be gently suctioned from the body using less pressure than with traditional liposuction. Ultrasound has been used throughout medicine in diagnostic procedures during pregnancy and to treat kidney stones, among others. Its applications in liposuction (fat reduction and body contouring) offers several patients benefits. Liquefying the fat first with ultrasound allows the surgeon to remove larger amounts of fat with less trauma to surrounding tissues and appears to improve skin contraction. This benefits patients since it allows skin to drape nicely. The ultrasound- assisted lipectomy is a useful tool in fibrous areas, such as upper abdomen, breast or back. These areas are easier to shape with this tool. Ultrasound can be used externally or internally at the tip of the suction cannula. Surgeons can perform liposuction on multiple sites at one time. The amount of fat that can be removed ranges from a few ounces to several pounds. In the case where larger areas are being suctioned, several treatments may be needed. Good candidates are healthy patients, with noticeable localized areas of fat. They also have good skin tone and elasticity.

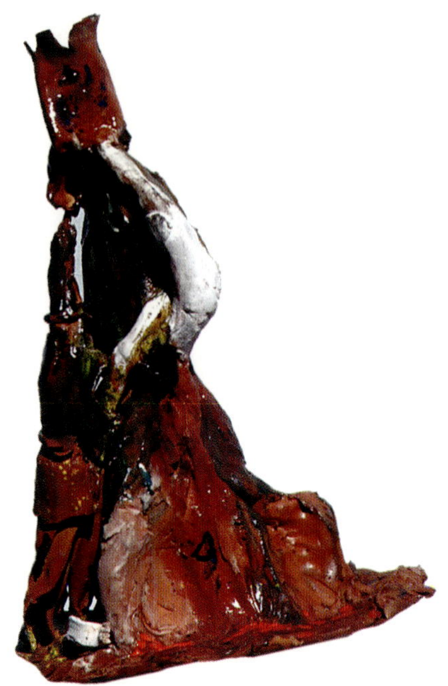

Length of Surgery

Liposuction is performed under general or local anesthesia with I.V. sedation or spinal anesthesia in the doctor's office, outpatient surgery facility or hospital. The procedure takes approximately one to two hours depending on the number of areas being suctioned. Following surgery, patients experience some discomfort including swelling and bruising, which will subside after two to six weeks. Numbness may persist for longer periods. Patients wear a snug dressing or a surgical "compression" garment for one week after surgery to promote healing, reduce swelling and increase comfort. In some cases, Magnetic therapy may aid patients by improving healing time. The unipolar magnets developed by Magnetherapy help in increasing blood circulation, while decreasing swelling.

In some cases, swelling may persist for longer periods. Besides numbness, swelling or bruising, rare complications may include blood clots, infection and pain. In some rare cases, the skin may look wavy and fails to contract. Patients are usually able to get out of bed the day of surgery and are up and around and return to work after a few days to a week.

Cellulite

Cellulite, that "cottage cheese" lumpy fat that forms on the sides and backs of the thighs and buttocks, cannot be corrected by liposuction. Newer techniques like Endomologie skin toning and conditioning offered by Nova Laser Light Cosmetic Centers appears to offer promise in reducing the "orange peel" and dimpling appearance of cellulite.

Most Common Questions

The question most often asked; does the fat return? The answer is no. The fat that is removed does not return once it is taken out. There will be permanent improvement to the areas, as long as there is no significant weight gain.

Another question patients ask involves thigh creams and cellulite removers. While these products can help to smooth out some lumpiness, they do not actually reduce the fat.

LIPOSUCTION

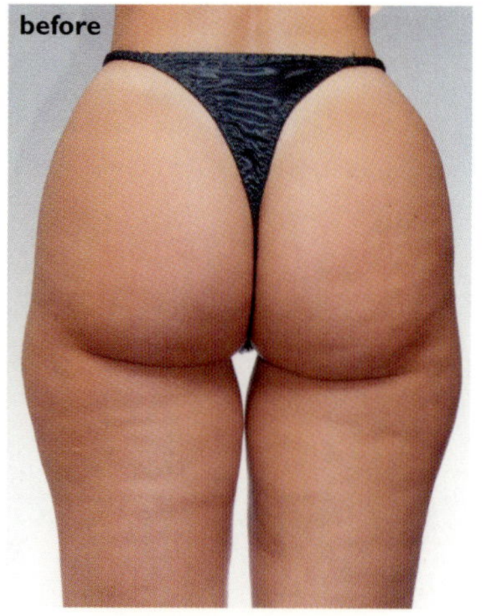

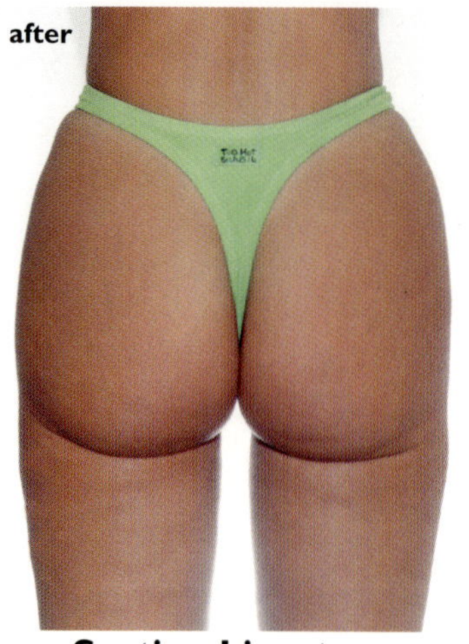

Suction Lipectomy

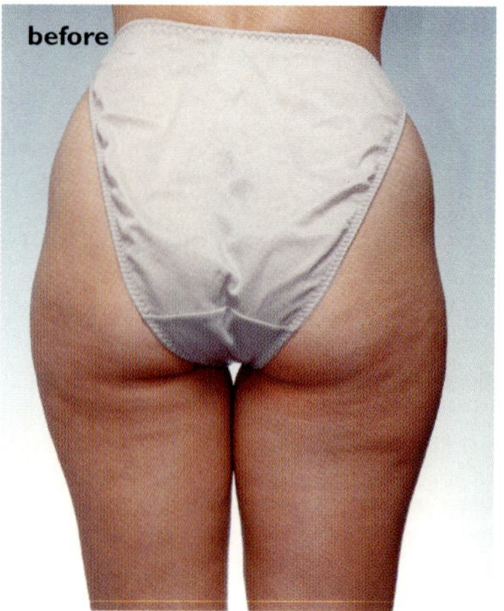

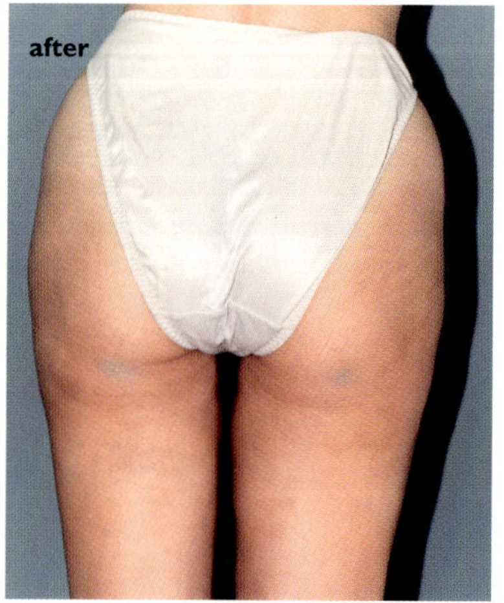

Suction Lipectomy

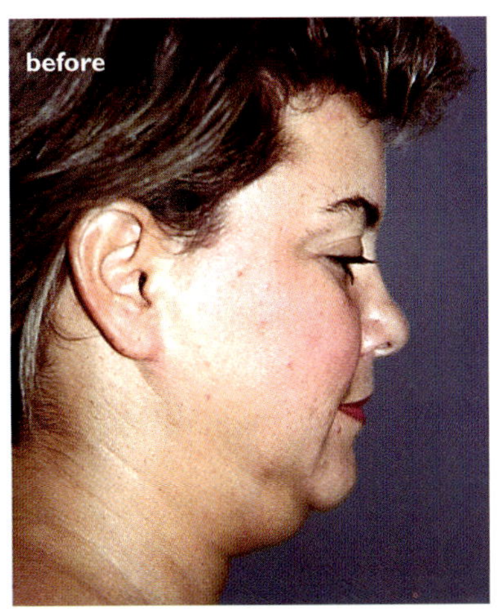

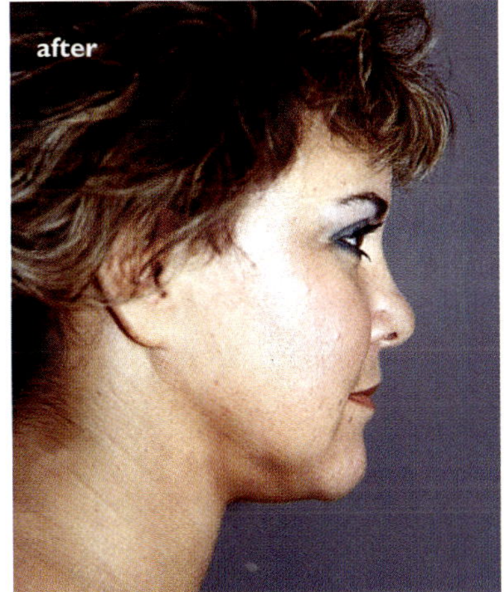

Suction Lipectomy of the neck

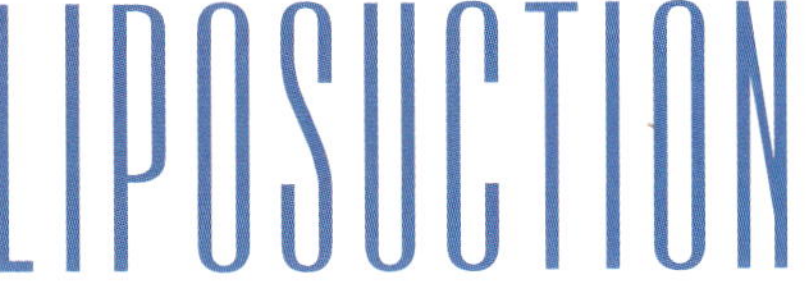

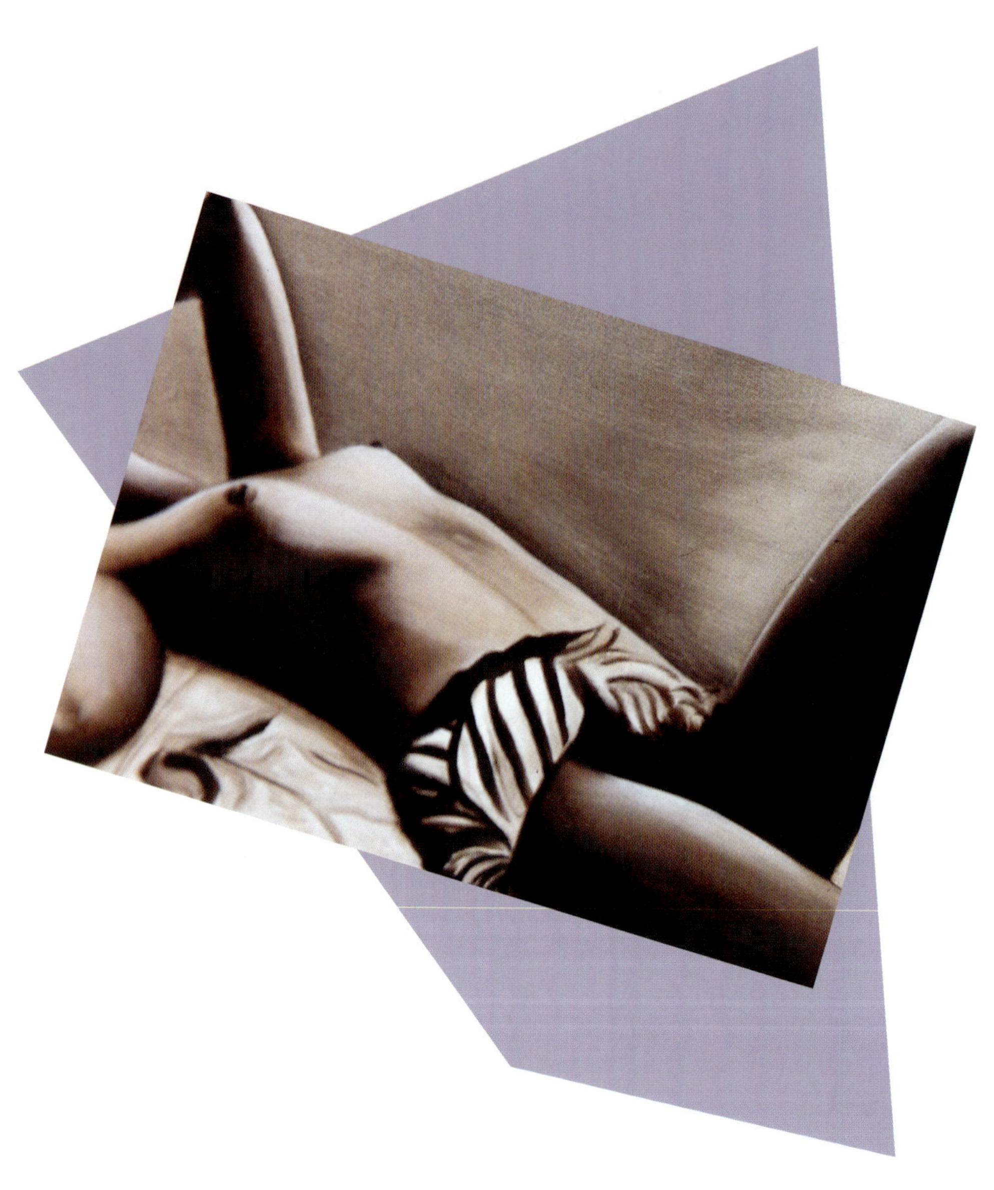

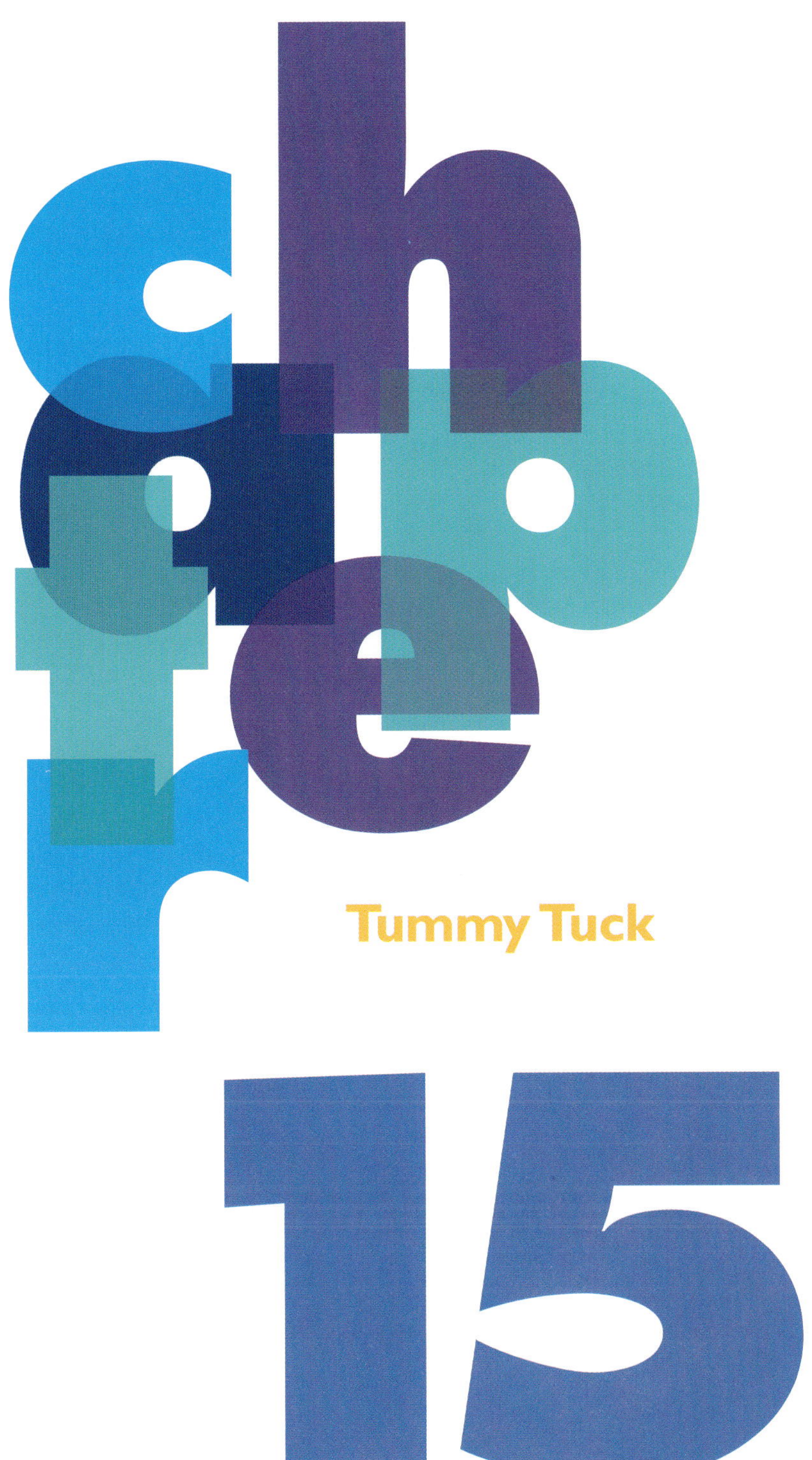

Chapter 15

Tummy Tuck

Tummy Tuck

Abdominoplasty is the surgical term for a tummy tuck, the procedure which tightens abdominal muscles, removes extra fat and skin and, in some cases, improves stretch marks. Those considering a tummy tuck are often women who have found that child-bearing has left them with fatty deposits, skin and loose muscles that don't respond to diet or exercise. Patients who have loss of skin elasticity and muscle tone and who have extra pounds are also excellent candidates.

Men, too, are having tummy tucks to

look better. Patients should be in good shape and average weight. Those patients who plan to lose a lot of weight or women who plan to get pregnant should postpone surgery.

Surgical Procedure

A tummy tuck is major surgery, which can be performed in the doctor's surgery facility, outpatient surgery center or the hospital. The procedure usually takes between two to four hours and consists of making a long incision just above the pubic area from hip to hip. The skin is separated from the abdominal wall up to the ribs, creating a skin flap. The two vertical abdominal muscles are tightened by positioning them closer together and stitching them into place. The skin flap is then pulled down, the excess skin removed, and the navel repositioned. The result is a firmer tummy and more narrow waistline. If most of the fat is below the belly button, then a "mini" tummy tuck can be performed. This procedure uses a much shorter incision and the navel may not have to be moved.

Tummy Tuck

Abdominoplasty

Purpose: *To flatten the stomach area, remove excess skin and fat, tighten abdominal muscles.*

Surgery Length: *2 – 4 hours depending on extent.*

Anesthesia: *General or spinal.*

Where: *Doctor's surgical facility, outpatient, surgery center or as an inpatient in a hospital.*

Recovery: *Back to work 1 – 2 weeks; avoid strenuous activity for 3 – 4 weeks. Patients wear a light support garment for few weeks.*

Risks: *Scarring, temporary swelling, infection, bleeding, blood clots, poor healing.*

Cost: *$3,700 – $9,500.*

**(Note: Prices may vary based on physician fees, anesthesia, surgical setting and number of procedures.. Data is based on a compilation of sources including Dr. Man.)*

Endoscopic Tummy Tuck

For many patients, the endoscope and liposuction may be an alternative to the traditional surgical method, eliminating 90 percent of the hip-to-hip scars left after traditional surgery. A small incision is made around the belly button and an endoscope inserted through which liposuction and other surgical tools are passed to suck out excess fat and tighten abdominal muscles. If hernia repair is needed, this can be done at the same time. After surgery the abdomen will be swollen and patients will experience discomfort. Patients usually wear a support garment for several weeks. Most return to work after one to two weeks, while others may need longer recovery. Vigorous exercise should be avoided initially. Scars will be permanent and may fade with time, though the newer endoscopic technique offers less scarring. This newer technique is suited for patients with minimal excess of loose skin.

TUMMY TUCK

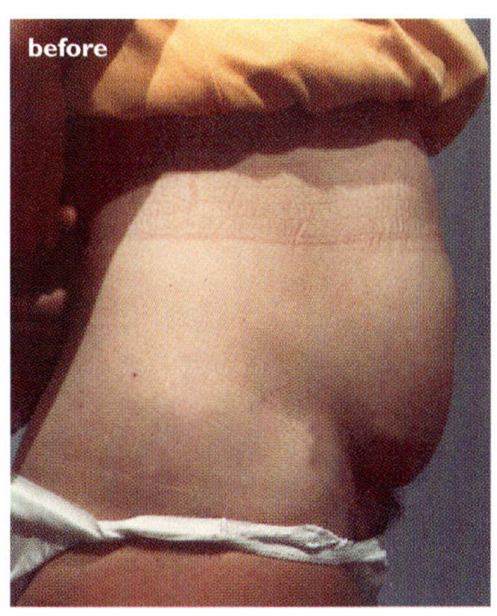

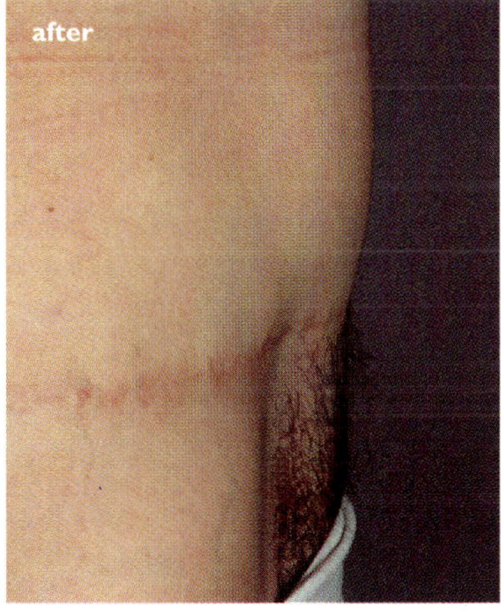

TUMMY TUCK

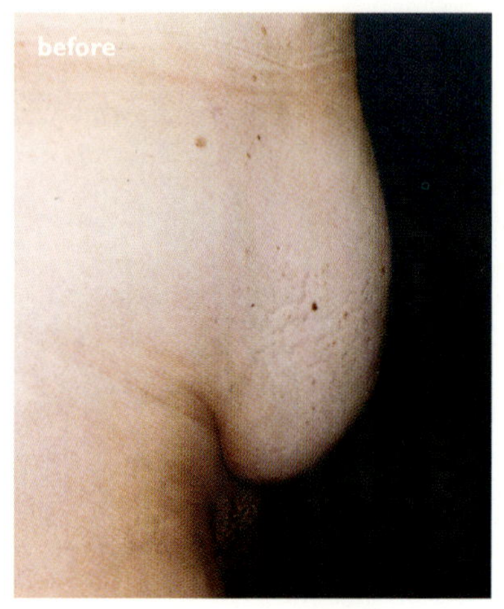

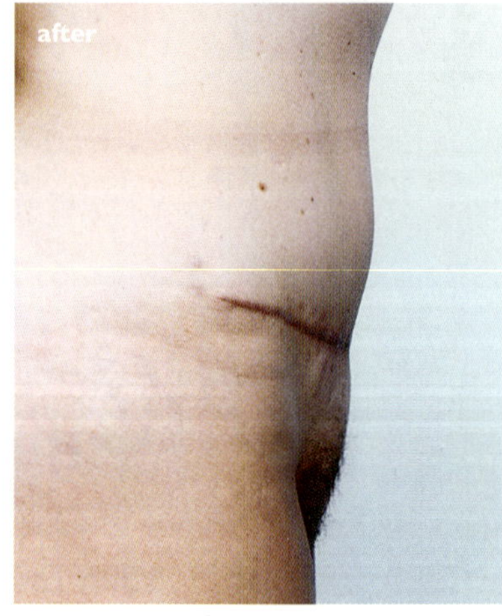

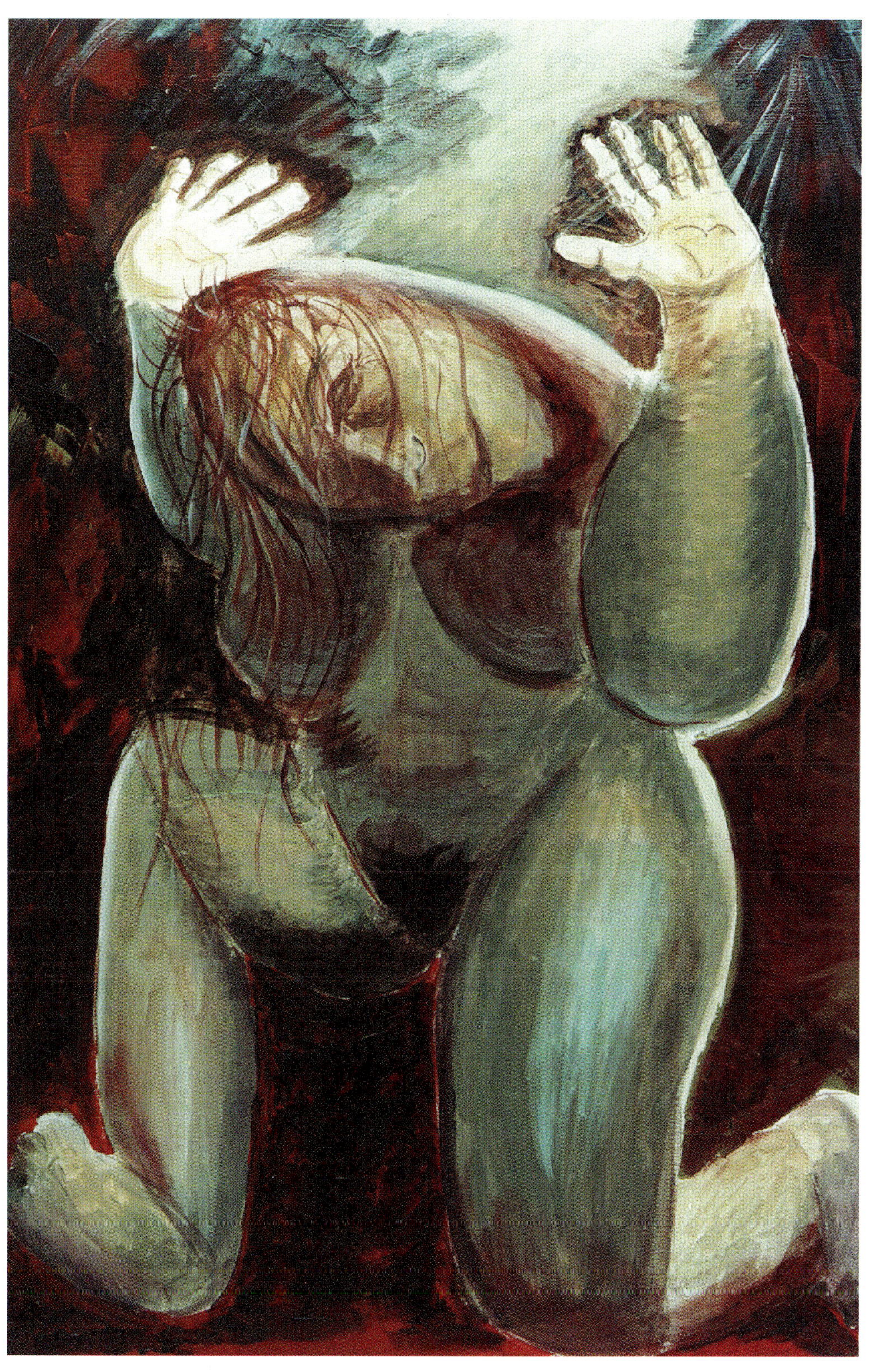

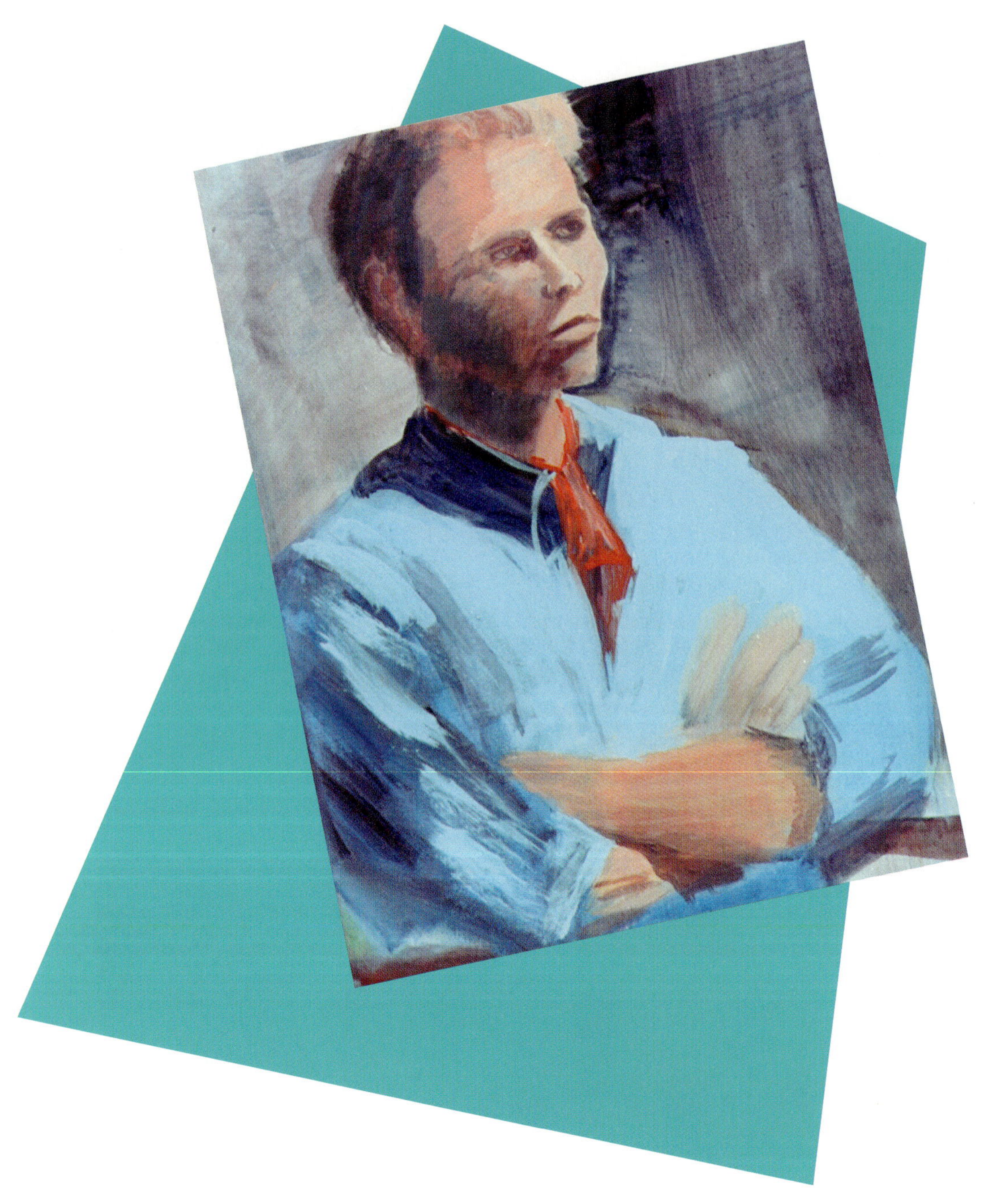

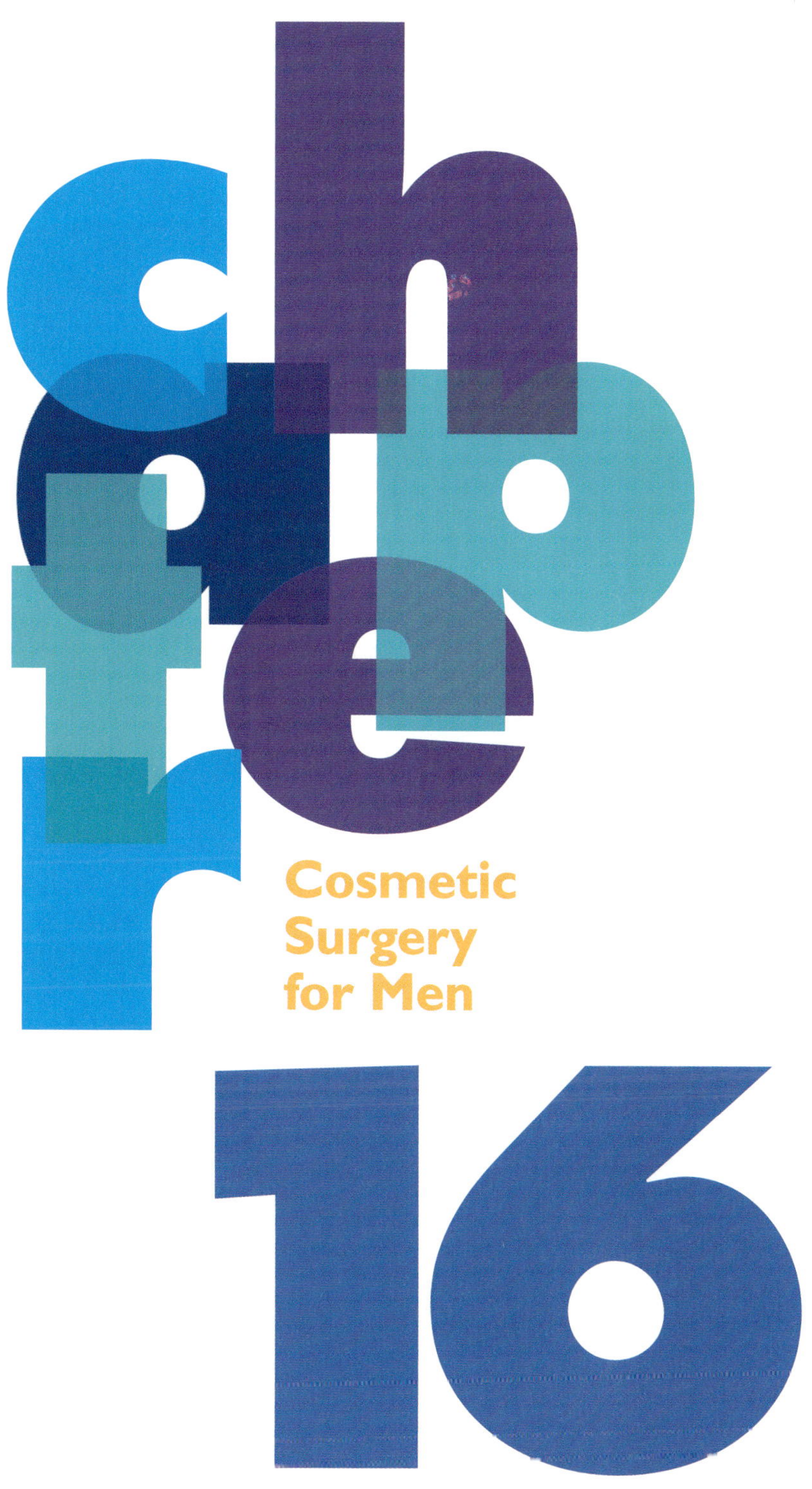

Chapter 16: Cosmetic Surgery for Men

Cosmetic Surgery for Men

Aging is just as much a concern for men as it is for women. Increasingly, men are looking at ways to improve their appearance. In our youth-oriented, competitive society much importance is placed on how you look, particularly in the corporate world, where men find they have to compete with a younger market.

A Change In Attitude

Today, there are very practical reasons for improving one's appearance through surgery. Gone is the stigma that plastic surgery is strictly vanity surgery. Wrinkles were once viewed as a sign of maturity and wisdom; now that attitude has changed. Men are recognizing that wrinkles, frown lines, crow's feet, droopy eyelids, baldness and double chins make them look tired, fatigued and less competitive on the job.

Men are now putting a "new face on their careers" with plastic surgery and discovering cosmetic products. Like their female counterparts, men are turning to hair coloring to lose the gray, going to hair stylists instead of barber shops, having facials, learning about moisturizers and makeup and they have even entered what was once the almost exclusive domain of women — plastic surgery. (*Wall Street Journal,* August 28, 1991; *New York Times,* June 9, 1996)

Why Do Men Do It?

One company president says his decision to have a facelift was 60 percent business and 40 percent personal. He is part of a growing number of business executives concerned with being more competitive on the job. Another segment Is in fear of getting the ax. Corporate downsizing has 45- to 54-year-olds living in fear of losing their jobs, according to the Bureau of Labor Statistics. Not surprisingly, this is the age group that is beginning to feel the effects of aging most, and it is the age group most frequently turning to plastic surgery.

Companies are getting lean and mean and they want their employees to look that way too. In a society that values youth, 50-year-old executives are competing with younger, fitter and more competitive 30-year-olds, who are often willing to work harder and for less money. One 40-year-old sales executive felt that his baggy eyelids and tired look affected his peers' perception of his ability and performance on the job. He said: "Every morning I would go to work and someone would ask if I was tired. In the business world the feeling is if you look tired or don't take care of yourself, people think you can't keep up."

A 59-year-old president of a multi-million dollar contracting company had a facelift and laser surgery to help him look younger. He travels around the world making presentations before county commissioners and hospital boards, "Why should I look 64 when I'm only 59?" he asked. "When I negotiate, I know I've got 30 seconds to make a good impression. I spend money on good suits, so why shouldn't I spend money to make my face look good, too?"

Not to be outdone by patients, physicians also recognize the importance of appearance. A hair transplant surgeon, Dr. C.P. Chambers of Delray Beach, Florida, did not like his profile. A frequent guest of television talk shows, he always stood facing the cameras so the audience couldn't see his side view. "I never let the camera tape me from the side," he said. His solution? Nose reshaping. "I don't have a bad side now. My surgery has also helped me to be more outgoing, which is important because I feel I can now relate better to my patients."

A Growing Trend

In 1980, only 10 percent of a plastic surgeon's patients were men. In 1994, that percentage more than doubled. Today, men can account for over 25 percent of a plastic surgeon's practice, and the number is growing. But, it's not just busy business executives in fear of losing their jobs who are filling the plastic surgeon's waiting room. On the homefront, men are also finding they want to keep pace with younger-looking wives. Following his wife's facelift, a retired executive put it like this, "Now that I have a young looking wife, I decided to take a look at myself."

Most Common Procedures For Men

What do men complain about the most? Baggy eyelids, receding hairlines, wrinkles, frown lines and sagging necks, to name a few. Hair transplants top the list of the most common procedures, followed by liposuction, nose surgery, eyelid surgery, collagen injections, face lifts, dermabrasion, ear tucks, chin implants and chemical peels. The advent of laser surgery is offering men more choices to remove lines, wrinkles, smooth aging, sun-damaged skin and repair baggy eyelids.

Liposuction is a very popular procedure requested by men to remove double chins, "spare tires" and "love handles" around the waist.

Men are also having pectoral implants to increase the size of their chests and calf implants to give their legs a more pleasing shape. Body toning and reshaping is also becoming widely used.

Top Ten Procedures

For Men

1. Nose Reshaping
2. Eyelid Surgery
3. Liposuction
4. Breast Reduction
5. Facelift
6. Ear Surgery
7. Dermabrasion
8. Chemical Peel
9. Chin Augmentation
10. Collagen Injections

(Source: 1994 Plastic Surgery Statistics, American Society of Plastic & Reconstructive Surgeons)

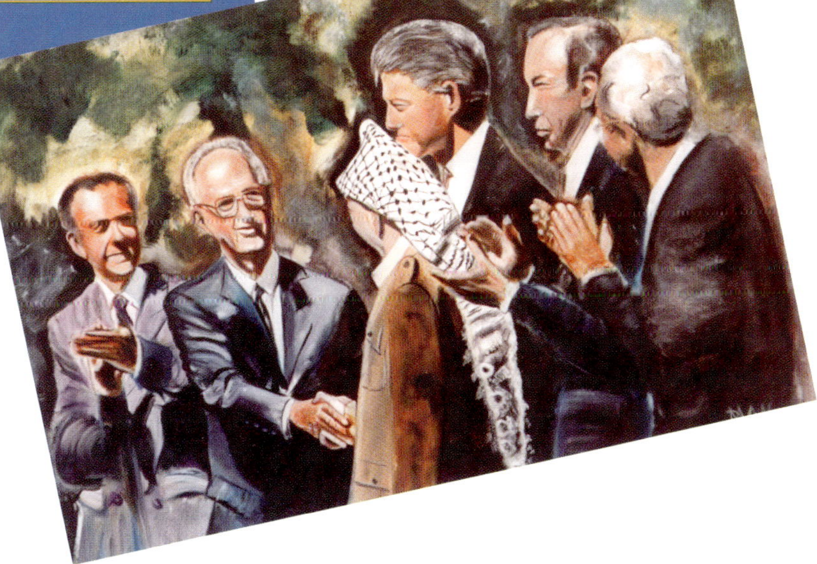

COSMETIC SURGERY FOR MEN

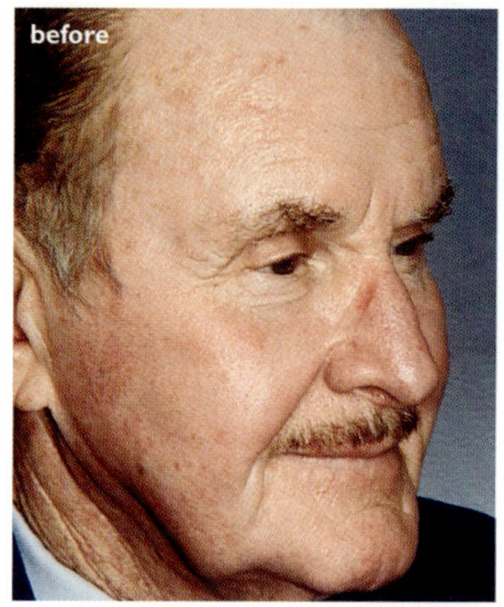

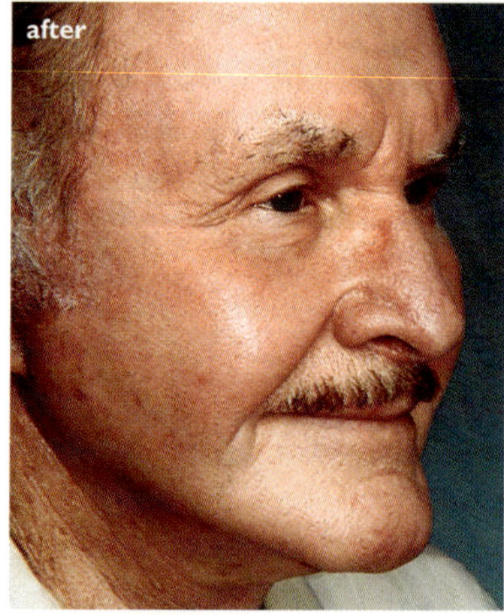

Face and Neck Lift & Full Face Laser.

PATIENT PORTRAITS

HERBERT RICHMAN
FACE, NECK & FOREHEAD LIFT; UPPER AND LOWER EYES; LASER
AGE: 62

I was starting to look like my father who had a turkey gullet. I had this mental picture of looking like him and I really wanted to do something to fix my own turkey gullet. I had gone to a doctor five years ago who explained to me that he would have to pull the skin up and back and tighten the muscles which would be better if I had it done with a facelift. I didn't think I needed a facelift. I was reluctant to do it.

I didn't like my eyes either which were beginning to get puffy and baggy. I had heard of some people having a facelift and being left with a surprised look. Finally, I decided it was time to do it and now, not when I was 70. So I started making inquiries. I interviewed plastic surgeons in Palm Beach and Boca Raton. I talked to one doctor's patients and they said they had no pain. I didn't know if their comments meant they had no pain with drugs or they had no pain without drugs. It didn't matter. I was definitely impressed about the no pain. I also was impressed because my doctor has a post–operation facility where I could stay several extra days and his staff would take care of me. I didn't want my wife to have to care for me while I was still swollen and had drains in.

Another thing I was impressed about was that the doctor sent a car for me. They also had a car drive me home when I was finished. I was surprised at how easy the surgery was. I went in on a Friday and didn't remember anything until Saturday morning. By next Thursday I felt good enough and looked good enough to have people over for dinner — even though I was still a little swollen. Within two weeks it was hard to tell I had any surgery at all. The doctor gave me some pills and I didn't have to take any of them. I'm a quick healer and my face healed very rapidly. But, I did hire a nurse for a few days to help me with my lotions and creams.

I was recently married and my friends who didn't know I had plastic surgery would say, "Marriage must agree with you. You look very relaxed." That makes me feel very good. You should also know that 15 years ago I had hair transplants. I guess that is why I've always been amenable to cosmetic surgery. The way I figured it, if you feel good, why not try to look as good as you can?

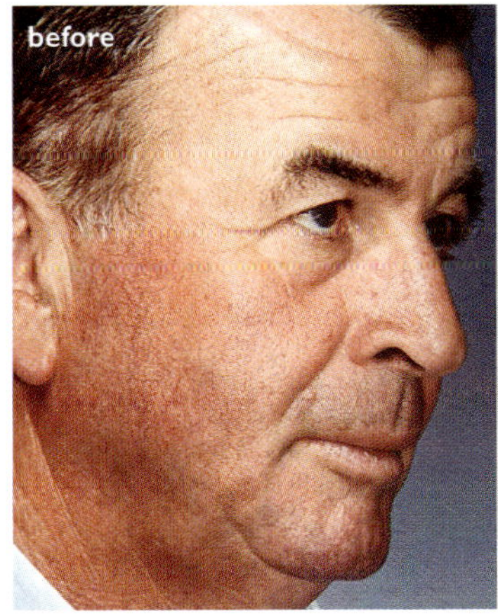
before

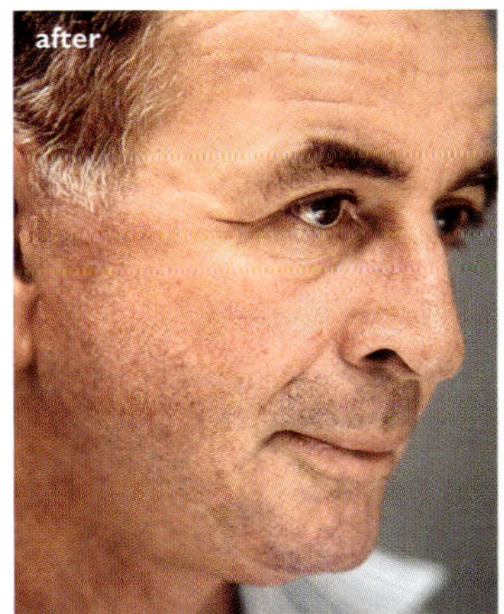
after

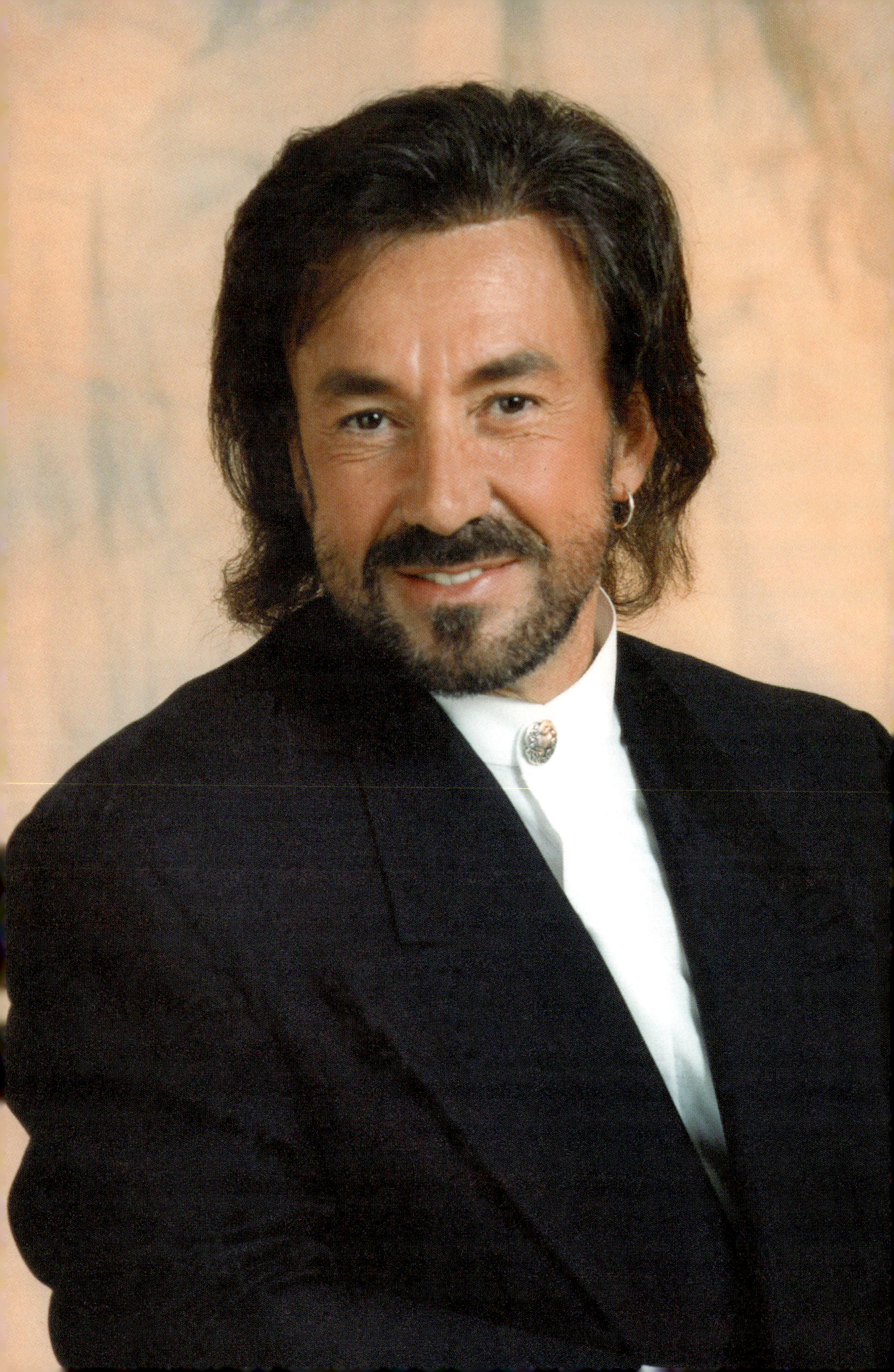

PATIENT PORTRAIT

JEAN MICHELE CRAVANZOLA
FACE & NECK LIFT, FOREHEAD LIFT, NOSE, LOWER EYE LIFT, SKIN REJUVENATION PEEL
AGE: 50

Everybody today wants to look beautiful and young. Self-image and first impressions are important. We should look as good as we can. When we do, we feel better about ourselves. Change helps us do that. So I always look for ways to improve myself. I didn't want to look 20 or 25. I just wanted to look good for my age.

I decided to have my nose fixed. I had broken it several times. Later I had my face and eyes done and then I had a peel. I also had a hair transplant by a specialist. The first time I changed (had surgery) people said, 'Why? You look good. You don't need surgery.' I said 'Yes, it is true. I look good, but that is not the problem. The problem is myself.' I wanted surgery because I like to improve myself and show people how it is possible to change themselves. I also changed how I live my life. I don't drink. I don't smoke. I exercise and go to the spa every morning. I try to keep my heart, my mind and my body strong. I start my day early, at 5 A.M. I work out. I play tennis. I lift weights. At 50, you need to work your body harder because your metabolism changes. Two years ago I competed in a body-building contest, and I won. I love to compete for the challenge. I want to live very long. And I want to look good doing it.

I am a designer. I sell clothes and jewelry in Boca Raton. I am also an interior decorator. It is very important that I look good for my work. I am also a father and a grandfather. I have two grandchildren and six children, three boys and three girls. No one believes me when I say I am a grandfather.

When I changed my face, my personality came out better. I feel good, more confident and more comfortable with myself. In my business it helps. It is very sad, but sometimes when I go to meetings, I notice younger businessmen sometimes don't listen to you because you are old. You look tired all the time. Now, they listen. I say, 'Do you know my age?' They think I'm 30. They do not know I'm 50.

Men are different from women. They are more shy. They want to change. But not too much. I believe to enjoy life, you must be comfortable with yourself. Surgery not only gives you a better appearance, it also gives you more self-esteem and a healthier look. I don't want to just look young. I want to look healthy.

You see yourself every day. If you're like me, one day you wake up and look in the mirror and say, 'Oh, wow, how can I look so bad? It's time for a change. Some say it is too expensive. I say, You spend money on a car, what you have after ten years is an old car. It is better to put money in yourself than in a big car. You put money away for vacation. At the end of the vacation you feel tired and broke. It's better to say no to a vacation for two years and spend the money on yourself.

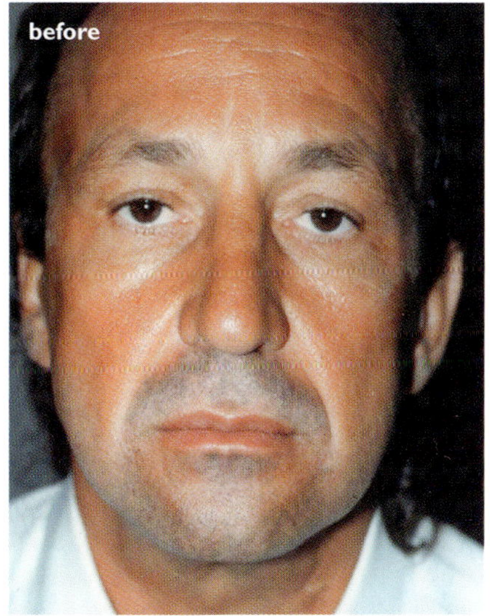

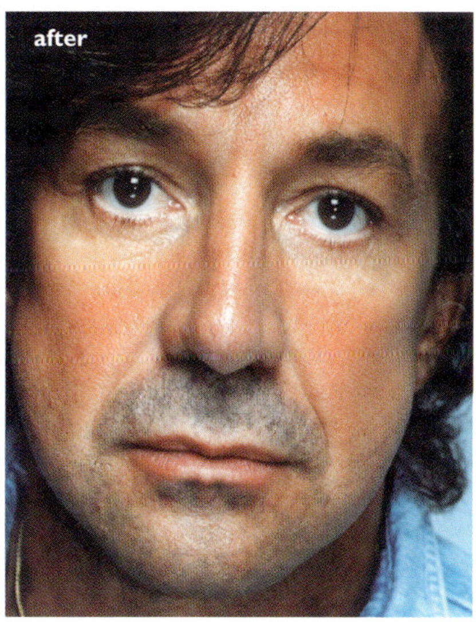

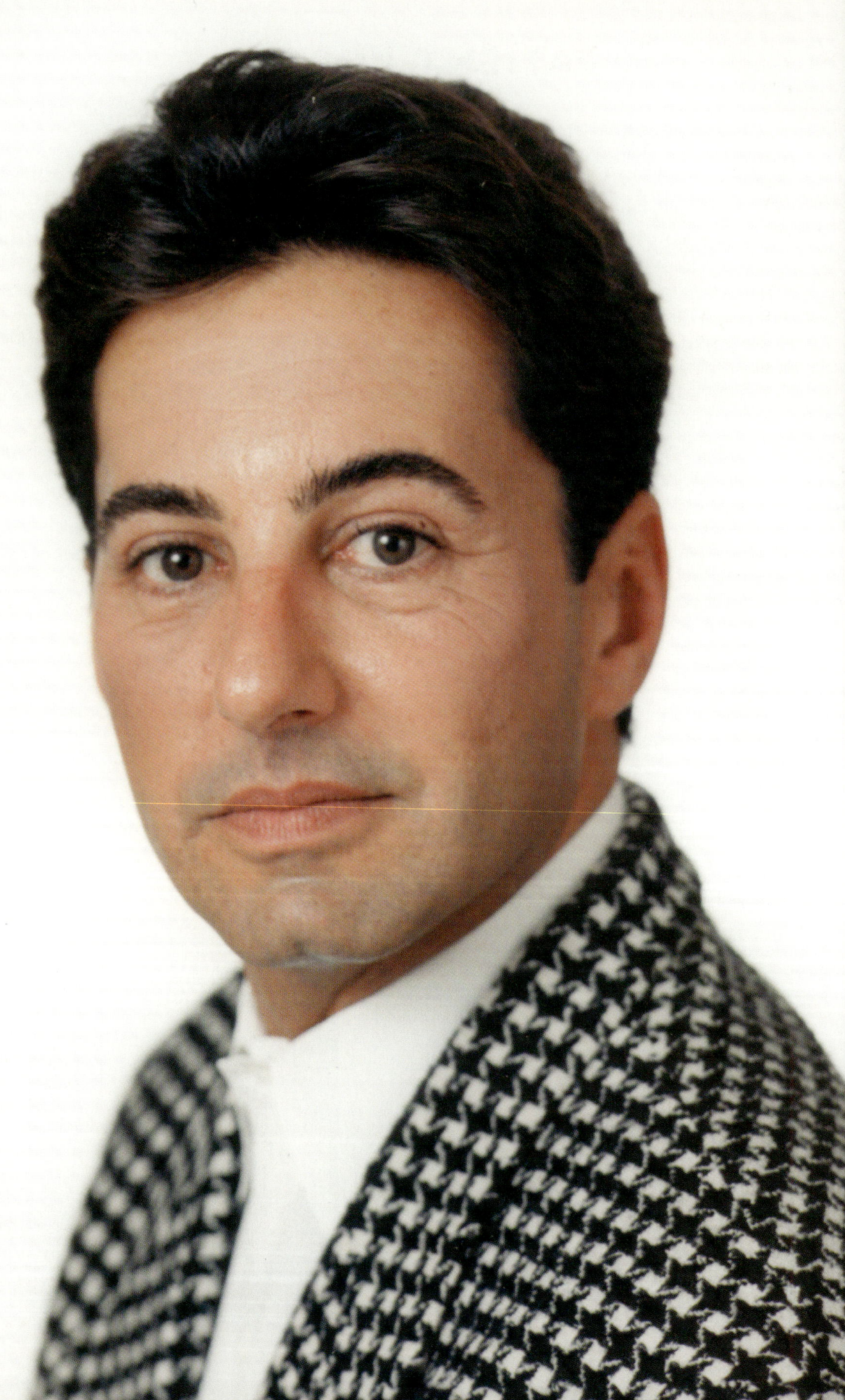

PATIENT PORTRAIT

STEPHEN NOCETI

FOREHEAD LIFT, UPPER & LOWER EYE LIFT, FAT INJECTIONS, BOTOX INJECTIONS, LASER

AGE: 40

I started working out a few years ago so I could have the body I wanted. I lost 40 pounds and went down six pants sizes. But my face didn't match my new look. I looked tired all the time, even when I was happy. So I decided to give myself a 40th birthday present.

The doctor did my forehead using the endoscope and laser, and he did my upper and lower eyelids and filled in the lines around my eyes — the crow's feet and the frown lines with fat injections.

What surprised me was that I had no black and blue marks and no pain. I never even opened the pain medication the doctor had prescribed for me just in case. I had heard that surgery was painful, and I expected to be black and blue and have headaches. That's what my friends said. But that didn't happen. I really never stopped working. I did have a little swelling, which was gone the next week.

People who know I had something done think I look ten years younger. People who don't know I had anything done think I lost weight. Or they might ask if I got my hair cut.

I'm a realtor. I sell ocean-front property in Aventura, which is an exclusive area in North Miami. Surgery has made me feel better about myself, and I think it has given me more confidence. Before, I used to wear sunglasses all the time to hide my eyes. Now, I don't do that any more. It really was the best birthday present I could give myself.

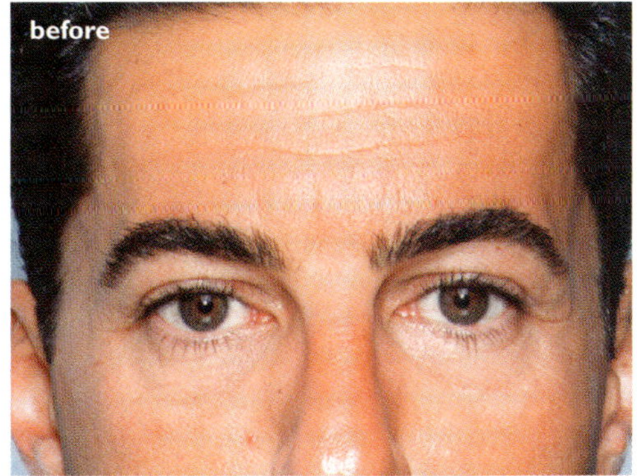
before

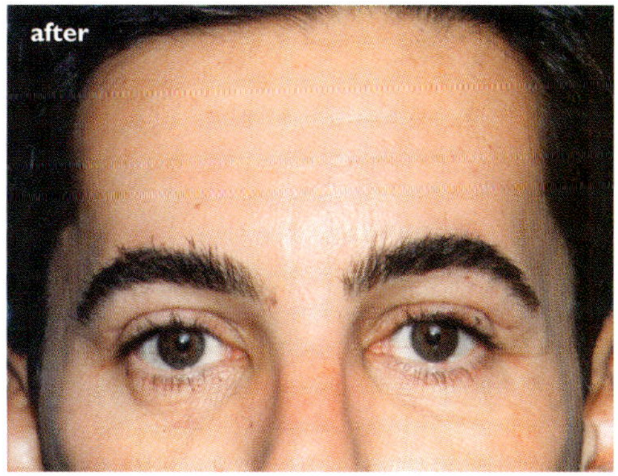
after

PATIENT PORTRAIT

PATRICK GERRITS
FACELIFT & NECKLIFT; FULL FACE LASER
AGE: 59

I think today that men should take a good hard look at themselves. It's not a question of trying to look 20 when you're 50. It makes sense to look as good as you can.

I'm 185 pounds and 6-feet, 1-inch tall. I can control my weight, so I let the plastic surgeon control my aging. Before I decided to have plastic surgery, I had to really rationalize my decision. I asked myself, 'Am I doing this for personal reasons because I'm vain and want to look good? Or, am I doing this for business reasons?' My answer was 60 percent business and 40 percent personal.

At 59, I don't want to look 64 when I step in front of a hospital or county commission board. Just like the book *Dress for Success* says, why not try to make a good impression and look as good as you can? I try to look nice and spend a lot of money on good suits. Why shouldn't I spend money to make my face look good, too?

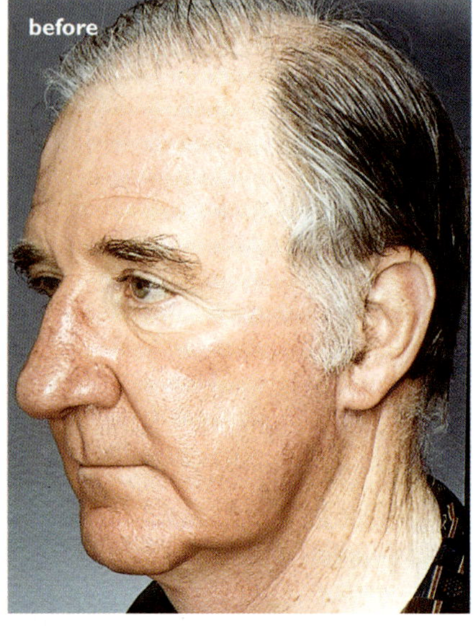

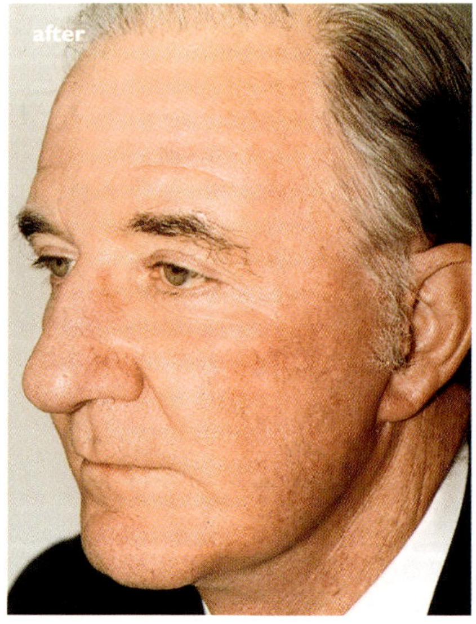

PATIENT PORTRAIT

CHARLIE GLYNN
RHINOPHYMA
AGE: 80

It started as a small spot on my nose. It had been there for years, as far back as I can remember. Suddenly, a few years ago it seemed to blossom out. It got bigger and bigger until it became this big bulky thing on my nose, flopping back and forth. It must have run in my family because my mother had the same thing and so did my grandmother before her.

It was awful. A lot of people think when you have a big nose that you're a big boozer. My close friends, of course, know I don't drink. But that didn't help. One experience that finally convinced me to do something was when I went to my class reunion. There were some remarks and people stared. They looked at me differently. Others were embarrassed and looked away. They couldn't believe it was me. I tried to tell myself I was the same old Charlie. But of course that wasn't true. The way people look at you can affect how you look at yourself. So I asked my doctor what I should do, and he suggested I go to a plastic surgeon.

Having surgery has made an awful lot of difference on my outlook. I feel better about myself and I know I'm not being looked at as a weird-looking person. I was clearing out my desk recently, and I saw a picture from when I graduated from college in 1940. My nose looks the same now as it did then, when I was in my 20s. People who see me now are truly amazed. I'm a lot more outgoing today.

Having surgery was also easier than I thought. I was in the hospital overnight and that was it. It didn't take long for me to recuperate at all. One of my daughters came down to look after me. But, after couple of days, I sent her home. I didn't need her.

I was fortunate because my surgery was covered by insurance. But even if it wasn't, that wouldn't have stopped me. I believe if it bothers you as an individual, you ought to do something about it. Otherwise, it can affect your personality. If you see people who have growths on their faces, you know they're unpleasant to look at. And, I know from experience that it's unpleasant for them to have it. So if you get rid of it, then life becomes pleasant.

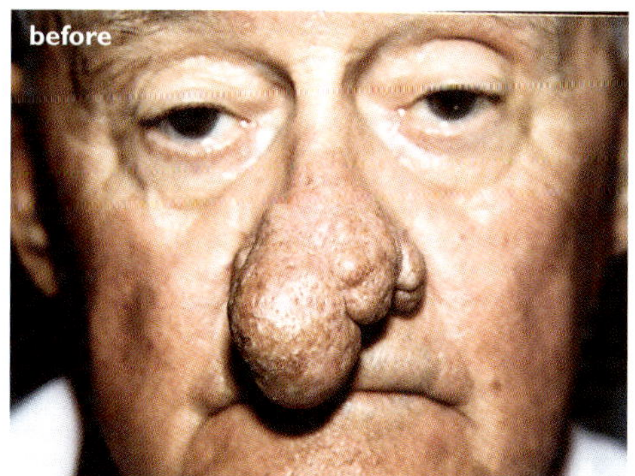

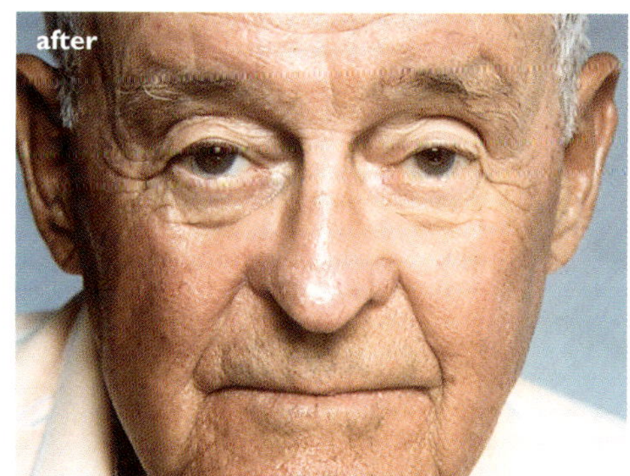

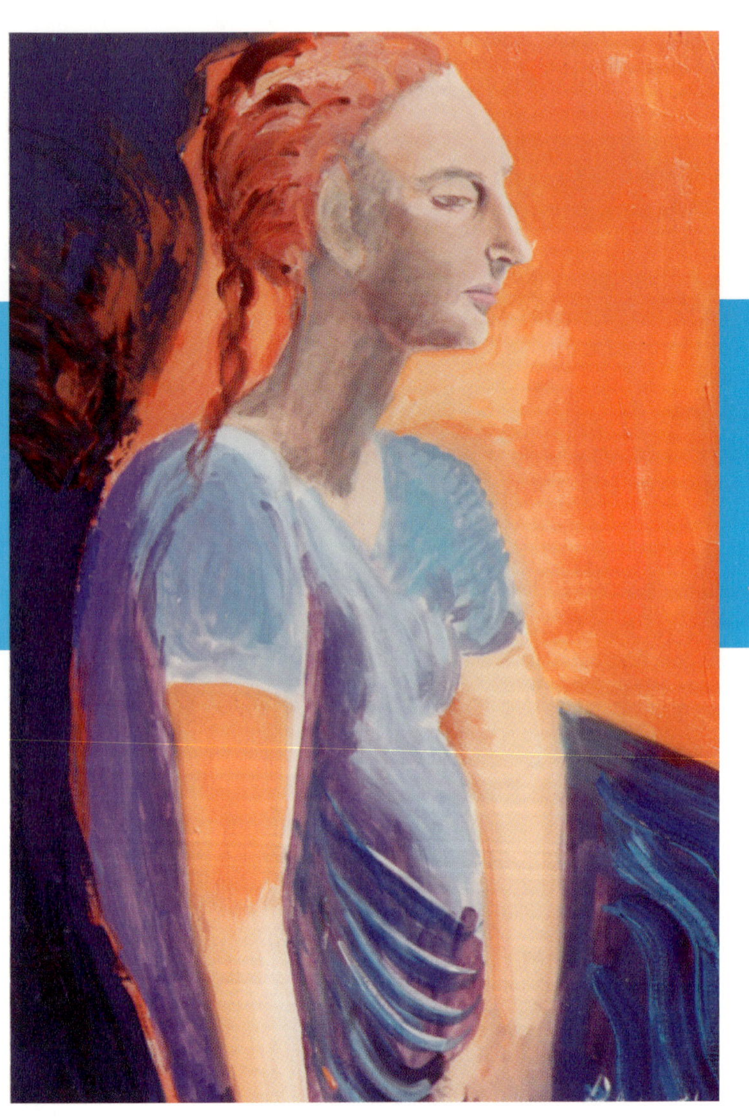

Part 3

Esthetics In Medicine

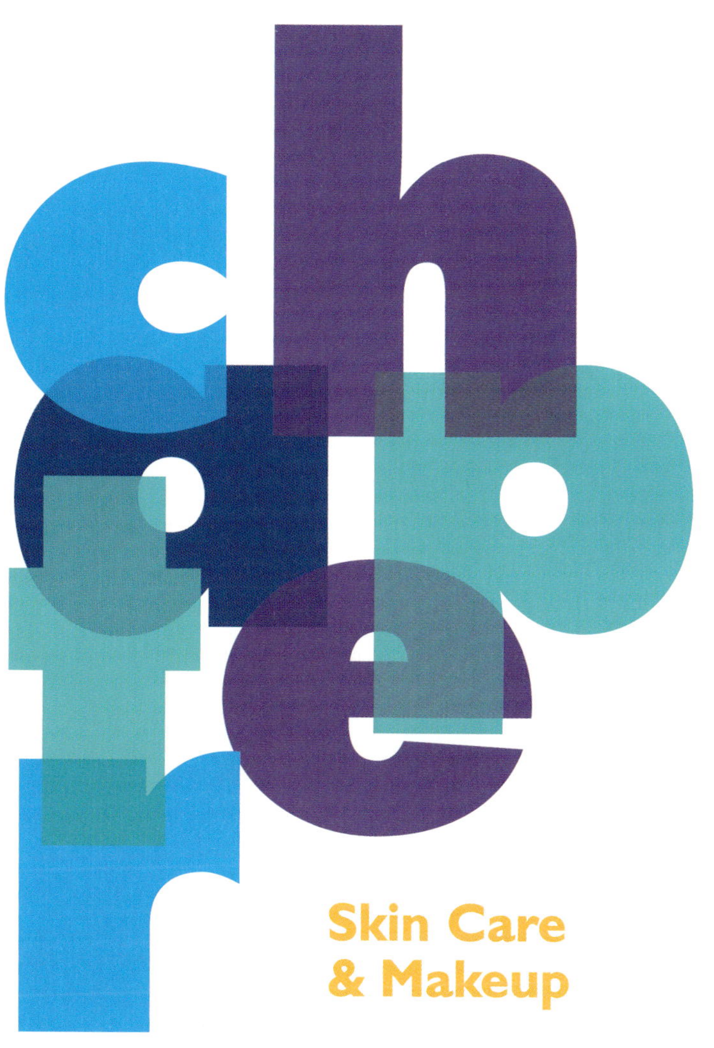

Skin Care & Makeup

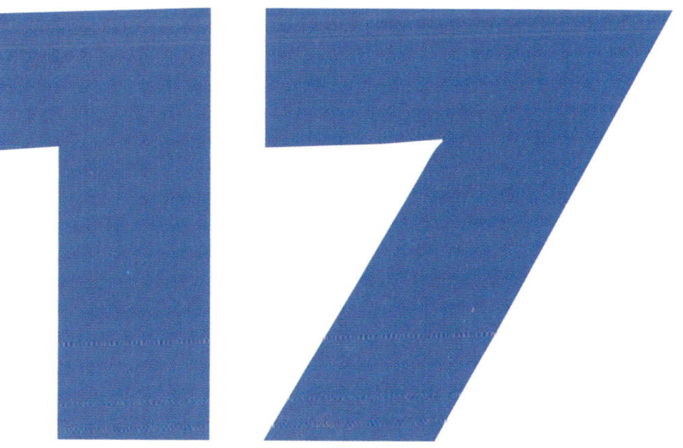

Skin Care & Makeup

Skin care and cosmetics are important components of plastic surgery. Few doctors had estheticians on their staff in the 1980s. Today, plastic surgeons and dermatologists recognize the valuable contributions of estheticians and their role in skin care. The esthetician's knowledge and skills contribute to the success of surgery by providing patient education and essential pre-and post-operative skin care, make-up and cover-up techniques.

Before surgery, the

esthetician will evaluate the condition of the skin. Especially in the cases of chemical peels and facelift surgery, the skin's condition is carefully considered. It is important that the skin be in the best condition possible to undergo the rigors of surgery.

The skin is the body's largest organ. It comprises over 20 square feet that protect and envelope the body. It gives many of the first clues as to how we are aging. Beautiful, healthy skin really begins within. This is why I ask patients to refrain from smoking and alcohol intake, get plenty of rest and drink plenty of water, preferably eight 8-ounce glasses each day. They should also eat a healthy diet, take antioxidant, vitamin and mineral supplements and exercise.

Proper pH

A proper pH is essential to maintaining balance and health of the skin, as well as the body. The pH helps our skin maintain its natural acidity, which forms a protective barrier against bacteria.

What is a proper pH? A proper pH level ranges from 5.5 to 6. Most over-the-counter soaps, cleansers, cosmetics and lotions have a pH level of 8, which strips the skin of its natural oils and moisture, leaving it vulnerable to a variety of problems, such as dryness and itchiness. For patients undergoing facelifts and peels, a proper pH level is even more essential.

Preparing The Skin For Surgery

Before undergoing facelift surgery, laser and peels, the skin will be carefully prepared with facial treatments that are specifically designed for the individual's needs — exfoliations, appropriate cleansers and hydration treatments. Lymphatic drainage may be prescribed by the doctor and the esthetician.

Six weeks before surgery, laser or peeling, the esthetic technician will prepare the skin with some of the following treatments: exfoliation of the dead skin cell build-up; deep pore cleansing of the face and neck, appropriate to the skin type and condition of the face and neck; massage to increase blood circulation and stimulate facial muscles; and lymphatic drainage to carry toxins away. Four weeks before surgery, patients follow the same routine as they do at six weeks, with the exception of exfoliation. If the exfoliation was missed at the first treatment, then it can be done at this time, otherwise no additional exfoliations or light peels should be done prior to

surgery or peeling. Two weeks prior to surgery patients undergo the same facial treatment as they did during the previous treatment. Adding glycolic acids and bleaching agents may be necessary.

Skin Beneficial Products

The esthetician will also recommend products that are healthy for the skin, as most over-the-counter soaps, creams, lotions and cosmetics contain many chemicals, dyes, fillers, fragrances and other ingredients that can even be harmful. For example, mineral oil, one of the most common ingredients found in store-bought cosmetics, foundations, cleansers and sun blocks, may be harmful to the skin, especially for facelift and peel patients.

The trend today is toward more natural health–promoting ingredients, containing vitamins and other nutrients and away from ingredients such as mineral oil, petrolatum, and talc. Mineral oil, petrolatum and petroleum jelly are by-products of petroleum, a flammable, liquid hydrocarbon from which gasoline, natural gas and kerosene are derived. The use of products containing these items causes a sealing of the skin so that the pores may get plugged. There may be times when the skin needs to be sealed, as in the case of dry skin to help retain moisture. People with acne or oily skin conditions are advised against oil-based products.

Beauty Begins Within

Science has recognized the importance of nutrition in aging, health, healing and in preventing diseases. Skin care products and cosmetics are now using "skin-beneficial and skin-rejuvenating" ingredients such as antioxidants, herbs and other nutrients.

The skin has the unique ability to absorb nutrients and other materials through the pores, which has proven advantageous for delivering medications. Common examples are heart patients and smokers who can receive medicines topically through small patches that are applied to the skin and absorbed into the body. Vitamin C applied topically is absorbed into the cells helping the new cells to become healthier and making the collagen and elastin fibers stronger.

A popular magazine called *Self* ran a headline "Skin Magic By The Mouthful," which reported on the new wave of "ingestible" beauty products that promote beauty from the inside out. They are the new rage among models.

Among their ingredients are antioxidants (which help prevent cell damage caused by free radicals), herbs and other nutrients. These also help maintain health and increase the rate of healing. Other examples include zinc picolinate, copper, vitamin A and vitamin B, vitamin C and vitamin E. Nutrients that reduce scar formation are vitamin E, the bioflavonoids and osteoprime forte. Other health-promoting products include enzymes such as pancreatin, bromelain and papaya which reduce tissue inflammation and tissue swelling. Arnica and vitamin K can help prevent bruising.

Antioxidant Role In Healing & Anti-aging

Studies have pointed to the role of antioxidants and phytonutrients in disease prevention and aging. Vitamin A, vitamin C, and vitamin E, in addition to many more nutrients from plants, provide essential disease fighting, healing and nutritional benefits. Food sources today do not contain many of these important nutrients. This is why supplementation is a good course, pre- and post-operatively to prepare the body and promote healing.

Antioxidants play a key role in wound healing and scar reduction. According to the *Journal of the American Society for Dermatologic Surgery*, antioxidants help fight damage to cell membranes and DNA by oxygen free radicals, which also impede healing.

Post-Operative Makeup & Coverups

Eliminating chemicals and fillers from cosmetics and skin care products is a new trend long overdue. The esthetician will recommend make-up and products that are best for the skin and benefit it. Other important ingredients such as sunblocks, vitamins and antioxidants will be recommended.

Most patients want to know when they can apply makeup after their surgery. Generally, makeup can be applied a few days after surgery. Camouflage makeup can be used to cover up incision marks, bruising, discoloration and swelling. Discolorations around the eyes can be covered with a fluid foundation rather than a concealer so there is no pulling or tugging on the skin. Neutral shades of eye shadow should be applied so as not to draw attention to the eyes.

After a facelift, the cheeks may also appear swollen. More defined cheekbones can be created by applying a highlighter foundation — one that is two shades lighter than your skin tone — along the top of the cheekbone. Apply a contour shadow foundation that is two shades darker than your normal skin tone in the hollow of the cheeks — the area just under and along the outside of the cheeks.

After facial surgery, laser or peeling, your skin care routine and makeup needs will change. It is important to remember that after surgery the skin will be sensitive and that the incisions should not be stressed or pulled. For the few weeks immediately following surgery when there is bruising and swelling, camouflage makeup can provide contouring and cover-ups for the discolorations that patients experience.

Facelift incisions are hidden behind the ear, inside the ear, and in the hairline. These fade with time and become almost imperceptible. During healing, concealing makeup can disguise these lines and cover up areas of discoloration. After nose surgery, discolorations are usually noticed around the eyes, particularly under the eyes, and the nose will appear swollen. This can be alleviated through contouring techniques. Applying foundation or concealer two shades darker than the skin along the sides of the nose can make it appear narrower, and a highlighter is then applied down the bridge (middle) of the nose.

Sometime in the future you may also want to consider the advantages of long-term makeup, such as permanent eyeliner or brow and lip coloring.

Sunscreens

The sun is the biggest contributor to aging of the skin and to skin cancer. Overexposure to ultraviolet (UV) radiation damages the cells and interferes with the ability to reproduce and repair. The skin's natural collagen (protein) fibers become less elastic, causing wrinkles.

The sun emits three types of ultraviolet rays — UVA, UVB and UVC. UVA rays, the long wave-length radiation, are the tanning rays. They accelerate the aging process and contribute to the formation of wrinkles. UVB, the medium wavelength rays, are the burning rays that penetrate the skin and have also been implicated in skin cancer. UVC rays are the strongest and most dangerous. They have ultra high-energy wavelength rates that are usually absorbed by the upper atmosphere's ozone layer. Because of the depletion of the ozone layer, scientists believe that these rays are penetrating the atmosphere with more frequency.

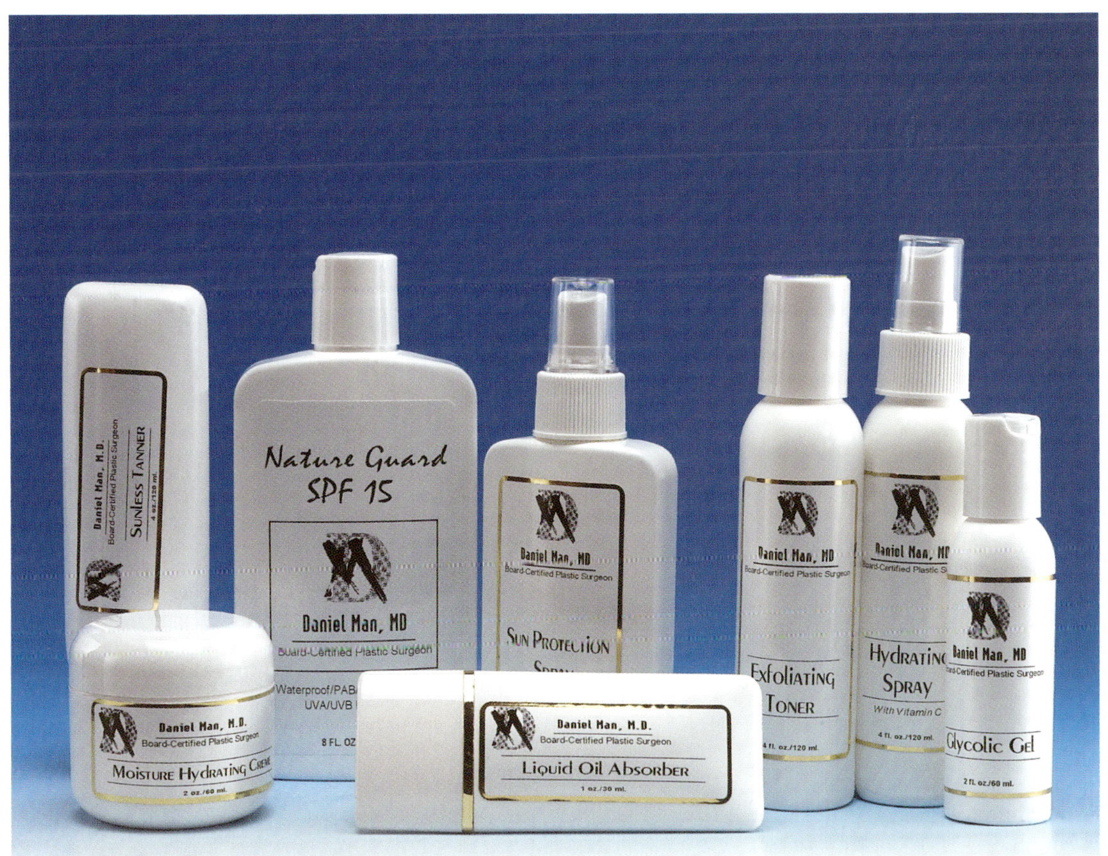

Which SPF Is Best?

Protecting the skin from these harmful rays can go a long way to keeping the skin healthy and reducing its aging. Sunblocks can provide protection from harmful rays and should be applied as part of a daily skin care regimen. The high rate of skin cancer and skin damage has also caused cosmetic manufacturers to add sunblocks to their products. They are now added to many skin care products, such as foundations and lipsticks. A Sun Protection Factor (SPF) of 15 blocks harmful rays. The best products use natural sun blocks such as titanium dioxide. An SPF of 15 will provide skin protection for four hours. SPFs of 20, 30 or higher have chemicals added to extend their life and may not be best since some people can be extremely sensitive to these added chemicals. It is always a good idea to check with the esthetician or your doctor before use.

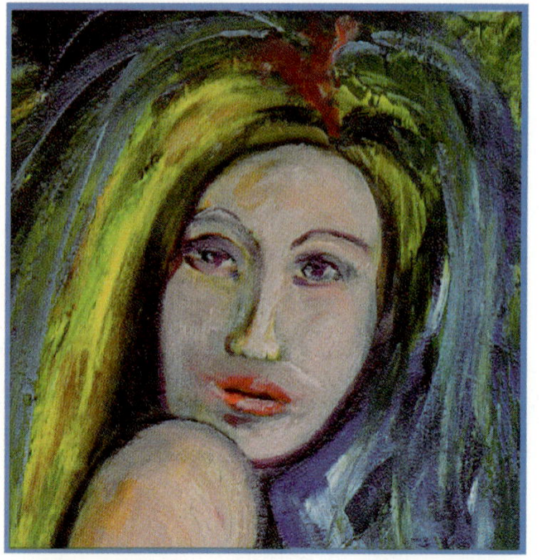

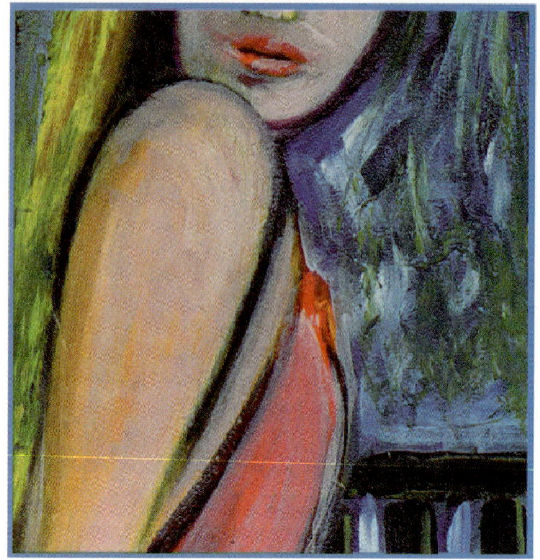

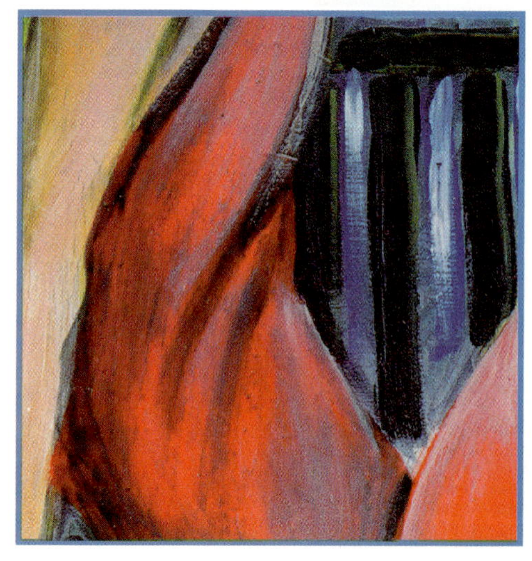

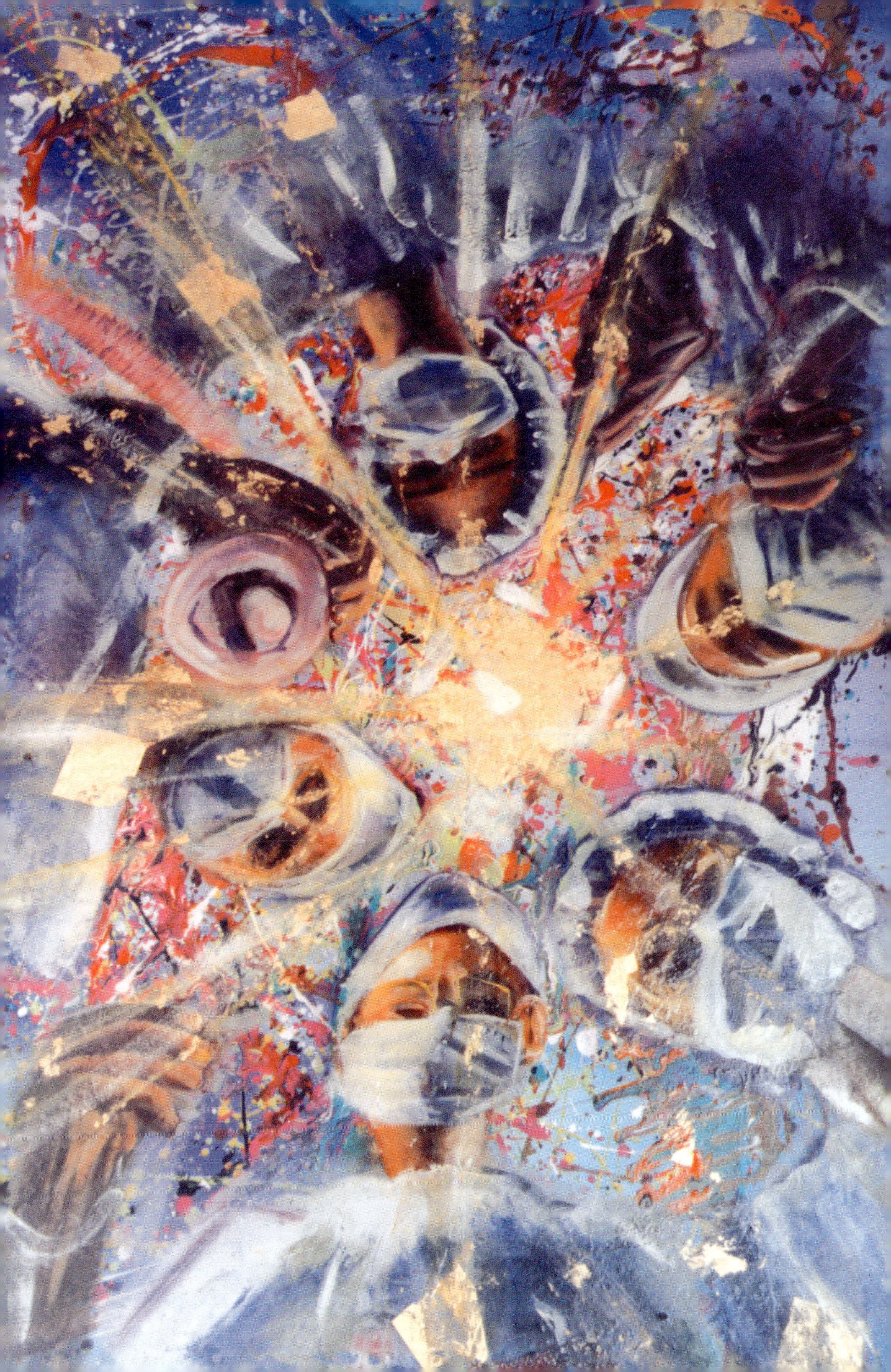

Part 4

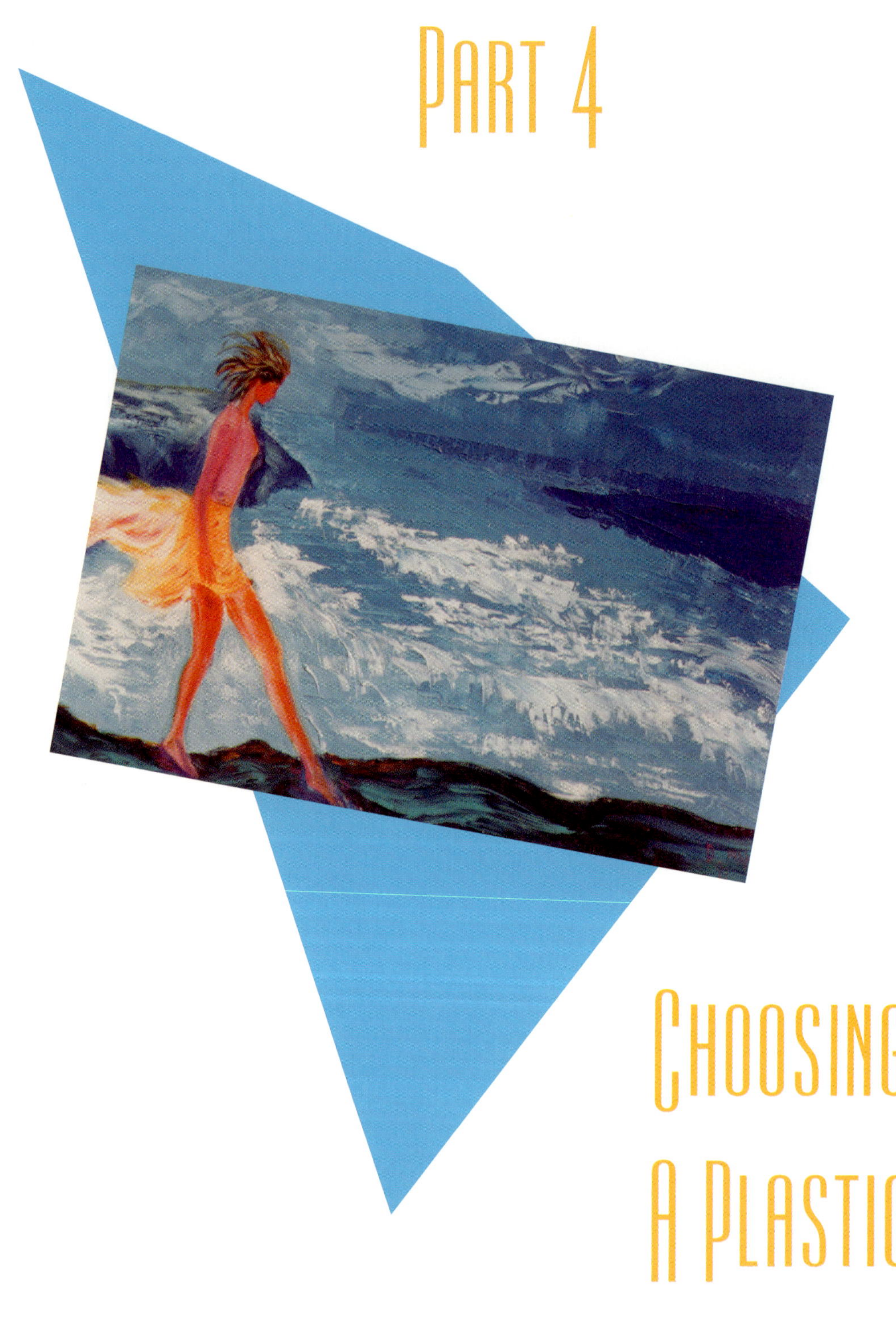

Choosing A Plastic Surgeon

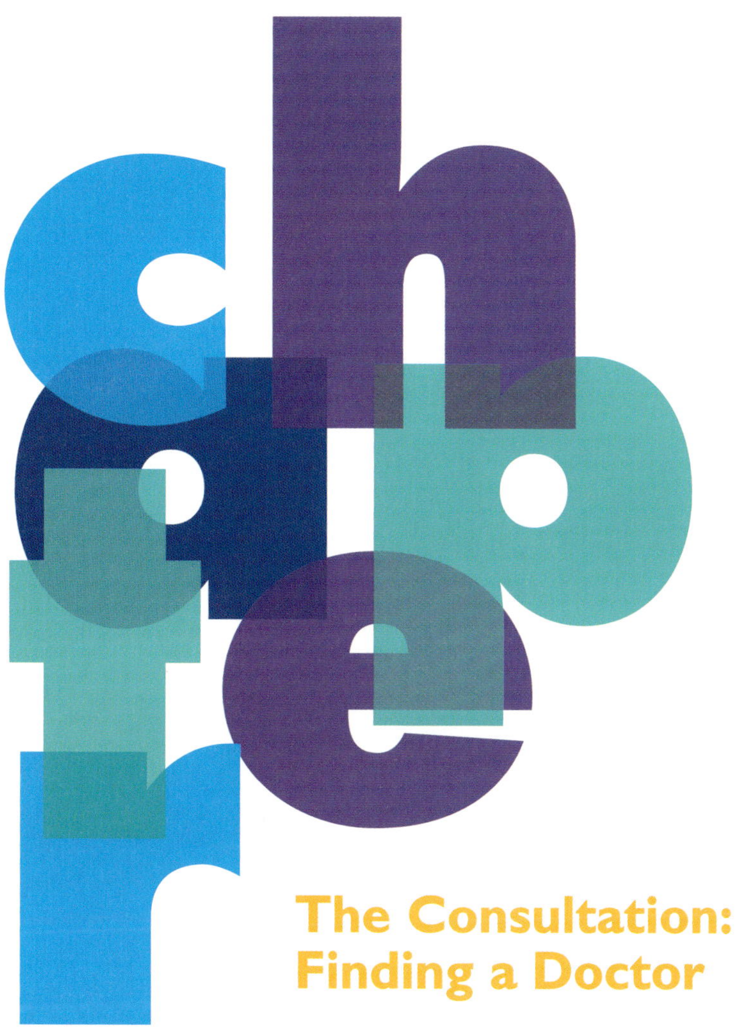

The Consultation: Finding a Doctor

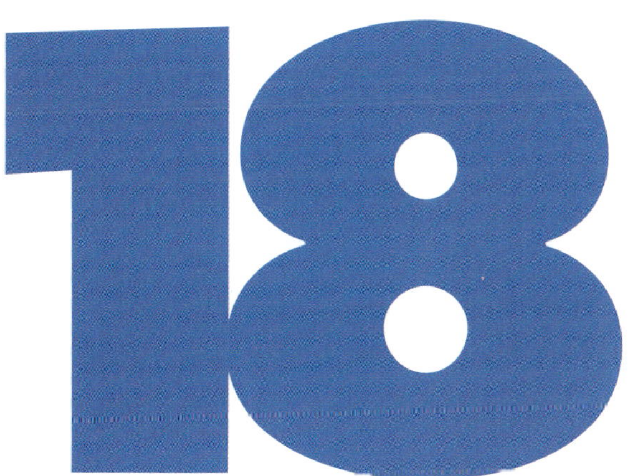

The Consultation: Finding a Doctor

Deciding to have plastic surgery is a major decision. How many of us have thought of changing our appearance? Most of us have, I'm sure. But, before you elect something as important as surgery, there are important considerations. There are questions you need to ask before your surgery. You will want to find a doctor whom you trust and who understands you. You need to be very candid about your feelings and what you expect from your surgery. If there is something about your appearance that you feel self-conscious about and you think about every day, then it is probably the right time to bring it up.

For some, the ravages of aging have severely altered their appearance. They may have lost their self-confidence and their ability to feel good about themselves. One patient explained her decision to have surgery this way, "My face literally fell in less than a year. I went from looking my age to looking older than my own mother. Living this way was unacceptable to me. That's why I decided to have plastic surgery."

Do It For Yourself

The best reason to have cosmetic surgery is to please yourself. Plastic surgery will not make someone fall in love with you or make people like you, but it can change your appearance. YOU have to do the rest.

Before you have surgery, it is a good idea to talk it over with someone else, a family member or close friend, who can help you examine your feelings and motives. Many people today are more open about plastic surgery and are willing to discuss their experiences. They may tell you in detail what surgery they had, what they didn't like, and whether they would do it again. However, though they may have achieved good results and met their expectations consider that this is only one person's experience. You should speak to several people. Ask your doctor if there are patients who would be willing to share their experiences and answer your questions. This can be very helpful, as many patients are willing to share the most intimate details of their surgery and will give you their honest opinion.

How to Find the Right Doctor

Finding the right doctor is the first step. You will want to be sure your doctor is one of the more than 5,000 physicians in the U.S. who are board certified in the specialty of plastic surgery. These physicians are specialists in the field of plastic surgery and certified by the American Board of Plastic Surgery (ABPS). This is the board of medical specialties set up by the American Medical Association that certifies and recognizes specialists in the practice of plastic surgery. Board certification signifies full-time plastic surgeons who have the skills and surgical judgment to perform a wide range of aesthetic and reconstructive procedures.

The ABPS sets the standards for physicians who wish to specialize in plastic surgery. In order to sit for the board's examination, a doctor is required to have graduated from an accredited medical school, and completed three or more years of approved residency training in general surgery, and two years of additional residency training in plastic surgery. The physician must also complete two years of full-time practice in plastic surgery and undertake extensive written and oral examinations. Only then is the physician able to use the distinction "board-certified plastic surgeon."

Board-certified plastic surgeons have no limitations on the areas of the body on which they can perform plastic surgery.

ASPRS

The American Society of Plastic and Reconstructive Surgeons (ASPRS) is the professional society that represents board-certified plastic surgeons in the U.S. It will provide a list of board-certified plastic surgeons in your area; call toll free 1-800-635-0635, or write 444 East Algonquin Road, Arlington Heights, Illinois 60005. Once you have a list, take it to your family doctor or dermatologist and ask if they are familiar with the names.

The yellow pages or a newspaper ad is not the best source for finding a doctor, since, the doctor is paying for the listing in the phone directory and for the advertisement in the newspaper.

Though the phone book does list doctors in your area who perform plastic surgery, check to make sure this list includes board-certified plastic surgeons.

Other medical professionals are also good sources for referrals. Local physicians often know the reputations of other surgeons from firsthand experience or from talking with other doctors. Nurses, for example, work with the doctors and the patients, so they have firsthand knowledge of the doctor's work and the patient's experience.

Another resource is your local library. The library carries reference books that lists physicians by their specialty. "The Official American Board of Medical Specialties" also called "ABMS Directory of Board-Certified Medical Specialists," published by the Research and Education Foundation of the American Board of Medical Specialties, gives the names, addresses and phone numbers of all medical specialists including plastic surgeons.

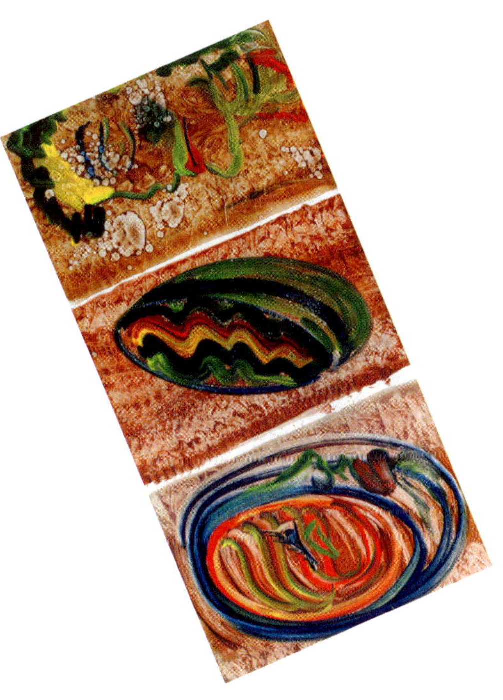

Local Medical Society

An easy method is to check with your local county medical society. It will tell you if the doctor is a member of the local society and whether he or she is board certified in the specialty of their practice. It will also tell you other information, including where the doctor graduated, and other schools where he or she received their medical training.

The Consultation

Once you have the names of several plastic surgeons, you will want to schedule a consultation. While there is a usually minimal fee for this consultation, it is well worth the time and money so that you can meet the doctor, learn about the practice and talk with patients.

During the consultation, you will want to be as candid as you can about your feelings, goals and expectations, and your medical history. If you have some medical condition that the doctor should know about, this is the time to reveal it. Remember, this is your opportunity to interview the doctor and establish rapport and understanding. Discuss your expectations. You may be told that they are not realistic. If they are not, this is the time to discover that, not after surgery.

If you find you don't have the right rapport or understanding with your doctor, then see the next one on your list. You might find you don't really like the doctor, or you might have a gut feeling or instinct that makes you unsure. Maybe you didn't really get the answers you wanted. Remember, it's your body.

10 Essential Questions To Ask Before Having Surgery

It is a good idea to bring a list of questions with you so you can be sure to ask the questions that are of most concern. Here is a list of questions you might want to include:

1. Ask if the doctor is in good standing with professional societies, in this case the American Society of Plastic and Reconstructive Surgeons (ASPRS).

ASPRS represents plastic surgeons who are certified by the American Board of Plastic Surgery, the only board that represents full-time plastic surgeons. You can reach ASPRS at 1-800-635-0635, or write: American Society of Plastic & Reconstructive Surgeons, 444 East Algonquin Road, Arlington Heights, Illinois 60005-4664. Is the board certification clearly displayed on the wall?

2. Ask about staff privileges at local hospitals. Where does the doctor serve on staff? You will want to make sure your doctor is on the staff of local hospital(s) and has similar operating privileges there.

3. You should ask about the doctor's experience: how many procedures has he or she performed of the type you are considering? Ask to see as many possible actual patient before and after photos.

4. You should also ask to speak to patients who have had the procedure that has been recommended to you. This is an excellent means of learning more about the procedure and finding out if patients were happy with their experience and if their expectations were met.

5. Ask about the surgery. Where will it be performed and who will perform it? Will it be done in the hospital, outpatient center or doctor's office? If the doctor has operating facilities, you will want to know if they are licensed and fully accredited. Ask how long it will take, what type of anesthesia will be used and who will administer it.

6. Ask about options to the procedure you are considering or that have been recommended to you. What you might think is the best procedure may not be what the doctor recommends based on your goals and expectations. Is this the best option for the results you expect? There may be medical reasons that preclude you from having one type of procedure but not another.

7. Ask what results can you realistically expect and how long these results will last? Will there be any scarring, and if so, where will they be and how can they be concealed with makeup?

8. Ask about the risks. Are there any complications? Ask if there will be any pain or discomfort? Inquire about such things as drainage tubes, dressings, bruising and swelling?

9. Ask when you will be able to go back to work and resume your normal activities. Will there be any physical limitations? When can you wear makeup?

10. Ask about the costs of the procedure, including fees for the surgeon, the anesthesiologist, the nurses, the operating room and follow-up visits? You'll also want to know how much of the cost of your surgery is covered by insurance, if any, and if there is any financing available.

Conclusion

I hope this book has in some way assisted readers in adding to their knowledge about plastic surgery and in discovering how it has helped others to change their lives. Plastic surgery is, for me, a journey into endless possibilities. Please feel free to let me know what you think. My door is always open. Call me at 1-800-232-5508. Or visit me on the internet at our web site at www.drman.com. You'll find even more important news on advances in plastic surgery, meet patients over the internet and keep updated with my seminars and speaking engagements, Please contact me at anytime or e-mail me your questions directly at info@drman.com.

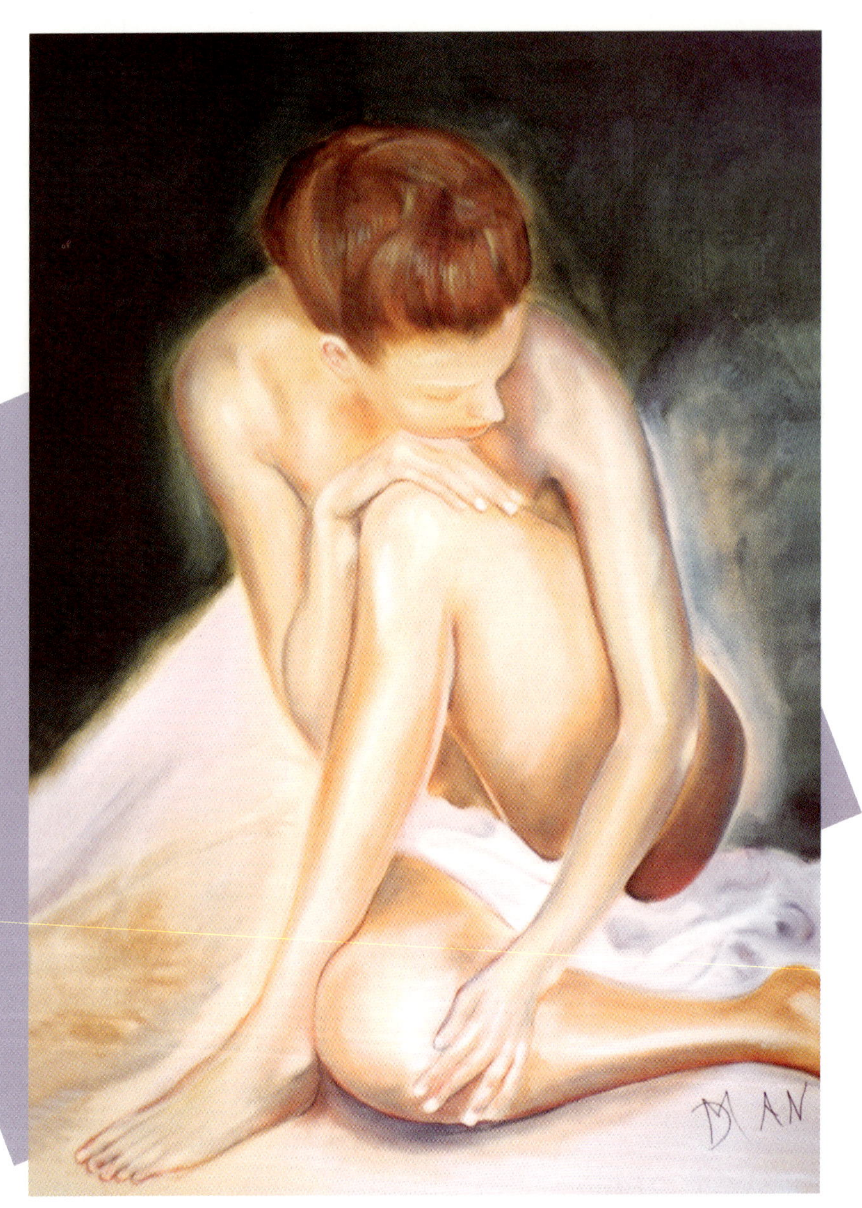

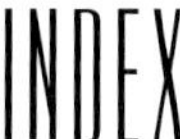

INDEX

INDEX TO PAINTINGS & SCULPTURES

**Paintings and Sculptures Depicted in "The Art of Man: Faces of Plastic Surgery are the work of Daniel Man, M.D. For additional information regarding Dr. Man's art please contact the Cunningham Artist's Gallery in Delray Beach, Florida (561) 265-0058.*

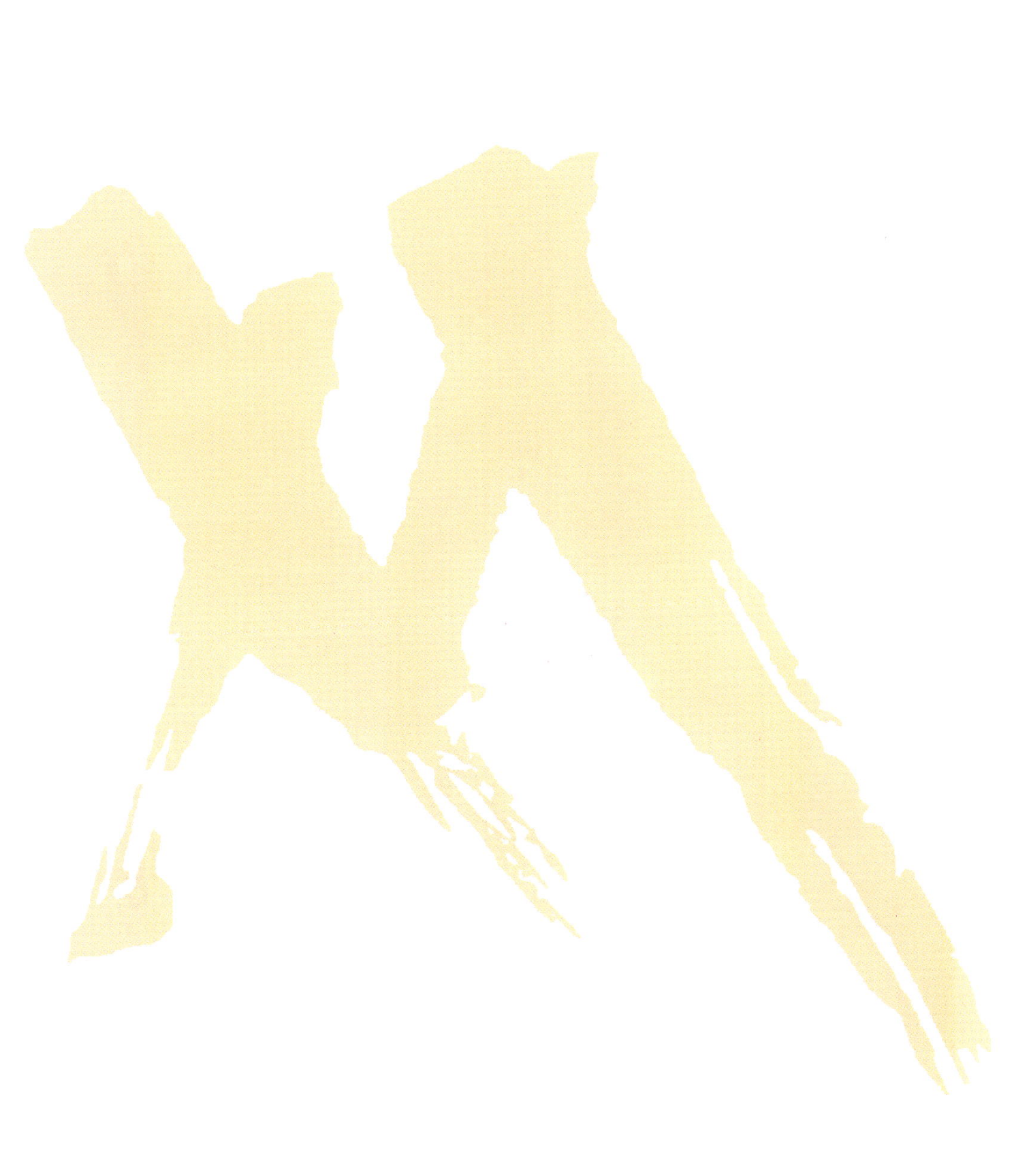

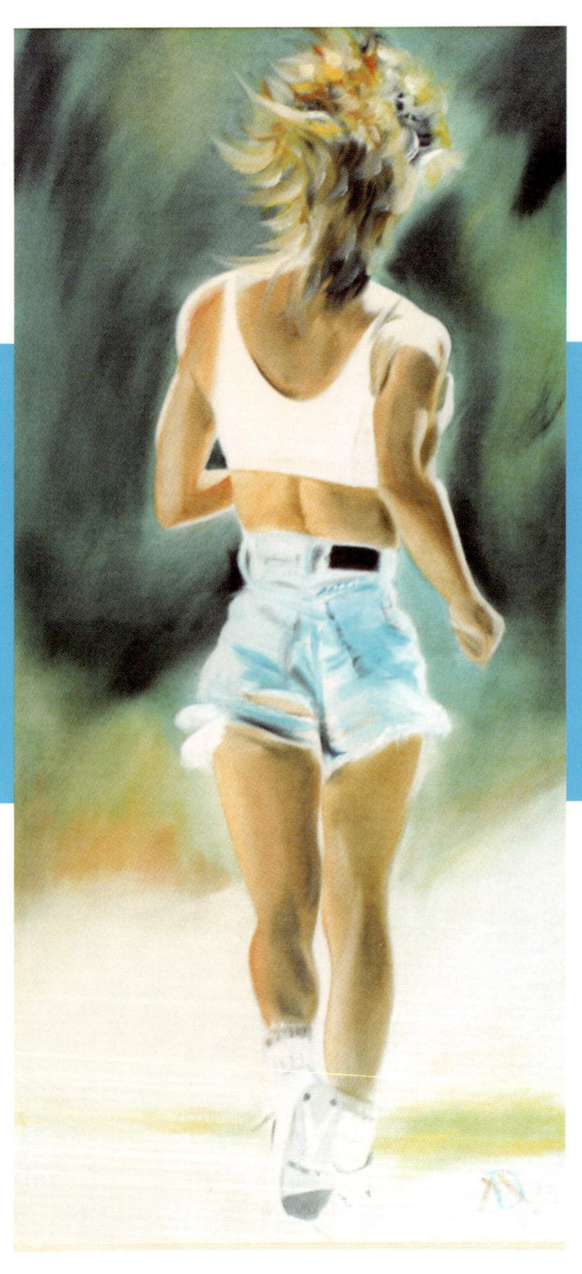

To order additional copies of

THE ART OF MAN
FACES OF PLASTIC SURGERY

Call 1-800-232-5508
or write:
Daniel Man, M.D.
851 Meadows Road, Suite 222
Boca Raton, Florida 33486
(561) 395-5508

email: info@drman.com

Please send me "The Art of Man: Faces of Plastic Surgery"

Name ______________________________ Phone ______________

Address ____

City, State, Zip ______________________________________

Please check:

❑ Enclosed is my check

❑ Please charge my credit card: ❑ VISA ❑ MasterCard ❑ DISCOVER

Account number ________________________

Signature ______________________________ Date ______________

I'd like to order ___ (Qty.) of Dr. Man's book at $29.95 each. __________

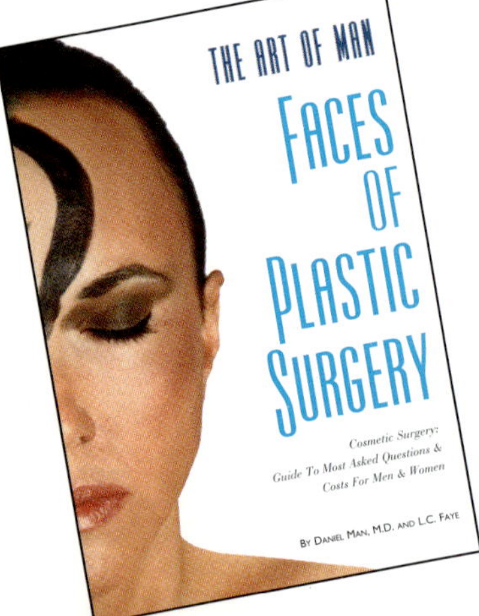

Shipping & Handling	$4.95 each
Subtotal	__________
Add 6% FL sales tax	__________
Total	__________

To order additional copies of

THE ART OF MAN
FACES OF PLASTIC SURGERY

Call 1-800-232-5508
or write:
Daniel Man, M.D.
851 Meadows Road, Suite 222
Boca Raton, Florida 33486
(561) 395-5508

email: info@drman.com

Please send me "The Art of Man: Faces of Plastic Surgery"

Name ____________________ Phone __________

Address ______________________________

City, State, Zip __________________________

Please check:

❑ Enclosed is my check

❑ Please charge my credit card: ❑ VISA ❑ MasterCard ❑ DISCOVER

Account number ____________________

Signature ____________________ Date __________

I'd like to order ___ (Qty.) of Dr. Man's book at $29.95 each. __________

THE ART OF MAN
FACES OF PLASTIC SURGERY
Cosmetic Surgery: Guide To Most Asked Questions & Costs For Men & Women
BY DANIEL MAN, M.D. AND L.C. FAYE

Shipping & Handling	$4.95 each
Subtotal	
Add 6% FL sales tax	
Total	